Recent Advances in Polymeric Delivery Vehicles for Controlled and Sustained Drug Release

Recent Advances in Polymeric Delivery Vehicles for Controlled and Sustained Drug Release

Ping Hu
Zheng Cai

MDPI

Basel • Beijing • Wuhan • Barcelona • Belgrade • Novi Sad • Cluj • Manchester

Ping Hu
College of Pharmacy
Jinan University
Guangzhou
China

Zheng Cai
School of Pharmaceutical
Sciences
Southern Medical University
Guangzhou
China

Editorial Office
MDPI AG
Grosspeteranlage 5
4052 Basel, Switzerland

This is a reprint of articles from the Special Issue published online in the open access journal *Pharmaceutics* (ISSN 1999-4923) (available at: www.mdpi.com/journal/pharmaceutics/special_issues/0WK2RBQOWE).

For citation purposes, cite each article independently as indicated on the article page online and using the guide below:

Lastname, A.A.; Lastname, B.B. Article Title. *Journal Name* **Year**, *Volume Number*, Page Range.

ISBN 978-3-7258-2152-5 (Hbk)
ISBN 978-3-7258-2151-8 (PDF)
https://doi.org/10.3390/books978-3-7258-2151-8

Contents

About the Editors

Ping Hu

Dr. Ping Hu ia currently working as Associate Professor in Jinan University. His research interests include broad topics including sustained drug release, hydrogels, stimuli-responsive drug delivery, and pharmacokinetics.

Zheng Cai

Prof. Zheng Cai is interested in the following research fields: controlled and sustained drug release; oral drug delivery systems; biopharmaceutics; pharmacokinetics; drug transporters. He has been an expert in these fields for more than 20 years.

pharmaceutics

MDPI

Editorial

Recent Advances in Polymeric Delivery Vehicles for Controlled and Sustained Drug Release

Hong Lu [1,2], Zheng Cai [3,*] and Ping Hu [1,2,*]

1 Department of Burns & Plastic Surgery, Guangzhou Red Cross Hospital, Faculty of Medical Science, Jinan University, Guangzhou 510006, China; luhong0910@foxmail.com
2 College of Pharmacy, Jinan University, Guangzhou 510006, China
3 School of Pharmaceutical Sciences, Southern Medical University, Guangzhou 510515, China
* Correspondence: caizheng@smu.edu.cn (Z.C.); inzahu@hotmail.com (P.H.)

1. Introduction

In the realm of modern therapeutics, the development of polymeric delivery vehicles has revolutionized drug administration, offering a sophisticated approach to controlled and sustained drug release. Polymeric drug delivery systems provide numerous advantages over traditional delivery methods, including the ability to improve drug stability, enhance bioavailability, and achieve targeted delivery to specific tissues or organs [1,2]. These systems are particularly vital in treating chronic diseases, where maintaining a consistent drug concentration within the therapeutic window is crucial for efficacy and patient compliance.

The concept of controlled drug release involves the gradual release of a drug over time, ensuring prolonged therapeutic effects and reducing the frequency of drug administration. This approach not only enhances patient convenience but also minimizes the risk of side effects associated with peak drug concentrations. Polymeric materials play a pivotal role in this process due to their versatile properties, such as biocompatibility, biodegradability, and tunable mechanical strength. These materials can be engineered to respond to various physiological stimuli, such as pH, temperature, or enzymatic activity, allowing for the precise control of drug release rates [3]. Among the most prominent polymeric systems are hydrogels, microspheres, nanoparticles, and micelles, each offering unique advantages depending on the therapeutic application. Hydrogels, for instance, are highly hydrated networks that can encapsulate a large amount of drug, providing a matrix for sustained release [4]. Microspheres and nanoparticles, on the other hand, offer the possibility of targeted delivery, where the drug is directed to a specific site within the body, thereby enhancing its therapeutic efficacy and reducing systemic exposure [5].

Recent advances in polymer science have led to the development of smart polymers, which can undergo reversible changes in response to environmental stimuli. These materials are particularly promising for creating drug delivery systems that can release their payload in response to specific triggers, such as a change in pH or temperature. This targeted approach not only improves the therapeutic outcomes but also reduces the risk of off-target effects, making these systems highly desirable in the treatment of complex diseases like cancer and neurological disorders [6,7].

Moreover, the integration of polymeric delivery systems with advanced technologies such as 3D printing and nanotechnology has opened up new avenues for personalized medicine. Three-dimensional printing, for example, allows for the fabrication of patient-specific drug delivery devices, tailored to the unique anatomical and physiological characteristics of the individual. This level of customization ensures optimal drug release profiles and improves patient outcomes [8]. Nanotechnology, on the other hand, has enabled the development of polymeric nanoparticles that can cross biological barriers, such as the blood–brain barrier, to deliver drugs to otherwise inaccessible sites. These nanoparticles can be functionalized with targeting ligands that recognize and bind to specific receptors

Citation: Lu, H.; Cai, Z.; Hu, P. Recent Advances in Polymeric Delivery Vehicles for Controlled and Sustained Drug Release. *Pharmaceutics* **2024**, *16*, 1184. https://doi.org/10.3390/pharmaceutics16091184

Received: 26 August 2024
Accepted: 4 September 2024
Published: 7 September 2024

on the surface of diseased cells, ensuring that the drug is delivered precisely where it is needed [9].

The growing body of research in polymeric drug delivery systems reflects the increasing recognition of their potential to address the limitations of traditional drug formulations. For instance, hydrophobic drugs, which are poorly soluble in water, can be encapsulated within polymeric matrices, thereby enhancing their solubility and bioavailability. Similarly, drugs with short half-lives can be formulated into sustained-release systems, reducing the frequency of administration and improving patient adherence.

As we delve into the specific advancements reported in the recent literature, it becomes evident that the field of polymeric drug delivery is on the cusp of significant breakthroughs. The following sections will provide a detailed examination of recent studies that highlight the diverse applications and innovative approaches being developed to enhance controlled and sustained drug release. These studies not only showcase the versatility of polymeric materials but also underscore the ongoing efforts to refine and optimize drug delivery systems for a wide range of therapeutic areas.

2. Overview of the Published Articles

The 11 papers in this Special Issue collectively highlight significant advancements in polymeric and nanoparticulate drug delivery systems, showcasing a wide range of innovative approaches aimed at enhancing therapeutic efficacy, stability, and targeted delivery. These studies represent a concerted effort to overcome the challenges associated with conventional drug delivery methods, pushing the boundaries of what is possible in terms of sustained release, targeting specific tissues, and improving the overall bioavailability of therapeutic agents.

Several papers focus on the development of long-acting injectable formulations, which are crucial for ensuring prolonged therapeutic effects and reducing the frequency of drug administration. For example, one study presents a water-free, PLGA-based depot gel designed for the sustained release of the peptide drug ACTY116 (contribution 1). This formulation not only demonstrates improved chemical and conformational stability of the peptide but also exhibits long-acting characteristics that make it an ideal candidate for in vivo sustained peptide delivery. Another study, employing a quality by design (QbD) approach, delves into the degradation mechanisms of peptides in long-acting injections (contribution 2). By conducting forced degradation studies, the researchers identify critical factors that influence peptide stability and implement strategic control measures to enhance the pharmacokinetic profile of the formulation, ensuring prolonged therapeutic efficacy.

In the realm of real-time drug release monitoring, a study utilizing fluorescence resonance energy transfer (FRET) technology makes significant strides (contribution 3). By encapsulating drugs within PLGA microspheres and tagging them with fluorescence markers such as Cy5 and Cy7, the researchers are able to correlate changes in FRET fluorescence with the drug release profile, offering a powerful tool for in vitro drug delivery studies. This method simplifies the analysis of drug release kinetics, providing valuable insights that could lead to better-designed delivery systems.

This Special Issue also emphasizes the development of targeted and responsive drug delivery systems. For instance, the creation of dual-targeted, pH-sensitive hybrid polymer micelles specifically for breast cancer treatment represents a significant advance in targeted therapy (contribution 4). These micelles, constructed from polymers modified with hyaluronic acid and folic acid, not only improve drug stability but also enhance the targeting of cancer cells, ensuring that the drug is released specifically in the tumor microenvironment. Another study introduces a thermo-responsive hydrogel system that encapsulates folate-targeted, curcumin-loaded nanoparticles (contribution 5). This innovative system offers the potential for highly localized drug delivery, especially in post-operative cancer treatment settings, where controlled and sustained release is critical.

Bone regeneration, another vital area of research, is addressed through the use of 3D-printed polycaprolactone (PCL) scaffolds enhanced with nano-topographically guided biomineralized coatings (contribution 6). These scaffolds demonstrate superior protein adsorption, ion release capacities, and the ability to guide the osteogenic differentiation of stem cells, making them a promising solution for bone regeneration therapies. Such advancements highlight the potential of integrating biomaterials with advanced manufacturing techniques to create next-generation therapeutic scaffolds.

Additionally, research exploring the influence of polymer composition on drug release profiles provides essential insights for the design of future delivery systems. One study, in particular, examines how varying the molecular weight and concentration of poly(ethylene) glycol diacrylate (PEGDA) affects the release of a model protein drug from photopolymerized systems (contribution 7). By manipulating these parameters, the researchers are able to modulate the swelling behavior and drug release profiles, thus offering a customizable approach to protein-loaded delivery systems.

This Special Issue also addresses the scalability of advanced drug delivery systems, as demonstrated in a pilot study on solid lipid nanoparticle-based metered-dose inhalers (SLN-MDIs) for lung disease treatment (contribution 8). This research not only demonstrates the successful fabrication of SLN-based MDIs with stable physicochemical properties but also highlights their potential for industrialization and clinical application, marking a significant step towards bringing these innovations from the lab to the marketplace.

Furthermore, the versatility and potential of biopolymer coatings in drug delivery are reviewed in a comprehensive analysis of cyclodextrin/citric acid (CD/CTR) biopolymers (contribution 9). This review underscores the environmentally friendly synthesis, biocompatibility, and effective controlled release mechanisms of CD/CTR-based systems, which hold promise for various drug delivery applications. Similarly, the application of the Box–Behnken design in optimizing tadalafil-loaded niosomal films for oral delivery represents a significant improvement in drug bioavailability and patient compliance, particularly for those with difficulty swallowing tablets (contribution 10).

Lastly, the use of engineered extracellular vehicles (EVs) for stroke therapy is explored, highlighting their unique advantages such as the ability to cross the blood–brain barrier, target specific cells, and maintain stability in circulation (contribution 11). This review provides a forward-looking perspective on the challenges and future prospects of EVs in clinical settings, especially for treating neurological disorders. Together, these papers underscore the tremendous progress being made in developing sophisticated drug delivery systems that are not only more effective but also precisely tailored to the specific needs of various therapeutic areas, paving the way for more personalized and targeted medical treatments in the future.

3. Conclusions/Future Directions

The advances in polymeric delivery vehicles, as evidenced by recent studies, underscore the transformative potential of these systems in modern medicine. From the development of long-acting injectable formulations to the exploration of 3D-printed scaffolds and smart hydrogels, researchers are continually pushing the boundaries of what is possible in controlled and sustained drug release. As the field progresses, the integration of new materials, technologies, and design strategies will likely lead to even more innovative solutions, addressing unmet medical needs and improving patient outcomes. The studies discussed here provide a glimpse into the future of drug delivery, where precision, efficiency, and patient-centered design will be at the forefront of pharmaceutical development.

Author Contributions: Conceptualization, P.H.; writing—original draft preparation, H.L. and P.H.; writing—review and editing, Z.C. and P.H. All authors have read and agreed to the published version of the manuscript.

Conflicts of Interest: The authors declare no conflicts of interest.

List of Contributions:

1. Xiong, Y.; Liu, Z.; Wang, Y.; Wang, J.; Zhou, X.; Li, X. Development and Evaluation of a Water-Free In Situ Depot Gel Formulation for Long-Acting and Stable Delivery of Peptide Drug ACTY116. *Pharmaceutics* **2024**, *16*, 620. https://doi.org/10.3390/pharmaceutics16050620.
2. Xiong, Y.; Wang, J.; Zhou, X.; Li, X. The Development of a Stable Peptide-Loaded Long-Acting Injection Formulation through a Comprehensive Understanding of Peptide Degradation Mechanisms: A QbD-Based Approach. *Pharmaceutics* **2024**, *16*, 266. https://doi.org/10.3390/pharmaceutics16020266.
3. Chen, Y.; He, Q.; Lu, H.; Yang, J.; Han, J.; Zhu, Y.; Hu, P. Visualization and correlation of drug release of risperidone/clozapine microspheres in vitro and in vivo based on FRET mechanism. *Int. J. Pharm.* **2024**, *653*, 123885. https://doi.org/10.1016/j.ijpharm.2024.123885.
4. Yang, D.; Li, Z.; Zhang, Y.; Chen, X.; Liu, M.; Yang, C. Design of Dual-Targeted pH-Sensitive Hybrid Polymer Micelles for Breast Cancer Treatment: Three Birds with One Stone. *Pharmaceutics* **2023**, *15*, 1850. https://doi.org/10.3390/pharmaceutics15061580.
5. Ertugral-Samgar, E.G.; Ozmen, A.M.; Gok, O. Thermo-Responsive Hydrogels Encapsulating Targeted Core-Shell Nanoparticles as Injectable Drug Delivery Systems. *Pharmaceutics* **2023**, *15*, 2358. https://doi.org/10.3390/pharmaceutics15092358.
6. Xing, F.; Shen, H.-Y.; Zhe, M.; Jiang, K.; Lei, J.; Xiang, Z.; Liu, M.; Xu, J.-Z.; Li, Z.-M. Nano-Topographically Guided, Biomineralized, 3D-Printed Polycaprolactone Scaffolds with Urine-Derived Stem Cells for Promoting Bone Regeneration. *Pharmaceutics* **2024**, *16*, 204. https://doi.org/10.3390/pharmaceutics16020204.
7. Rekowska, N.; Wulf, K.; Koper, D.; Senz, V.; Seitz, H.; Grabow, N.; Teske, M. Influence of PEGDA Molecular Weight and Concentration on the In Vitro Release of the Model Protein BSA-FITC from Photo Crosslinked Systems. *Pharmaceutics* **2023**, *15*, 1039. https://doi.org/10.3390/pharmaceutics15041039.
8. Shu, L.; Wang, W.; Ng, C.-i.; Zhang, X.; Huang, Y.; Wu, C.; Pan, X.; Huang, Z. A Pilot Study Exploiting the Industrialization Potential of Solid Lipid Nanoparticle-Based Metered-Dose Inhalers. *Pharmaceutics* **2023**, *15*, 866. https://doi.org/10.3390/pharmaceutics15030866.
9. Escobar, K.; Garrido-Miranda, K.A.; Pulido, R.; Naveas, N.; Manso-Silvan, M.; Hernandez-Montelongo, J. Coatings of Cyclodextrin/Citric-Acid Biopolymer as Drug Delivery Systems: A Review. *Pharmaceutics* **2023**, *15*, 296. https://doi.org/10.3390/pharmaceutics15010296.
10. Abla, K.K.; Mneimneh, A.T.; Allam, A.N.; Mehanna, M.M. Application of Box-Behnken Design in the Preparation, Optimization, and In-Vivo Pharmacokinetic Evaluation of Oral Tadalafil-Loaded Niosomal Film. *Pharmaceutics* **2023**, *15*, 173. https://doi.org/10.3390/pharmaceutics15010173.
11. Ahmed, W.; Kuniyan, M.S.; Jawed, A.M.; Chen, L. Engineered Extracellular Vesicles for Drug Delivery in Therapy of Stroke. *Pharmaceutics* **2023**, *15*, 2173. https://doi.org/10.3390/pharmaceutics15092173.

References

1. Varde, N.K.; Pack, D.W. Microspheres for controlled release drug delivery. *Expert Opin. Biol. Ther.* **2004**, *4*, 35–51. [CrossRef]
2. Ding, D.; Zhu, Q. Recent advances of PLGA micro/nanoparticles for the delivery of biomacromolecular therapeutics. *Mater. Sci. Eng. C Mater. Biol. Appl.* **2018**, *92*, 1041–1060. [CrossRef]
3. Cheng, R.; Meng, F.; Deng, C.; Klok, H.-A.; Zhong, Z. Dual and multi-stimuli responsive polymeric nanoparticles for programmed site-specific drug delivery. *Biomaterials* **2013**, *34*, 3647–3657. [CrossRef] [PubMed]
4. Merino, S.; Martin, C.; Kostarelos, K.; Prato, M.; Vazquez, E. Nanocomposite Hydrogels: 3D Polymer-Nanoparticle Synergies for On-Demand Drug Delivery. *ACS Nano* **2015**, *9*, 4686–4697. [CrossRef] [PubMed]
5. Jacob, J.; Haponiuk, J.T.; Thomas, S.; Gopi, S. Biopolymer based nanomaterials in drug delivery systems: A review. *Mater. Today Chem.* **2018**, *9*, 43–55. [CrossRef]
6. Hajebi, S.; Rabiee, N.; Bagherzadeh, M.; Ahmadi, S.; Rabiee, M.; Roghani-Mamaqani, H.; Tahriri, M.; Tayebi, L.; Hamblin, M.R. Stimulus-responsive polymeric nanogels as smart drug delivery systems. *Acta Biomater.* **2019**, *92*, 1–18. [CrossRef]
7. Sabourian, P.; Tavakolian, M.; Yazdani, H.; Frounchi, M.; van de Ven, T.G.M.; Maysinger, D.; Kakkar, A. Stimuli-responsive chitosan as an advantageous platform for efficient delivery of bioactive agents. *J. Control. Release* **2020**, *317*, 216–231. [CrossRef] [PubMed]

8. Jakus, A.E.; Geisendorfer, N.R.; Lewis, P.L.; Shah, R.N. 3D-printing porosity: A new approach to creating elevated porosity materials and structures. *Acta Biomater.* **2018**, *72*, 94–109. [CrossRef]
9. Zou, Y.; Sun, X.; Yang, Q.; Zheng, M.; Shimoni, O.; Ruan, W.; Wang, Y.; Zhang, D.; Yin, J.; Huang, X.; et al. Blood-brain barrier-penetrating single CRISPR-Cas9 nanocapsules for effective and safe glioblastoma gene therapy. *Sci. Adv.* **2022**, *8*, eabm8011. [CrossRef] [PubMed]

pharmaceutics

Article

Quantification of Microsphere Drug Release by Fluorescence Imaging with the FRET System

Yuying Chen [1], Huangjie Lu [1], Qingwei He [1], Jie Yang [1], Hong Lu [1], Jiongming Han [2], Ying Zhu [1] and Ping Hu [1,*]

[1] College of Pharmacy, Jinan University, Guangzhou 511436, China; cyy19981209@stu2021.jnu.edu.cn (Y.C.); tyxx70126@stu2021.jnu.edu.cn (H.L.); heqingwei524@163.com (Q.H.); msjieyang@163.com (J.Y.); luhong0910@foxmail.com (H.L.); 17670960705@163.com (Y.Z.)
[2] International School, Jinan University, Guangzhou 511436, China; 18203931589@163.com
* Correspondence: inzahu@hotmail.com or pinghu@jnu.edu.cn; Tel.: +86-18581483142

Abstract: Accurately measuring drug and its release kinetics in both in vitro and in vivo environments is crucial for enhancing therapeutic effectiveness while minimizing potential side effects. Nevertheless, the real-time visualization of drug release from microspheres to monitor potential overdoses remains a challenge. The primary objective of this investigation was to employ fluorescence imaging for the real-time monitoring of drug release from microspheres in vitro, thereby simplifying the laborious analysis associated with the detection of drug release. Two distinct varieties of microspheres were fabricated, each encapsulating different drugs within PLGA polymers. Cy5 was selected as the donor, and Cy7 was selected as the acceptor for visualization and quantification of the facilitated microsphere drug release through the application of the fluorescence resonance energy transfer (FRET) principle. The findings from the in vitro experiments indicate a correlation between the FRET fluorescence alterations and the drug release profiles of the microspheres.

Keywords: drug release; PLGA; microspheres; clozapine; risperidone; FRET

check for updates

Citation: Chen, Y.; Lu, H.; He, Q.; Yang, J.; Lu, H.; Han, J.; Zhu, Y.; Hu, P. Quantification of Microsphere Drug Release by Fluorescence Imaging with the FRET System. *Pharmaceutics* **2024**, *16*, 1019. https://doi.org/10.3390/pharmaceutics16081019

Academic Editor: Juan Torrado

Received: 13 June 2024
Revised: 26 July 2024
Accepted: 27 July 2024
Published: 31 July 2024

1. Introduction

Schizophrenia, an intense psychiatric condition, is distinguished by psychosis, resulting in substantial impairment across personal, familial, social, educational, and occupational spheres. Atypical antipsychotic medications [1], exemplified by risperidone (Ris) and clozapine(Clo), constitute pivotal elements in the management of this disorder [2,3]. Risperidone plays the role of a highly selective antagonism of 5-hydroxytryptamine 2A receptors and dopamine D2 receptors [4], which effectively control the positive symptoms of schizophrenia, such as hallucinations and delusions, while also improving negative symptoms like cognitive impairment and emotional apathy. Adherence to a consistent daily regimen of these pharmacotherapies is essential for symptom management, as discontinuation due to physical factors can lead to reduced efficacy and poor patient compliance [5]. Consequently, there exists a pressing necessity to innovate novel formulations to tackle this challenge.

A diverse array of extended release formulations has been developed to address the requirements of patients for enhanced compliance and sustained dosing [6]. Microsphere formulations are typically formed by active pharmaceutical ingredients (APIs) dispersed as molecules or small clusters in a polymer matrix [7,8]. Poly (lactic-co-glycolic acid) (PLGA) has become extensively utilized in creating microsphere formulations. Its widespread use is due to its highly favorable properties as a carrier for controlled drug release, particularly owing to its excellent biocompatibility and degradability [8,9]. The FDA has approved several PLGA microspheres for slow and controlled release formulations. Risperidone microsphere formulations are available, and there are several generic versions of risperidone microspheres in development [10]. However, the following factors influence the drug release effect of microspheres, including the lactic acid/glycolic acid ratio (LA/GA), molecular weight of PLGA, and variations in the preparation process, all of which can impact the in vivo drug release profile and safety [11,12]. Therefore, further comprehensive investigation into the relationship between drug release kinetics and manufacturing processes is essential to thoroughly investigate the connection between drug release kinetics and manufacturing processes to advance and evaluate both innovative and generic microsphere formulations.

The primary method for monitoring drug release remains the combination of in vitro drug release assays and in vivo blood concentration measurements [13]. However, these testing methods are cumbersome and cannot provide overall data on drug release conveniently. Methods such as scanning electron microscopy (SEM) only provide a static snapshot of the sample and do not capture its dynamic processes [14]. We would like to have a functional tool that can fully reveal and quantify the process of drug release from microspheres. Recently, fluorescent bioimaging has increasingly been used to track nanocarriers, and the routine characterization involves the use of various fluorescent probes. Although common fluorescent probes offer stable and robust signals, they are usually ineffective in providing information on drug release and are optically unstable and prone to photobleaching [15]. Fluorescent dyes with an aggregation-induced burst (ACQ) effect and aggregation-induced luminescence (AIE) properties pose challenges in achieving efficient near-infrared fluorescent probes and have the limitations of fluorescence bursting or reluminescence, making them unsuitable for monitoring the kinetics of drug release from long-acting injectable formulations like microspheres [16,17].

Optical imaging modalities enable the detection of Förster resonance energy transfer (FRET) channels, whose principle is the molecular interaction between donor and acceptor dyes [18]. This method is widely utilized for characterizing the properties of biological and nanomaterials and their responses to biological environments. FRET is highly distance-sensitive, making the encapsulation of both the donor and acceptor within a micrometer carrier essential for achieving high FRET efficiency [19]. The anticipated outcome upon the discharge of the drug from the microspheres into the medium is the diminishment of the FRET signal, with its absence indicating complete release of the drug substance. In addition, when FRET occurs between two fluorescent dyes, a double emission of donor and FRET can be obtained, which opens the possibility of quantitative ratio measurements using fluorescence detection in two different optical windows. To monitor potential drug leakage and microsphere degradation, Cy5 and Cy7 dyes were selected for this study. The dyes were commercially available as cyanine fluorescent dyes, which have advantages such as high penetration in the near-infrared range (700–900 nm). This facilitates increased penetration depth at the excitation wavelength thereby reducing interference of in vivo imaging.

The objective of this study is to establish a platform for quantifying drug release from microspheres in vitro using the Förster resonance energy transfer principle, enabling real-time assessment of drug release [20], a new quantitative technique developed for analyzing drug release from microspheres. As illustrated in Scheme 1, we propose to use the FRET effect relationship between Cy5 and Cy7 to realize drug release quantification when risperidone or clozapine drugs are released from microspheres. The results show that the FRET principle successfully enables the visualization and quantitative monitoring of microspheres. The fit of the in vitro release pattern and the FRET alteration pattern showed superior congruence for Clo-FRET-PLGA/M compared to Ris-FRET-PLGA/M. These results highlight the utility of the FRET principle in therapeutic diagnostic drug delivery with the potential in using fluorescence readout for quantitative monitoring of the drug release process.

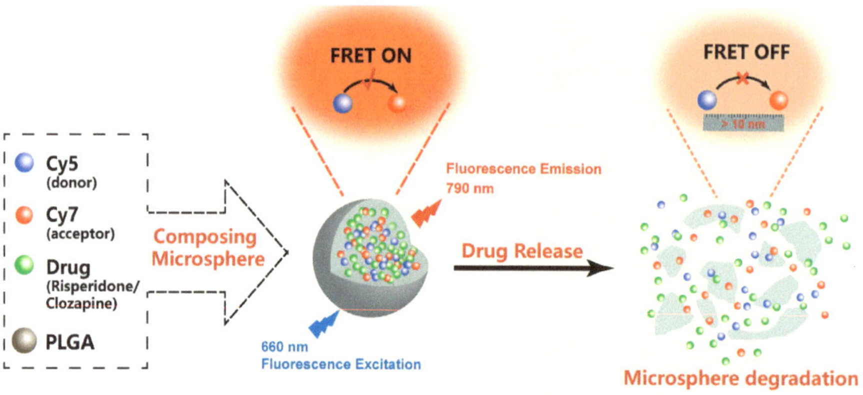

Scheme 1. Quantification and visualization of drug release by PLGA microspheres during in vitro drug release using the FRET principle.

2. Materials and Methods

2.1. Materials

Poly (D,L-lactic acid-glycolic acid copolymer) (PLGA) copolymer (molecular weight: 30k Da) was purchased from Jinan Daigang Bioengineering Co., Ltd. (Jinan, China) with a PLA/PGA ratio of (*w*/*w*) 75:25. Poly(vinyl alcohol) (87–89% hydrolyzed) was purchased from Acmec Biochemistry Co., Ltd. (Shanghai, China); Cy5 was purchased from Shanghai Yuanye Bio-technology Co., Ltd. (Shanghai, China); Cy7 was obtained from Nanjing Guye Ltd. (Nanjing, China). Trifluoroacetic acid (TFA), formic acid (HCOOH), acetonitrile (CH_3CN), and the drugs (i.e., risperidone and clozapine) were purchased from Shanghai McLean Biochemical Co. (Shanghai, China). Dichloromethane and dimethyl sulfoxide (DCM, DMSO) were purchased in analytical grade Shanghai Anergy Co., Ltd. (Shanghai, China). ddH_2O was used for any required steps.

2.2. Preparations of Clo-FRET-PLGA/M and Ris-FRET-PLGA/M

The emulsification solvent volatilization method was utilized for the preparation of microspheres. PLGA with a molecular weight of 30k Da was specifically selected for this purpose, with a PLGA to model drug (risperidone and clozapine) ratio of 5:1. The ratio of PLGA to fluorescent dye was 1000:1. Fluorescent dyes, pharmaceuticals, and PLGA were dissolved in dichloromethane to form the organic phase, and a volume ratio of 1:14 was maintained between the oil phase and the aqueous phase. Utilizing a homogenizer operating at a speed of 3400 rpm/min for 2 min, the organic phase was gradually introduced into a specified volume of 1% PVA in the aqueous phase, yielding an O/W primary emulsion under the controlled delivery of the organic phase by a syringe pump.

The emulsion underwent transfer into an aqueous PVA solution of 0.5% (*w*/*v*), at a volume three times that of the emulsion, with stirring at 1000 rpm [21]. A vacuum was subsequently applied to the aqueous phase for 4 h at 1000 rpm to facilitate the evaporation of methylene chloride and the solidification of the microspheres. Following this, the resulting suspension was transferred to a 50 mL centrifuge tube and centrifuged at 4000 rpm for 5 min. The microspheres were then subjected to three washes with 20 mL of deionized water and dried using a freeze dryer [14]. The resultant white powder, signifying the completion of the microsphere preparation process, was stored at 4 °C until further use [22].

2.3. Determination of Drug Loading and Encapsulation Efficiency of Clo-FRET-PLGA/M and Ris-FRET-PLGA/M

For the formulation of drug-loaded microspheres, approximately 5 mg of both Clo-FRET-PLGA/M and Ris-FRET-PLGA/M was accurately measured and dissolved in 2.5 mL of dimethyl sulfoxide (DMSO). Following the complete disruption of the microspheres, the solution was moved to a 10 mL volumetric flask and adjusted to its final volume using methanol. The mixture was subjected to ultrasonic agitation in an ultrasonic cleaner until dissolution was confirmed. Filtration was performed using a Millex® HV, 0.22 μm polyvinylidene fluoride (PVDF) syringe filter to ensure clarity [23].

The drugs encapsulated within the microspheres were quantified through high-performance liquid chromatography (HPLC). Employing an Agilent 1260 HPLC system, coupled with a SuperLu C18-AQ column (250 × 4.6 mm, 5 μm, 100 Å), facilitated the establishment of a drug concentration profile for risperidone and clozapine. The concentration of risperidone in Ris-FRET-PLGA/M was ascertained with a mobile phase of acetonitrile and water/trifluoroacetic acid (TFA) in a ratio of 30/70/0.1 ($v/v/v$), at a flow rate of 1 mL/min and a detection wavelength set at 275 nm. Similarly, the concentration of clozapine in Clo-FRET-PLGA/M was determined using a mobile phase of methanol and water/TFA in a ratio of 65/35/0.5 ($v/v/v$), with a consistent flow rate of 1 mL/min and a detection wavelength set at 254 nm [24].

Subsequent to the HPLC analysis, the concentrations of risperidone and clozapine were deduced from the established standard curves. These data enabled the calculation of drug loading (DL) and encapsulation efficiency (EE) for the microspheres. To ensure accuracy and reproducibility, each formulation underwent triplicate analysis, with the outcomes expressed as mean values accompanied by standard deviations.

$$\text{Encapsulation efficiency } (\%) = \frac{\text{actual amount of encapsulated drug of microspheres}}{\text{theoretical amount of encapsulated drug of microspheres}} \times 100 \quad (1)$$

$$\text{Drug loading } (\%) = \frac{\text{weight of drug contained in microspheres}}{\text{weight of microspheres}} \times 100 \quad (2)$$

2.4. *In Vitro Drug Release*

To ascertain the release of risperidone or clozapine from the microspheres, 5 mg of Ris-FRET-PLGA/M and Clo-FRET-PLGA/M was weighed and dispersed in 4 mL of phosphate-buffered saline (PBS, pH 7.4) containing 0.05% NaN_3 as preservative and 0.02% (w/v) Tween 80. The release experiment was carried out under sink conditions, and 0.02% Tween 80 served to increase the wettability and prevent the microspheres from floating. The microspheres were placed in a thermostatic oscillator (ZD-85, manufactured by Xuri Experimental Instrument Factory Co., Ltd., Changzhou, China), and the microspheres were kept at 37 °C and a shaking rate of 100 rpm. On the initial day 0, day 1, and every two days, 3 mL of samples was taken in 4 mL Eppendorf microtubes and centrifuged at 4000 rpm for 5 min at predetermined time points. To determine the drug content of the samples, 3 mL of supernatant was withdrawn and replaced with 3 mL of fresh release medium in the released samples. A plot of cumulative percent release versus time, calculated using the following equation, allowed us to assess the cumulative drug release of risperidone or clozapine from the microspheres [25]. Each formulation was also analyzed in triplicate, and the mean and standard deviation were reported. The calculation formula was (3):

$$\text{Release rate of microspheres} (\%) = \frac{\text{cumulative release of drug from microspheres}}{\text{total content of drug in microspheres}} \times 100 \quad (3)$$

2.5. *Detection of Fluorescence Intensity*

During the in vitro release experiment described in Section 2.4., the fluorescence intensity was measured by aspirating the whole solution and microspheres on the initial day 0, day 1, and every two days thereafter until the fluorescence intensity disappeared completely.

A fluorescence spectrometer (FS5, Edinburgh Instruments, Livingston, UK) was utilized to measure the fluorescence intensity under the excitation wavelength of 640 nm, and the absolute values of emitted fluorescence intensity at 690 nm and 790 nm were subsequently recorded. The decreasing trend of FRET fluorescence for each measurement was calculated using F/D using day 0 of the initial phase as a 100% reference.

The calculation formula was (4) [26].

$$F/D = \frac{F_{FRET}}{F_{Donor}} \tag{4}$$

F_{FRET}: the FRET fluorescence intensity, (Ex = 640 nm, Em = 790 nm); F_{Donor}: the donor fluorescence intensity, (Ex = 640 nm, Em = 690 nm).

Equations (5) and (6) were used as a 100% reference using day 0 of the initial phase and each subsequent time after ratio processing from the absolute value of the measured fluorescence intensity:

$$\text{FRET change rate } (\%) = \frac{F/D}{F0/D_0} \times 100\% \tag{5}$$

$$\text{FRET remaining rate } (\%) = (1 - \frac{F/D}{F0/D_0}) \times 100\% \tag{6}$$

2.6. *Determination of Weight Loss of PLGA Microspheres*

The weight of the microspheres (W_0) was recorded before putting them in 4 mL of release medium for the release of Ris-FRET-PLGA/M on days 1, 4, 7, 14, 18, and 26. Similarly, after placing Clo-FRET-PLGA/M in the release medium for 1, 4, 7, 14, 22, and 30 days, the microspheres and medium were vacuum-filtered through a 0.8 μm microporous filter membrane rinsed with a small quantity of purified water. The resulting microspheres underwent drying in a vacuum drying oven at 30 °C for a duration of 24 h until they were completely dry. The weight of the dried microspheres was recorded as W_2 [27]. The weight loss of the microspheres was calculated as follows (7):

$$\text{Mass Loss } (\%) = \frac{(W_0 - W_2)}{W_0} \times 100\% \tag{7}$$

2.7. *Determination of Water Absorption of PLGA Microspheres*

Ris-FRET-PLGA/M was released in the release medium on days 1, 4, 7, 14, 18, and 26. Similarly, after days 1, 4, 7, 14, 22, and 30 of Clo-FRET-PLGA/M exposure to the release medium, the microspheres and the release medium were filtered with a 0.8 μm microporous filter membrane under vacuum filtration. Subsequently, a minimal quantity of distilled water was applied, saturating the microspheres, which were then subjected to vacuum drying for 1 min to eliminate surface moisture, and the moisture content of the microspheres was weighed immediately This weight, representing the water-containing microspheres, was recorded as W_1. The resulting microspheres underwent drying in a vacuum drying oven at 30 °C for a duration of 24 h until the weight of the microspheres was constant and not decreasing, and the weight of the dried microspheres was weighed and recorded as W_2. Then, the difference in the weights between the wet microspheres and the dried microspheres was used for the estimation of the interparticle water ratio (W_i) at time t, which was defined as (8):

$$W_{i(t)} = \frac{\left(W_{1(t)} - W_{2(t)}\right)}{W_2(t)} \tag{8}$$

2.8. *Confocal Laser Microscopy Scanning*

The release medium conditions for both microspheres were the same as in Section 2.4, with three samples taken from each of the seven time points, 1 d, 4 d, 7 d, 14 d, 18 d, and 26 d for Ris-FRET-PLGA/M. Similarly, Clo-FRET-PLGA/M took three samples out at each of the six time points of 1 d, 4 d, 7 d, 14 d, 22 d, and 30 d. After the samples were filtered through a 0.8 μm microporous membrane filter and subsequently rinsed with a modest quantity of purified water, the resulting microspheres were placed in a vacuum drying oven (DZF-6050AB, Shanghai Li-Chen Bangxi Instrument Technology Co., Ltd., Shanghai, China) for drying, and the fluorescence changes in the microspheres were obtained as a graph of changes in fluorescence over time.

The collected microspheres were imaged using an ultrafast laser confocal microscope (FV3000, Olympus Corporation, Tokyo, Japan) [28]. The conditions of the instrument were set as follows: 1. Donor channel: Ex = 640 nm, Em = 690 nm. 2. FRET channel: Ex = 640 nm, Em = 790 nm.

2.9. Scanning Electron Microscope (SEM)

In order to investigate the changes in the morphological characteristics of the two microspheres over time, three samples of Ris-FRET-PLGA/M were taken out at each of the seven time points, 1 d, 4 d, 7 d, 14 d, 18 d, and 26 d, after incubation in PBS at 37 °C. Similarly, three samples of Clo-FRET-PLGA/M were taken out at each of the six time points of 1 d, 4 d, 7 d, 14 d, 22 d, and 30 d for SEM evaluation. Conductive double-sided adhesive tape was adhered to a standard sample carrier stage. Following this, a limited quantity of microspheres earmarked for testing were positioned on the conductive tape. Any unattached microspheres were expelled using a high-speed airflow. The microsphere samples were then sputter-coated with gold before the carrier stage was introduced into a high-resolution scanning electron microscope (SU1000, Hitachi, Tokyo, Japan) for observation of the microspheres' surface morphology [29].

2.10. Relation Study

The risperidone or clozapine release curves measured in vitro were compared with their corresponding (1-F/D) curves; the f_2 similarity factor was calculated; the correlation between the two curves from the same microspheres was established by using Origin software (Version 9.1, OriginLab Corporation, Northampton, MA, USA) and fitted equations were obtained. The drug release from microspheres was predicted by determining f_2 for the similarity coefficient when ($f_2 > 50$ is considered as valid value) [30].

3. Results

3.1. Preparations and Characterizations of Ris-FRET-PLGA/M and Clo-FRET-PLGA/M

The experimentally determined drug loadings of Ris-FRET-PLGA/M and Clo-FRET-PLGA/M in this study were 18.52 ± 1.26% (*w*/*w*) and 16.40 ± 1.21% (*w*/*w*), respectively. The encapsulation rates were all similar, approximately 73% for both samples. SEM images of Ris-FRET-PLGA/M and Clo-FRET-PLGA/M are shown in Figure 1. The microspheres exhibited spherical shapes with uniformly smooth surfaces across all samples. Their particle sizes were measured and are shown at around 70 μm.

Fluorescent dyes Cy5 and Cy7 were selected as FRET pairs for encapsulation into microspheres. Their chemical structures and physical properties are depicted in Figure S1 and Table S1. These dyes were chosen due to their similar log *p* values with the model drugs and their ideal in vivo imaging spectral properties. The fluorescence spectra of the fluorescent dyes under methanol solution were recorded as in Figure 2A, with strong emission bands at 650–750 nm for Cy5. As shown in Figure 2B, Cy7 has a strong emission band at 750–850 nm. As depicted in Figure 2C, the absorption spectrum of Cy5 aligns precisely with the emission spectrum of Cy7, while its emission in the near-infrared region at 780 nm is completely separated from that of Cy5; thus, theoretically, the energy of Cy5 can be efficiently transferred to the Cy7 fluorescent dye with the generation of the FRET effect, which makes this pair of combinations perfectly suited for ratiometric FRET imaging. As illustrated in Figure 2D, Cy5 and Cy7 were encapsulated into microspheres resulting in emission peaks corresponding to the donor channel, as well as remarkably intense FRET peaks. The results confirm that the microspheres exhibiting the FRET effect were successfully prepared.

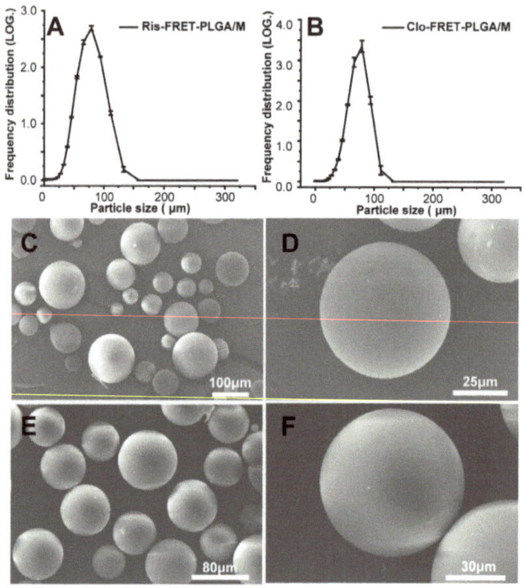

Figure 1. (**A**,**B**) Particle size distribution measurement of Ris-FRET-PLGA/M and Clo-FRET-PLGA/M; (**C**,**D**) Scanning electron microscopy images of Ris-FRET-PLGA/M; (**E**,**F**) Scanning electron microscopy images of Clo-FRET-PLGA/M.

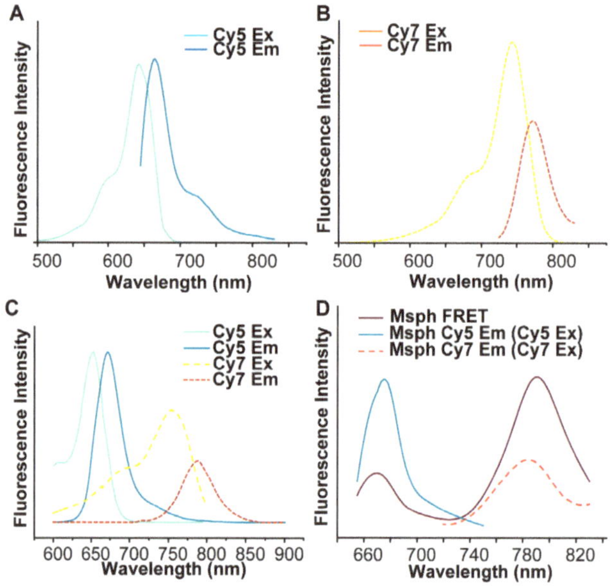

Figure 2. (**A**) Excitation and emission spectra for Cy5 were recorded in a methanol solution; (**B**) Excitation and emission spectra for Cy7 were recorded in a methanol solution; (**C**) Excitation and emission spectra for Cy5 and Cy7 were recorded in a methanol solution; (**D**) Spectral emission analysis was conducted for Cy5 microspheres (Msph) and Cy7 microspheres, as well as for the combination of Cy5 and Cy7 encapsulated within PLGA microspheres, using an excitation wavelength of 640 nm.

3.2. In Vitro Drug Release

The in vitro release profiles of both microspheres, conducted under simulated physiological conditions mimicking in vivo environments, demonstrated an initial burst release (within 24 h) of risperidone and clozapine, which accounted for less than 5% of the total release [31]. Subsequently, sustained drug release was observed, as illustrated in Figure 3A. The release rate of risperidone exhibited slow–fast–slow phases, finally reaching a plateau of 94% release by day 32. Figure 3B illustrates the donor and FRET fluorescence intensities obtained from Ris-FRET-PLGA/M, as measured using a fluorescence photometer. On day 2, both donor and FRET fluorescence intensities began to increase, followed by a continuous decline after day 6. This phenomenon might be due to the fact that the concentrations of donors and acceptors were relatively high within the microspheres, which causes quenching by the aggregation of fluorescent dyes, followed by a decrease in fluorescence concentration within the microspheres due to the beginning of the release of the drug and fluorescent dyes from the microspheres, and the quenching effect is diminished. The microspheres show a reluminescence phenomenon, and the fluorescence intensity value increases. The phenomenon suggests that the concentrations of fluorescent dyes could be further optimized to obtain a more ideal FRET change profile in future studies.

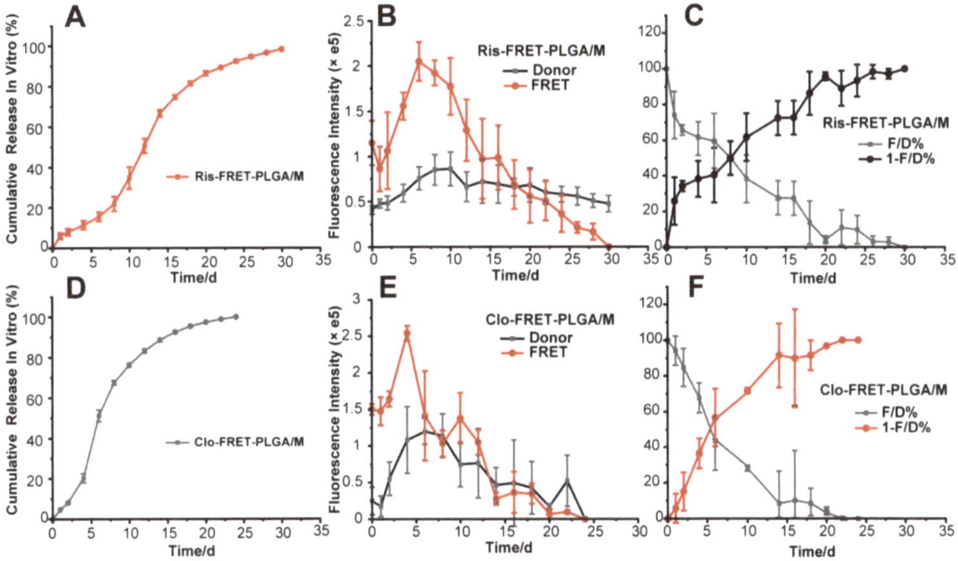

Figure 3. (**A**) Drug release profiles of Ris-FRET-PLGA/M in pH = 7.4 release medium; (**B**) Absolute values of fluorescence intensity of Ris-FRET-PLGA/M measured in vitro; (**C**) F/D and 1-F/D% values of Ris-FRET-PLGA/M after ratio treatment; (**D**) Clo-FRET-PLGA/M in PH = 7.4 release medium drug release profile; (**E**) Absolute values of fluorescence intensity of Clo-FRET-PLGA/M measured in vitro; (**F**) F/D and 1-F/D% values of Clo-FRET-PLGA/M after ratio treatment.

Despite the decreasing trend observed in the later stages, the absolute fluorescence intensities of the dyes fluctuated due to instrumental and other interferences. Therefore, through the computation of the FRET fluorescence intensity ratio to that of the donor fluorescence intensity (F/D), depicted in Figure 3C, the fluctuations in FRET of risperidone microspheres remained minimal, illustrating a consistent downward trend. Therefore, compared to the absolute fluorescence intensities of the donor and FRET channels, the FRET changes in the microspheres were more accurately characterized after applying the F/D ratio. Figure 3D indicates that clozapine's release was obviously faster, reaching 50% by day 6, after which the release rate significantly slowed down until complete release on day 26. Figure 3E presents the donor and FRET fluorescence intensities measured for Clo-FRET-PLGA/M. On day 2, both donor and FRET fluorescence intensities began to increase, followed by a steady decline starting on day 4. This pattern is analogous to the FRET change results observed with risperidone, although the fluorescent intensities for Clo-FRET-PLGA/M declined faster compared to Ris-FRET-PLGA/M. Figure 3F shows that after F/D calculation, a more stable decreasing trend in FRET change for clozapine microspheres was obtained [32].

Figure 4A,B depict the comparison of fluorescence changes and drug release for Ris-FRET-PLGA/M and Clo-FRET-PLGA/M, revealing that the similarity for clozapine is superior to that of risperidone microspheres. This similarity was calculated and is shown as the f_2 value, which was 59.79 for clozapine (Table 1), confirming that the FRET change in clozapine has a better fit with its drug release compared to risperidone.

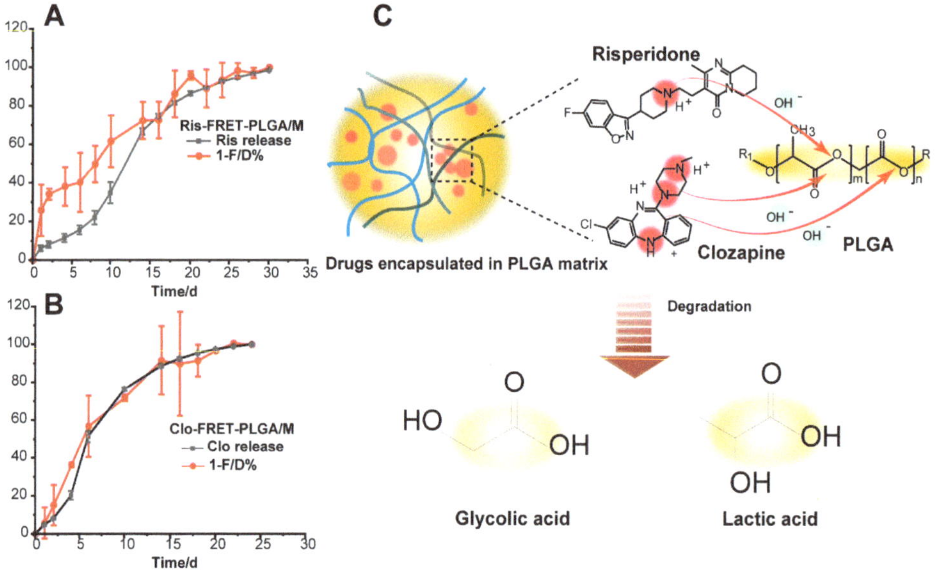

Figure 4. (**A**) Comparison between the in vitro drug release rate and the residual percentage of the FRET ratio (1 − F/D%) for Ris-FRET-PLGA/M and (**B**) Clo-FRET-PLGA/M (n = 3); (**C**) The proposed mechanism of PLGA degradation accelerated by the tertiary amine groups on risperidone and clozapine.

Table 1. f_2 factor analysis of the microspheres in vitro.

Microsphere	Total Drug Absorbed/Released In Vitro (%)	1 − A/D (%)	f_2
Ris-FRET-PLGA/M	98.39	100	39.10
Clo-FRET-PLGA/M	100	100	59.70

While risperidone had a lower log p value than clozapine, risperidone exhibited a slower release profile compared to clozapine. The degradation mechanism of PLGA involves chemical hydrolysis and enzyme-catalyzed hydrolysis [33]. The pH value of the environment greatly influences the hydrolysis and degradation of PLGA molecules. The water solution of risperidone or clozapine appears to be alkaline due to their chemical structures, and the hydrolysis of PLGA is accelerated in an alkaline environment. As in Figure 4C, the protonated amine groups on drugs can induce alkaline catalysis and accelerate the degradation of PLGA. More precisely, the tertiary amine molar concentration of risperidone is calculated to be 0.00277 g/mol, while that of clozapine is 0.00573 g/mol, which suggests that clozapine is a more effective catalyst for PLGA polymer degradation. Finally, due to its molecular weight being around 100 Da smaller than risperidone, clozapine molecules could diffuse more easily through the microspheres' networked pores, which lead to a faster release profile.

3.3. Determination of Weight Loss and Water Absorption of PLGA Microspheres

Microspheres require water absorption to initiate hydrolytic degradation. The expedited release observed in the release phase under specific conditions is believed to be associated with the ingress of water into the hydropore network of the microspheres. As depicted in Figure 5A,B, notable disparities were observed in the water uptake profiles of Ris-FRET-PLGA/M and Clo-FRET-PLGA/M. They both showed a gradual increase in water absorption over time, although clozapine absorbs water more rapidly. This trend is similar to the in vitro drug release results.

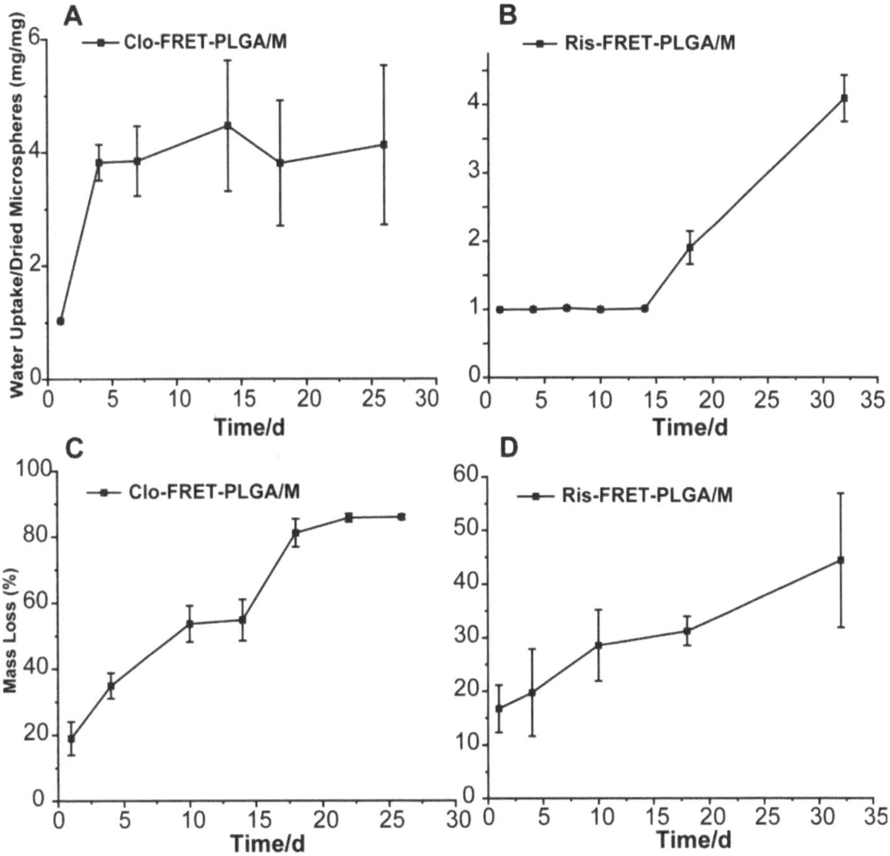

Figure 5. (**A**) In vitro kinetics of water uptake of Clo-FRET-PLGA/M (n = 3); (**B**) In vitro kinetics of water uptake of Ris-FRET-PLGA/M (n = 3); (**C**) In vitro mass loss of Clo-FRET-PLGA/M (n = 3); (**D**) In vitro mass loss of Ris-FRET-PLGA/M (n = 3).

The dissolution of polymers represents a crucial mechanism influencing the release of drugs from PLGA microspheres. Assuming erosion as the primary release mechanism and the drug is uniformly dispersed within the microspheres, the rate of drug release would be similar to the rate of polymer erosion (i.e., the rate of polymer mass reduction) [21,34]. Data depicting the mass loss during the in vitro release for Ris-FRET-PLGA/M and Clo-FRET-PLGA/M are presented in Figure 5C,D. The Ris-FRET-PLGA/M dissolved significantly slower than Clo-FRET-PLGA/M in the in vitro environment. When risperidone was completely released, the mass loss of microspheres reached 45%. In contrast, the mass loss of Clo-FRET-PLGA/M continued to increase with time and finally reached 90%.

3.4. Degradation of Ris-FRET-PLGA/M and Clo-FRET-PLGA/M over Time by Scanning Electron Microscope (SEM)

The morphological changes in degraded Ris-FRET-PLGA/M and Clo-FRET-PLGA/M are illustrated in Figure 6. At day 0 and day 1, both microspheres maintained smooth surfaces and exhibited spherical shapes. Subsequently, the Clo-FRET-PLGA/M displayed earlier morphological changes, as some of the microspheres showed initial degradation. This process is due to the hydrolysis of PLGA molecules and is expedited by the presence of the amine groups on clozapine, wherein PLGA hydrolyzed to lactic acid and glycolic acid under humid conditions [35]. In contrast, risperidone microspheres only exhibited cracks and pores on day 7 with a wrinkled surface, while maintaining their intact spherical shape. Over time, the risperidone microspheres showed an increase in pore size by day 14, and the particle size seemed to increase due to water absorption and swelling, accompanied by the appearance of some fragments. By day 30, the microspheres demonstrated increased surface porosity, consistent with the in vitro drug release results.

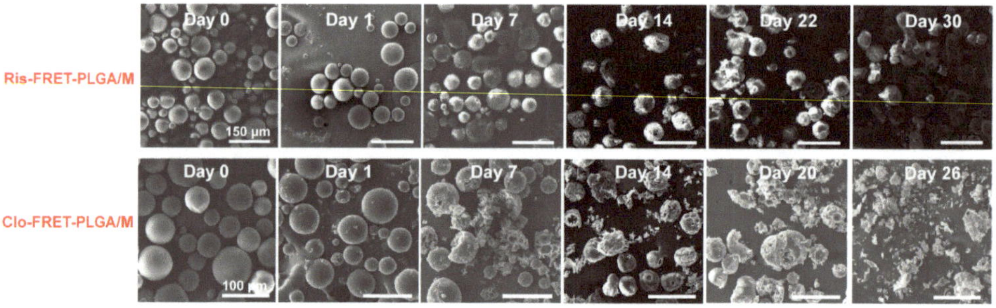

Figure 6. SEM revealed the degradation process for Ris-FRET-PLGA/M over a period of 30 days and for Clo-FRET-PLGA/M across 26 days in the release medium.

3.5. Degradation of Ris-FRET-PLGA/M and Clo-FRET-PLGA/M over Time by Confocal Laser Microscopy Scanning

Subsequently, confocal imaging was employed to observe the changes in the FRET effect with microsphere degradation, as depicted in Figure 7. Both donor and FRET channels were observed and recorded. The results demonstrate the presence of the FRET effect of the two types of microspheres. The fluorescence intensity of donor channels and FRET channels of both microspheres decreased with time. By the seventh day, some microspheres displayed cavities and uneven fluorescence distributions. Furthermore, a gradual decrease in fluorescence and loss of spherical shape were noted, especially for clozapine microspheres, which degraded at a faster rate than risperidone. Ratiometrically processed images indicate that the final FRET/D signal change closely mirrored the in vitro drug release, which was related to the PLGA degradation and microsphere fragmentation. These observations confirm the visualization and quantification of changes in FRET fluorescence, correlating with drug release from the microspheres.

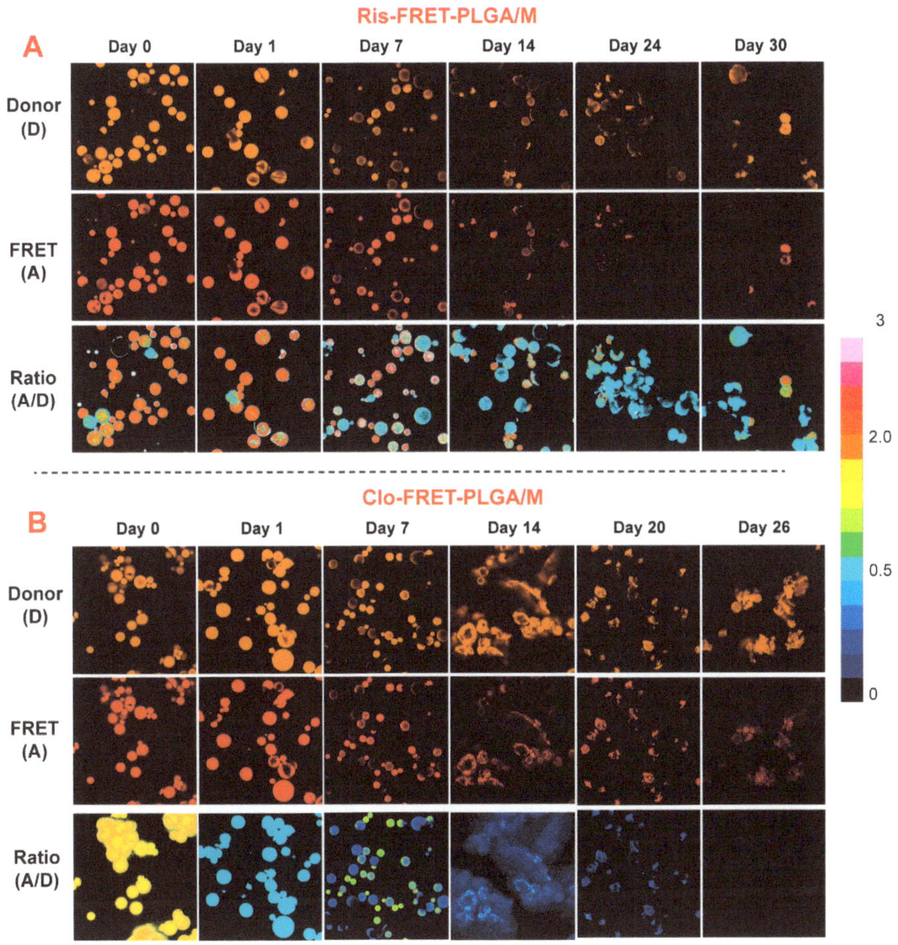

Figure 7. Extended in vitro observation through confocal microscopy for (**A**) Ris-FRET-PLGA/M over 30 days and (**B**) Clo-FRET-PLGA/M over 26 days.

3.6. Correlation and Prediction Studies

A series of in vitro experiments demonstrated the relationship between FRET changes in microspheres and in vitro drug release. By fitting the FRET changes to drug release data, we developed equations that provided a better quantitative understanding of this relationship. Figure 8A,C show a one-to-one linear relationship between the in vitro drug release and FRET changes for both types of microspheres. The correlation for Clo-FRET-PLGA/M was more significant with an R2 value of 0.983. Using the correlation formulas derived from our analysis (Table 2), FRET change data can be used to predict the drug release profiles in vitro. Figure 8B,D depict the actual and predicted in vitro drug release profiles of both microspheres. The trends of these predicted release data closely align with their observed data. Our analysis of the f_2 values indicates that a more accurate in vivo drug release profile could be obtained using the FRET change data and the correlation equation, particularly for Clo-FRET-PLGA/M, which showed a stronger correlation. Furthermore, the findings also lend quantitative backing to the theory that FRET alterations can indicate in vitro drug release from microspheres.

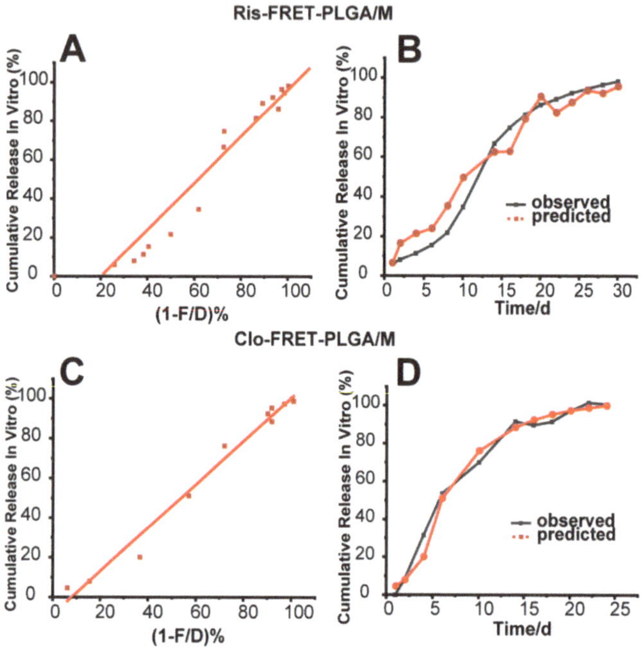

Figure 8. (**A**) The relationship between the drug release in vitro and the fluorescence variation in Ris-FRET-PLGA/M.; (**B**) Predicted and actual in vitro drug release patterns of Ris-FRET-PLGA/M; (**C**) The association between the in vitro release of the drug and the alteration in fluorescence of Clo-FRET-PLGA/M; (**D**) Comparison between the anticipated and actual drug release profiles of Clo-FRET-PLGA/M in vitro.

Table 2. Analytical comparison and forecast of in vitro drug release for Ris-FRET-PLGA/M and Clo-FRET-PLGA/M.

	Microsphere	Correlation Equation	R^2	f_2 Observed/Predicted
In vitro	Ris-FRET-PLGA/M	a = −24.480 + 1.204 × b	0.932	47.1
	Clo-FRET-PLGA/M	a= −8.2214 + 1.089 × b	0.983	73.0

4. Conclusions

In conclusion, this study represents a novel approach to quantify released drug from microspheres based on FRET principle. Our research successfully shows the preparation of PLGA microspheres encapsulating two fluorescent dyes, Cy5 and Cy7, along with two model drugs (risperidone and clozapine) to leverage the FRET concept in imaging microsphere drug release applications. The application utilized the fluorescence ratio of FRET and donor to characterize the FRET fluorescence changes within the microspheres, enabling accurate, sensitive, and reproducible quantitative analysis. Successful mitigation of interferences in common fluorescence imaging was achieved, and a reliable calibration of the results was obtained. Furthermore, this study compared the results of different drug release profiles, revealing that clozapine microspheres and the selected FRET pairs exhibited superior correlation, whose in vitro correlation between fluorescence changes and drug release reached 0.98. This work significantly contributes to the assessment and advancement of the drug release from PLGA microspheres, and expands avenues for further investigation into the mechanisms of PLGA-based long-acting products.

Supplementary Materials: The following supporting information can be downloaded at https://www.mdpi.com/article/10.3390/pharmaceutics16081019/s1, Figure S1: Chemical Structures of Risperidone, Clozapine, and Cyanine dyes. Table S1: Molecular Weights and Log P values of Risperidone, Clozapine, and Cyanine dyes.

Author Contributions: Y.C.: Methodology, Investigation, Formal analysis, and Writing—original draft. Q.H., H.L. (Huangjie Lu), J.Y., H.L. (Hong Lu), J.H., and Y.Z.: Investigation and Formal analysis. P.H.: Conceptualization, Formal analysis, and Writing—review and editing. All authors have read and agreed to the published version of the manuscript.

Funding: This work was supported by the National Natural Science Foundation of China (No. 82071367), Natural Science Foundation of Guangdong Province of China (Nos. 2021A1515220047 and 2023A1515011135).

Institutional Review Board Statement: The study was conducted in accordance with the Declaration of Helsinki, and approved by the Institutional Review Board of Jinan University (Protocol code 20200314-07, 13 March 2020).

Informed Consent Statement: Not applicable.

Data Availability Statement: The data presented in this study are available in this article and Supplementary Material.

Conflicts of Interest: The authors declare no conflict of interest.

References

1. Alvarado, A.T.; Rojas-Macetas, A.; Medalla-Garro, G.; Saravia, M.; Losno, R.; Valderrama-Wong, M.; Pariona, R. Potential polymorphic CYP1A2 and CYP2D6-mediated pharmacokinetic interactions between risperidone or olanzapine and selected drugs intended to treat COVID-19. *Drug Metab. Lett.* **2022**, *16*, 6–13. [CrossRef] [PubMed]
2. Liu, X.; Sun, H.; Zhang, Y.; Sun, Y.; Wang, W.; Xu, L.; Liu, W. Clozapine affects the pharmacokinetics of risperidone and inhibits its metabolism and P-glycoprotein–mediated transport in vivo and in vitro: A safety attention to antipsychotic polypharmacy with clozapine and risperidone. *Toxicol. Appl. Pharmacol.* **2021**, *422*, 115560. [CrossRef] [PubMed]
3. Sulejmanpasic, G.; Bise, S. Clozapine augmented with risperidone in treatment-resistant schizophrenia. *Eur. Psychiatry* **2017**, *41*, S385. [CrossRef]
4. Chopko, T.C.; Lindsley, C.W. Classics in Chemical Neuroscience: Risperidone. *ACS Chem. Neurosci.* **2018**, *9*, 1520–1529. [CrossRef]
5. Gee, S.; Taylor, D. Alternative Routes of Administration of Clozapine. *CNS Drugs* **2022**, *36*, 105–111. [CrossRef] [PubMed]
6. Puri, S.; Mazza, M.; Roy, G.; England, R.M.; Zhou, L.; Nourian, S.; Anand Subramony, J. Evolution of nanomedicine formulations for targeted delivery and controlled release. *Adv. Drug Deliv. Rev.* **2023**, *200*, 114962. [CrossRef]
7. Patel, M.; Jha, A.; Patel, R. Potential application of PLGA microsphere for tissue engineering. *J. Polym. Res.* **2021**, *28*, 214. [CrossRef]
8. Rahmani, F.; Naderpour, S.; Nejad, B.G.; Rahimzadegan, M.; Ebrahimi, Z.N.; Kamali, H.; Nosrati, R. The recent insight in the release of anticancer drug loaded into PLGA microspheres. *Med. Oncol.* **2023**, *40*, 229. [CrossRef] [PubMed]
9. Bee, S.-L.; Hamid, Z.A.A.; Mariatti, M.; Yahaya, B.H.; Lim, K.; Bee, S.-T.; Sin, L.T. Approaches to Improve Therapeutic Efficacy of Biodegradable PLA/PLGA Microspheres: A Review. *Polym. Rev.* **2018**, *58*, 495–536. [CrossRef]
10. Kohno, M.; Andhariya, J.V.; Wan, B.; Bao, Q.; Rothstein, S.; Hezel, M.; Wang, Y.; Burgess, D.J. The effect of PLGA molecular weight differences on risperidone release from microspheres. *Int. J. Pharm.* **2020**, *582*, 119339. [CrossRef]
11. Szlęk, J.; Pacławski, A.; Lau, R.; Jachowicz, R.; Kazemi, P.; Mendyk, A. Empirical search for factors affecting mean particle size of PLGA microspheres containing macromolecular drugs. *Comput. Methods Programs Biomed.* **2016**, *134*, 137–147. [CrossRef]
12. Zawbaa, H.M.; Szlęk, J.; Grosan, C.; Jachowicz, R.; Mendyk, A. Computational Intelligence Modeling of the Macromolecules Release from PLGA Microspheres-Focus on Feature Selection. *PLoS ONE* **2016**, *11*, e0157610. [CrossRef]
13. Andhariya, J.V.; Jog, R.; Shen, J.; Choi, S.; Wang, Y.; Zou, Y.; Burgess, D.J. In vitro-in vivo correlation of parenteral PLGA microspheres: Effect of variable burst release. *J. Control. Release* **2019**, *314*, 25–37. [CrossRef]
14. Gu, B.; Sun, X.; Papadimitrakopoulos, F.; Burgess, D.J. Seeing is believing, PLGA microsphere degradation revealed in PLGA microsphere/PVA hydrogel composites. *J. Control. Release* **2016**, *228*, 170–178. [CrossRef]
15. Zhang, Y.; Ju, J.; Wang, D.; Yuan, H.; Hao, L.; Tan, Y. Aggregation-induced emission for the visualization of the structure and properties of polymers. *J. Mater. Chem. C* **2021**, *9*, 11484–11496. [CrossRef]
16. Zhan, R.; Pan, Y.; Manghnani, P.N.; Liu, B. AIE Polymers: Synthesis, Properties, and Biological Applications. *Macromol. Biosci.* **2016**, *17*, 1600433. [CrossRef]
17. Qi, J.; Hu, X.; Dong, X.; Lu, Y.; Lu, H.; Zhao, W.; Wu, W. Towards more accurate bioimaging of drug nanocarriers: Turning aggregation-caused quenching into a useful tool. *Adv. Drug Deliv. Rev.* **2019**, *143*, 206–225. [CrossRef] [PubMed]
18. Kaur, A.; Dhakal, S. Invited Review: Recent applications of FRET-based multiplexed techniques. *Trends Anal. Chem.* **2019**, *123*, 115777. [CrossRef]

19. Charron, D.M.; Zheng, G. Nanomedicine development guided by FRET imaging. *Nano Today* **2018**, *18*, 124–136. [CrossRef]
20. Stenken, J.A. Introduction to Fluorescence Sensing. *J. Am. Chem. Soc.* **2009**, *131*, 10791. [CrossRef]
21. Fredenberg, S.; Wahlgren, M.; Reslow, M.; Axelsson, A. The mechanisms of drug release in poly(lactic-co-glycolic acid)-based drug delivery systems—A review. *Int. J. Pharm.* **2011**, *415*, 34–52. [CrossRef] [PubMed]
22. Alexis, F. Factors affecting the degradation and drug-release mechanism of poly(lactic acid) and poly[(lactic acid)-co-(glycolic acid)]. *Polym. Int.* **2005**, *54*, 36–46. [CrossRef]
23. Shi, C.; Yan, P.; Wang, K.; Chen, R. Inhibition of Fusarium graminearum growth and deoxynivalenol production by geocarpospheric bacterial strains. *J. Earth Sci.* **2010**, *21*, 306–308. [CrossRef]
24. Yang, Q.; Bian, Y.; Ren, G.; Hong, M. Insight into the Behavior Regulation of Drug Transfer of Nimodipine Loaded PLGA Microspheres by Emulsion Evaporation Method. *Colloids Surf. A Physicochem. Eng. Asp.* **2023**, *670*, 131569. [CrossRef]
25. Hu, X.; Zhang, J.; Tang, X.; Li, M.; Ma, S.; Liu, C.; Gao, Y.; Zhang, Y.; Liu, Y.; Yu, F.; et al. An Accelerated Release Method of Risperidone Loaded PLGA Microspheres with Good IVIVC. *Curr. Drug Deliv.* **2017**, *15*, 87–96. [CrossRef] [PubMed]
26. He, H.; Xie, Y.; Lv, Y.; Qi, J.; Dong, X.; Zhao, W.; Wu, W.; Lu, Y. Bioimaging of Intact Polycaprolactone Nanoparticles Using Aggregation-Caused Quenching Probes: Size-Dependent Translocation via Oral Delivery. *Adv. Healthc. Mater.* **2018**, *7*, e1800711. [CrossRef]
27. Yicheng, F.; Nan, Z.; Qi, L.; Jianting, C.; Subin, X.; Weisan, P. Characterizing the release mechanism of donepezil-loaded PLGA microspheres in vitro and in vivo. *J. Drug Deliv. Sci. Technol.* **2019**, *51*, 430–437. [CrossRef]
28. Zolnik, B.S.; Burgess, D.J. Effect of acidic pH on PLGA microsphere degradation and release. *J. Control. Release* **2007**, *122*, 338–344.
29. Aart, A.v.A.; van Manen, H.-J.; Jeroen, M.B.; Joost, D.d.B.; Clemens, A.v.B.; Cees, O. Raman Imaging of PLGA Microsphere Degradation Inside Macrophages. *J. Am. Chem. Soc.* **2004**, *126*, 13226–13227. [CrossRef]
30. D'Souza, S.; Faraj, J.A.; Giovagnoli, S.; Deluca, P.P. IVIVC from Long Acting Olanzapine Microspheres. *Int. J. Biomater.* **2014**, *2014*, 407065. [CrossRef]
31. An, T.; Choi, J.; Kim, A.; Lee, J.H.; Nam, Y.; Park, J.; Sun, B.K.; Suh, H.; Kim, C.-J.; Hwang, S.-J. Sustained release of risperidone from biodegradable microspheres prepared by in-situ suspension-evaporation process. *Int. J. Pharm.* **2016**, *503*, 8–15. [CrossRef]
32. Ji, X.; Cai, Y.; Dong, X.; Wu, W.; Zhao, W. Selection of an aggregation-caused quenching-based fluorescent tracer for imaging studies in nano drug delivery systems. *Nanoscale* **2023**, *15*, 9290–9296. [CrossRef] [PubMed]
33. Ford Versypt, A.N.; Pack, D.W.; Braatz, R.D. Mathematical modeling of drug delivery from autocatalytically degradable PLGA microspheres—A review. *J. Control. Release* **2012**, *165*, 29–37. [CrossRef] [PubMed]
34. Antonios, V.; Georgia, K.; Evangelia, B.; Vasileios, D.; Theocharis, K.; Myrika, S.; Nikolaos, D.B.; Evi, C.; Ioanna, K.; Evangelos, K.; et al. Poly(Lactic Acid)-Based Microparticles for Drug Delivery Applications: An Overview of Recent Advances. *Pharmaceutics* **2022**, *14*, 359. [CrossRef] [PubMed]
35. Busatto, C.; Berkenwald, E.; Mariano, N.; Casis, N.; Luna, J.; Estenoz, D. Homogeneous hydrolytic degradation of poly(lactic-co-glycolic acid) microspheres: Mathematical modeling. *Polym. Degrad. Stab.* **2015**, *125*, 12–20. [CrossRef]

pharmaceutics

MDPI

Article

Development and Evaluation of a Water-Free In Situ Depot Gel Formulation for Long-Acting and Stable Delivery of Peptide Drug ACTY116

Yingxin Xiong [1,†], Zhirui Liu [2,†], Yuanqiang Wang [3], Jiawei Wang [3], Xing Zhou [4,*] and Xiaohui Li [1,5,*]

1 Institute of Materia Medica and Department of Pharmaceutics, College of Pharmacy, Army Medical University, Chongqing 400038, China; yx.xiong@gmail.com
2 Department of Pharmacy, Xinan Hospital, Army Medical University, Chongqing 400038, China; zhirui_liu@tmmu.edu.cn
3 Chongqing School of Pharmacy and Bioengineering, Chongqing University of Technology, Chongqing 400054, China; wangyqnn@cqut.edu.cn (Y.W.); wangjiawei0423@gmail.com (J.W.)
4 Yunnan Key Laboratory of Stem Cell and Regenerative Medicine, Science and Technology Achievement Incubation Center, Kunming Medical University, Kunming 650500, China
5 Engineering Research Center for Pharmacodynamics Evaluation, College of Pharmacy, Army Medical University, Chongqing 400038, China
* Correspondence: zhouxing@kmmu.edu.cn (X.Z.); lpsh008@aliyun.com (X.L.)
† These authors contributed equally to this work.

Abstract: In situ depot gel is a type of polymeric long-acting injectable (pLAI) drug delivery system; compared to microsphere technology, its preparation process is simpler and more conducive to industrialization. To ensure the chemical stability of peptide ACTY116, we avoided the use of harsh conditions such as high temperatures, high shear mixing, or homogenization; maintaining a water-free and oxygen-free environment was also critical to prevent hydrolysis and oxidation. Molecular dynamics (MDs) simulations were employed to assess the stability mechanism between ACTY116 and the pLAI system. The initial structure of ACTY116 with an alpha helix conformation was constructed using SYBYL-X, and the copolymer PLGA was generated by AMBER 16; results showed that PLGA-based in situ depot gel improved conformational stability of ACTY116 through hydrogen bonds formed between peptide ACTY116 and the components of the pLAI formulation, while PLGA (Poly(DL-lactide-co-glycolide)) also created steric hindrance and shielding effects to prevent conformational changes. As a result, the chemical and conformational stability and in vivo long-acting characteristics of ACTY116 ensure its enhanced efficacy. In summary, we successfully achieved our objective of developing a highly stable peptide-loaded long-acting injectable (LAI) in situ depot gel formulation that is stable for at least 3 months under harsh conditions (40 °C, above body temperature), elucidating the underlying stabilisation mechanism, and the high stability of the ACTY116 pLAI formulation creates favourable conditions for its in vivo pharmacological activity lasting for weeks or even months.

Keywords: peptide; in situ depot gel; long-acting injectable; stability; molecular dynamics

Citation: Xiong, Y.; Liu, Z.; Wang, Y.; Wang, J.; Zhou, X.; Li, X. Development and Evaluation of a Water-Free In Situ Depot Gel Formulation for Long-Acting and Stable Delivery of Peptide Drug ACTY116. *Pharmaceutics* **2024**, *16*, 620. https://doi.org/10.3390/pharmaceutics16050620

Academic Editors: Duncan Craig and Alyssa Panitch

Received: 20 March 2024
Revised: 26 April 2024
Accepted: 29 April 2024
Published: 5 May 2024

1. Introduction

Peptides are a unique class of molecules that show diverse biological activities, rendering them appealing for therapeutic applications. Insulin, the pioneering peptide therapeutic developed for diabetes treatment [1], approved for medical use in the early 1920s, has been playing a pivotal role in diabetes management [2]. The success of insulin paved the way for peptide therapeutics, yet challenges persist. Peptides are susceptible to protease degradation in the gastrointestinal tract, limiting their oral bioavailability, and their size and hydrophilicity hinder cellular membrane penetration, often necessitating injection.

Moreover, rapid renal clearance and enzymatic degradation lead to short half-lives, requiring frequent administration and incurring compliance and cost issues. Peptides also face chemical and conformational instability, compromising their efficacy and safety [3,4]. Formulating stable and long-acting peptide dosage forms is a complex task.

Cardiac hypertrophy is a common cardiac disease characterised by an increase in cardiomyocyte volume and ventricular wall thickness, impairing cardiac function, which may include chest pain, dyspnea, syncope, arrhythmia, etc., and may even lead to heart failure or sudden death in severe cases. ACTY116 is a peptide designed to mimic the carboxyl terminus of Gαq protein [5,6], which can inhibit Gαq-mediated signal transduction and attenuate or reverse cardiac hypertrophy induced by pressure overload. ACTY116 has advantages such as high activity, low toxicity, and multiple effects, making it a promising candidate for anti-cardiac hypertrophy therapy [7,8]. As a 29-amino acid peptide (MW: 3424, its structure is depicted in Figure 1a), it faces the same challenges as other peptides, with extremely low oral bioavailability, poor stability, and a short in vivo half-life. Considering that cardiac hypertrophy is a chronic disease that requires long-term treatment, the objective of this study was to develop a stable long-acting injectable (LAI) formulation of peptide ACTY116 for sustained delivery.

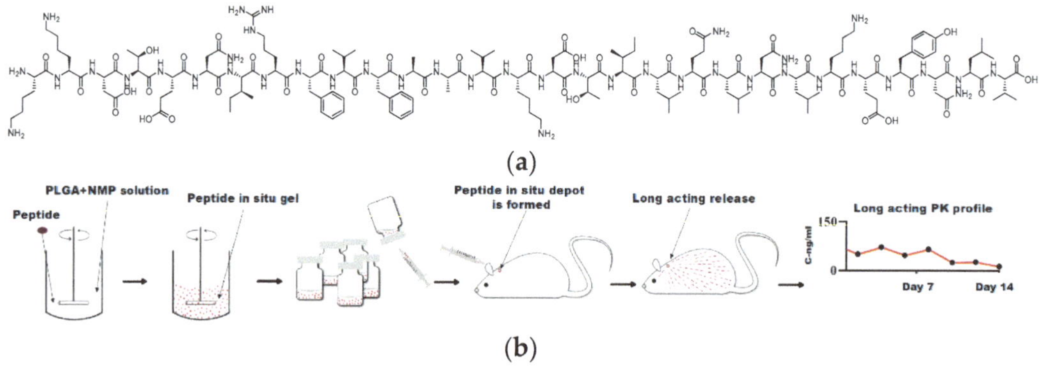

Figure 1. (**a**) Structure of peptide ACTY116; (**b**) schematic illustration of in situ depot gel preparation and in vivo long-acting performance.

The polymeric long-acting injectable (pLAI) formulations based on biodegradable polymers are widely utilised to extend the half-life of an active pharmaceutical ingredient (API). These formulations primarily encompass two forms: microspheres and in situ depot gels, with microspheres being the most extensively researched [9–13]. Approved microsphere LAIs for peptide delivery can exhibit prolonged in vivo residence time; Lupron Depot (leuprorelin acetate), Sandostatin LAR Depot (octreotide acetate), and Trelstar (triptorelin pamoate) are good examples [14,15]. Peptides are chemically unstable molecules, and achieving long-term stability at body temperature (37 °C) over several months poses a significant challenge. Thus, this study aimed to design, screen, and optimise a pLAI formulation capable of stabilising peptide ACTY116 for extended release in the human body.

Given the inherent susceptibility of peptide molecules to hydrolysis, this study aimed to develop a water-free in situ depot gel formulation [16,17] for ACTY116, and its stability was compared to that of ACTY116 microspheres. Stability assessments were conducted under challenging (40 °C, above body temperature) and long-term storage (25 °C) conditions, and in vitro release, in vivo pharmacokinetics, and pharmacological efficacy of ACTY116pLAI in situ depot gel were also evaluated (Figure 1b).

2. Materials and Methods

2.1. Materials

ACTY116 was synthesised by a contract research organization (HLXK, Beijing, China), PLGA was purchased from Evonik (Darmstadt, Germany) and Tanshtech (Guangzhou, China), N-methylpyrrolidone (NMP) and dichloromethane (DCM) were purchased from Chengdu Kelong Chemical Co., Ltd. (Chengdu, China), mannitol was purchased from Roquette (Lestrem, France), the NT-proBNP enzyme-linked immunosorbent assay (ELISA) kit was purchased from Elabscience Biotechnology (Wuhan, China), the BNP and β-MHC antibody immunohistochemical kit and diaminobenzidine (DAB) chromogenic agent were purchased from Servicebio (Wuhan, China), and norepinephrine (NE) was purchased from Sigma (Shanghai, China).

The moist heat autoclave (XD1-D, Xinhua, Shandong, China), IKA digital mixer (RW20, IKA, Staufen, Germany), polarizing microscope (BK-POL, Aote Optical Instrument, Chongqing, China), thermostatic oscillator (SHA-C, GY2016-SW, Changzhou, China), digital rotary viscometer (NDJ-8S, Fangrui, Shanghai, China), laser diffraction particle size analyzers (Mastersizer 3000, Malvern, Worcestershire, UK), ultra-high performance liquid chromatograph (e2695-2998, Waters, Milford, MA, USA), LC-MS/MS (6460, Agilent, Santa Clara, CA, USA), refrigerated centrifuge (Legend Micro 17R, Thermo, Waltham, MA, USA), microplate reader (infinite M200 pro, Tecan, Grödig, Austria), slide scanner (3D HISTECH, Budapest, Hungary), and Leica microscope (DM500, Leica, Wetzlar, Germany) were also procured.

2.2. Animals

BALB/C mice (20–25 g) were purchased from Army Medical University, China; SD rats (200–250 g) were purchased from Ensiweier Biotechnology, China. All animals had free access to a standard diet and drinking water and were housed in a room maintained at 22.0 ± 3 °C and with a 12:12 h cyclic lighting schedule. All animal experiments were approved by Laboratory Animal Welfare and Ethics Committee of Army Medical University (approval no.: AMUWEC20203377), and all the experiments were performed in accordance with the National Institutes of Health guidelines for the care and use of laboratory animals.

2.3. Method

2.3.1. Preparation of Different Dosage Forms

Preparation of ACTY116 Solution

Two milligrams (2 mg) of ACTY116 were weighed and added into 20 mL saline solution, stirring till dissolved (pH was 5.35), and ACTY116 saline solution was filled into vials (F1).

Preparation of ACTY116 PLGA Microspheres

The double emulsion–solvent extraction/evaporation method (Figure 2) was adopted due to the high hydrophilicity of ACTY116 [18]. ACTY116 (2 mg) was weighed and dissolved in 200 μL of water for injection (WFI) as water phase (W1 phase), 300 mg of PLGA (with a ratio of lactide to glycolide at 50:50, MW:7000–17,000, acid-terminated) was dissolved in 2 mL of DCM as oil phase, and a hydrophilic drug solution (W_1 phase) was emulsified in the organic polymer solution (O phase) under 15,000 rpm high shear mixing for 5 min to form the primary water-in-oil (W_1/O) emulsion. The obtained W_1/O emulsion was subsequently added into 200 mL of 1% PVA solution (W_2 phase) under 25,000 rpm high shear mixing for 10 min to form double emulsion (W_1/O/W_2). Evaporation of DCM was performed under 50 ± 1 °C, 100 rpm continuous shaking condition for 4 h, the microsphere suspension was centrifuged at 5000 rpm for 2 min (4 °C), and then dispersed with 10 mL of WFI for washing PVA and the unencapsulated ACTY116. The washing step was repeated for 5 cycles. Finally, the microspheres were dispersed in 10% mannitol solution, filled into vials, and lyophilised (F2) with the process as below (Table 1).

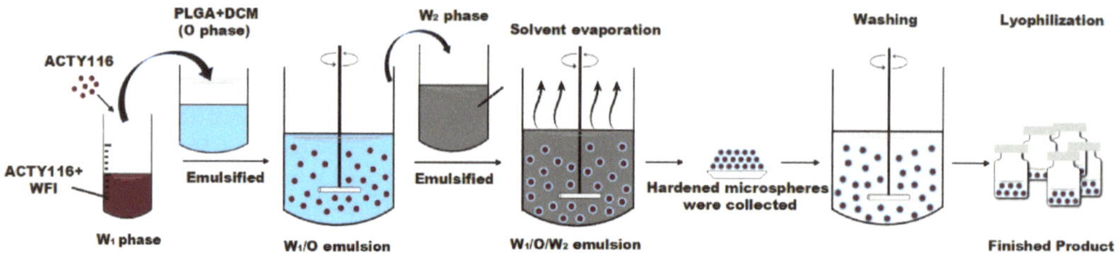

Figure 2. Schematic illustration of double emulsion–solvent extraction/evaporation technique for microsphere preparation.

Table 1. Lyophilization process for ACTY116 PLGA microspheres.

Temperature (°C)	Duration (min)	Pressure (Pa)
−40	30	—
−40	180	—
−20	120	10–16
−20	270	10–16
0	180	10–16
25	120	10–16
25	600	10–16

Evaluation of Microspheres

ACTY116 microspheres were dispersed in 10 mL of purified water to obtain a suspension, which was dropped onto the glass slide for polarising microscopic observation. Particle size was determined using laser diffraction particle size analysers, in which 2 mL of suspension was dispersed in 250 mL purified water, and instrument parameters were set to background measurement duration for 10 s, sample measurement duration for 30 s, obscuration range as 5.0–10.0%, and stirrer speed at 1000 rpm.

Encapsulation efficiency (EE): 40 mg of microspheres were weighed into a 5 mL centrifuge tube. Subsequently, 4 mL of purified water was added, and the mixture was shaken to ensure uniform dispersion of the microspheres. After centrifuging at 10,000 rpm for 5 min, the supernatant was collected to measure unencapsulated peptide. The microspheres that had settled at the bottom were transferred to a 25 mL volumetric flask using DMSO, the centrifuge tube was rinsed with DMSO for five times, and the rinses were pooled in the same volumetric flask; the mixture was then diluted to volume and thoroughly mixed, and the encapsulated peptide (ACTY116) was quantified using HPLC. Encapsulation efficiency was calculated using the following expression:

$$\text{Encapsulation efficiency (EE)\%} = \frac{\text{Encapsulated peptide}}{\text{Unencapsulated peptide} + \text{Encapsulated peptide}} \times 100\% \quad (1)$$

Preparation of ACTY116 pLAI In Situ Depot Gel

Following an extensive review of the literature, we designed the pLAI in situ depot gel formulation using PLGA (with a ratio of lactide to glycolide at 50:50, MW:7000–17,000, acid-terminated) as the sustained-release matrix [9,17,19,20]. An amount of 660 mg of PLGA was first dissolved into 1280 mg of NMP, and then 56 mg of ACTY116 was added and stirred for about 10 min until a suspension was visually observed, and the suspension was filled into vials for use (F3).

2.3.2. Stability Evaluation of Different Dosage FormFs

Assay Method for ACTY116

In the HPLC assay method for ACTY116, a C18 chromatographic column (150mm × 4.6 mm, 5 μm) was utilised, and the analysis was performed at a wavelength of 220 nm, maintaining a column temperature of 40 °C, and a constant flow rate of 1 mL/min was employed, with an injection volume of 5 μL. The gradient elution process is shown below (Table 2), with the mobile phase transitioning from A (water and 0.1% trifluoroacetic acid) to B (acetonitrile and 0.1% trifluoroacetic acid) over a specified time period.

Table 2. The gradient elution process.

Time/min	A (%)	B (%)
0	70	30
7	40	60
8	70	30
13	70	30

Chemical Stability for Different Dosage Forms

To investigate the chemical stability of ACTY116 during the preparation of different dosage forms, assay values were analysed and compared between different stages of preparation, and a short-term stability was performed under 40 °C for 5 days and 10 days.

Determination of Secondary Structure of ACTY116 Using Circular Dichroism

The secondary structure of ACTY116 before and after preparation in different dosage forms (solution (F1), microspheres (F2), and pLAI in situ depot gel (F3)) were tested, and a short-term secondary structure stability under 40 °C for both 5 days and 10 days were also tested, respectively. Samples were diluted to 0.05 mg/mL of ACTY116 and then transferred into the quartz cell (1 mm) for a circular dichroism (CD) spectra measurement, which was carried out on a computer-assisted Chirascan qCD circular dichroism spectrometer. The CD spectra were recorded from 185 to 280 nm with bandwidth of 1 nm and step size of 1 nm.

2.3.3. Formulation Optimization of ACTY116 pLAI In Situ Depot Gels

Acid-terminated PLGA (with a ratio of lactide to glycolide at 50:50, MW: 7000–17,000) was used in the study.

Evaluation of the impact of NMP on ACTY116 stability in pLAIs was performed by varying the ratio of NMP to ACTY116, and the formulations are provided in Table 3. The different formulations were filled into 7 mL vials and sealed with stoppers, respectively. The filled vials were autoclaved under 121 °C for 8 min and then tested for assay value by a HPLC method.

Table 3. Formulation compositions with different NMP quantities.

Formulation	F4	F5	F6	F7	Ingredient Function
ACTY116 (mg)	10	10	10	10	Active
PLGA (mg)	30	30	30	30	Control release polymer
NMP (mg)	200	300	400	500	solvent
NMP:ACTY116	20:1	30:1	40:1	50:1	——

Evaluation of the impact of PLGA quantity on ACTY116 stability in pLAIs was also performed by varying the ratio of PLGA to ACTY116, and the formulations are provided in Table 4. The quantities of NMP and ACTY116 were kept constant while the PLGA quantity was varied to make the ratios of PLGA: ACTY116 range from 0:1 to 15:1. The different formulations were filled into 7 mL vials and sealed with rubber stoppers. The filled vials were autoclaved under 121 °C for 8 min and then tested for assay values.

Table 4. Formulation compositions with different PLGA quantities.

Formulation	F8	F9	F10	F11	F12	F13
ACTY116 (mg)	10	10	10	10	10	10
PLGA (mg)	0	10	20	50	100	150
NMP (mg)	200	200	200	200	200	200
PLGA:ACTY116	0:1	1:1	2:1	5:1	10:1	15:1

Evaluation of the impact of vial diameter on the ACTY116 stability in pLAIs was performed using Formulation F11 (Table 4). The suspension was filled into glass vials with different inner diameters (4, 10, and 19 mm) and sealed with rubber stoppers. The filled vials were autoclaved under 121 °C for 8 min and then tested for assay value.

Evaluation of the impact of residual oxygen in the headspace on ACTY116 stability in pLAIs was performed using formulation F11, as shown in Table 4. The formulation was filled into 10 mm-diameter vials, and residual oxygen in the headspace was controlled between 0.1% and 5.0%. The filled vials were autoclaved under 121 °C for 8 min and then tested for assay values.

2.3.4. Stability Study of ACTY116 pLAI In Situ Depot Gel

The stability evaluation of the selected ACTY116 pLAI in situ depot gel was performed using formulation F11, as shown in Table 4. The formulation suspension was filled into 4 mm-diameter vials, headspace oxygen was controlled to be not more than 0.1% and sealed with rubber stoppers. The samples for stability study were stored under the harsh condition (40 °C/75% RH) and the long-term storage condition (25 °C/65% RH), respectively. Critical quality attributes such as assay, headspace oxygen, viscosity, and polarizing microscope observation were tested at predetermined time intervals.

Viscosity of the ACTY116 in situ depot gel was determined with a digital rotary viscometer, 3.0 rpm for 2 min [21]. The ACTY116 in situ depot gel was dropped onto the glass slide for polarizing microscopic observation [22,23].

2.3.5. Conformational Stability by Computer Molecular Dynamics (MDs) Simulations

The initial structure of ACTY116 with an alpha helix conformation was constructed using SYBYL-X 1.3 [24], and the copolymer PLGA was generated by AMBER 16 [25] employing GAFF2 force fields. The 12 units of ACTY116 were dissolved in water and set to periodic boundary within 10 Å, then heated to 373.15 K, and subjected to 100 ns production MDs simulations using the AMBER 16 package with ff14SB [26]. After density adjustment and equilibrium, the complex obtained a stable conformation while the root mean square deviation (RMSD) fluctuated steadily over 20 ns. Similarly, the ensemble of the complex with ACTY116 and PLGA (molar ratio of ACTY116:PLGA is about 1:2 in F11) was manually constructed, then dissolved in NMP within 10 Å to the edge of the periodic boundary; after density adjustment and equilibrium using AMBER 16, MDs simulations were performed under 373.15 K for 100 ns by AMBER 16. The average structure was extracted from the latest 20 ns for analysis. All visualisations were presented using Pymol 2.5 [27].

2.3.6. Evaluation of ACTY116 Formulations for Pharmacological Activity in Mice with Cardiac Hypertrophy Induced by Norepinephrine

Peptide ACTY116 was designed to treat cardiac hypertrophy (CH). An animal model of cardiac hypertrophy in mice induced by norepinephrine (NE) has been reported and was used in this study to evaluate the pharmacological action of ACTY116 (F1) solution and pLAI in situ depot gel (F11) [28]. BALB/C mice were randomly divided into 5 groups (6 mice/group) as follows:

Group 1: Vehicle-control mice received subcutaneous injection of a solution containing 5% glucose and 0.1% vitamin C, 20 mL/kg/d, bid, for 14 successive days.

Group 2: NE-treated mice received subcutaneous injection of NE (3.0 mg/kg/d) bid, for 14 successive days to induce cardiac hypertrophy.

Group 3: NE-treated mice also received subcutaneous injection of ACTY116 solution at a dose of 1.0 mg/kg, bid, for 14 successive days.

Group 4: NE-treated mice also received subcutaneous injection of ACTY116 pLAI at a dose of 7 mg/kg, once a week on day 0 and day 7.

Group 5: NE-treated mice also received subcutaneous injection of ACTY116 pLAI at a single dose of 14 mg/kg on day 0.

The dose regime is illustrated in Figure 3.

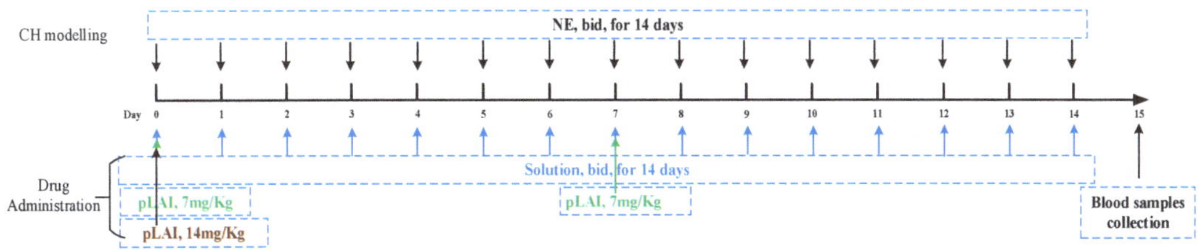

Figure 3. CH modelling and drug administration.

At the day 15, blood samples for all mice were collected from the retrobulbar venous plexus, and the plasma was separated by refrigerated centrifuge at 4 °C. The biomarker for cardiac hypertrophy, i.e., NT-Pro-brain natriuretide (NT-pro BNP) was analysed with an ELISA kit [29,30]. The heart tissues were harvested from mice, and cardiac morphology was then observed and recorded. Subsequently, the heart weight, body weight and tibial length were measured [31]. The heart weight to body weight ratio (HW/BW) and heart weight to tibial length (HW/TL) were then calculated and evaluated with statistical analysis. The heart tissues were dissected, and part of these tissues were fixed in 4% buffered formalin for 48 h, then dehydrated, embedded in paraffin, and sectioned. BNP and β-MHC immunohistochemical analysis were performed: diaminobenzidene chromogenic reaction was performed after BNP and β-MHC antibody incubation, respectively, and the positive expression of BNP and β-MHC was brownish yellow. H&E and WGA staining were performed, and the images were scanned and observed using a slide scanner [32–34]. Thereafter, the pathological changes and the cross-sectional areas of cardiomyocytes in heart tissues were measured by using ImageJ software (version 1.8.0.172, NIH, Bethesda, MD, USA).

2.3.7. In Vitro Release Testing for ACTY116 PGLA In Situ Depot Gel Formulations

Impact of both quantity and type of PLGA in the in situ depot gels on in vitro ACTY116 release was performed using different formulations. Formulations with different quantities of PLGA (L:G = 75:25, MW: 10,000–20,000) are provided in Table 5 while formulations with different type of PLGA are listed in Table 6. An accelerated method was used to test in vitro release of ACTY116 PLGA in situ depot gel. An elevated temperature around the glass transition (Tg) of PLGA was adopted as a method to accelerate peptide release from the PLGA matrix. When the PLGA is close to/above Tg, the polymer is in the rubbery state, where mobility of the polymer results in significant acceleration of peptide release via diffusion, and hydration/degradation is also accelerated when compared to the glassy state [35,36]. An accelerated method by elevating the temperature was used to test in vitro release of ACTY116 pLAI in situ depot gel. Briefly, about 30–50 mg of ACTY116 pLAI in situ depot gel was pipetted into the 20 mL vial dissolution device containing 20 mL purified water as release medium at 50 ± 1 °C and under 100 rpm continuous shaking conditions. An aliquot of 200 μL of the release medium was sampled at 2, 5, 24, 48, 72, 96, 120, 144, and 168 h, respectively, and the released peptide ACTY116 was analysed by the bicinchoninic acid (BCA) method [37].

Table 5. Formulations with different PLGA:ACTY116 ratios.

	F14	F15	F16
ACTY116 (mg)	10	10	10
PLGA (L:G = 75:25) (mg)	30	40	50
NMP (mg)	200	200	200
PLGA:ACTY116	3:1	4:1	5:1

Table 6. Formulations with different PLGA types.

	F17	F18	F19	F20
ACTY116 (mg)	10	10	10	10
PLGA (mg)	50	50	50	50
NMP (mg)	200	200	200	200
PLGA type (L:G)	50:50	65:35	75:25	85:15
Molecular weight	7000–17,000	24,000–38,000	10,000–20,000	190,000–240,000

2.3.8. Pharmacokinetics of ACTY116 Solution and pLAI In Situ Depot Gels in Rats

ACTY116 solution (F1) was injected subcutaneously in rats for pharmacokinetic (PK) behaviour as an immediate release formulation. Six (6) rats received ACTY116 solution at a dose of 1.0 mg/kg, bid, and blood samples were collected from the retrobulbar venous plexus at minutes 10, 20, 40, 60, 90, 120, and 180 after subcutaneous administration; then, plasma was separated by refrigerated centrifuge, and the level of ACTY116 was analysed with a LC-MS/MS method.

Formulations (F14, F15, and F16 in Table 5) were used to evaluate the impact of PLGA quantity on in vivo pharmacokinetics in rats. Eighteen rats were randomly divided into 3 groups (6 rats/group), and each group of rats received different ACTY116 pLAI formulations at a single SC dose of 14 mg/kg. The blood samples were collected from the retrobulbar venous plexus at hours 1, 2, 4 and on days 1, 3, 5, 7, 9, 11, 13, 15, 17, 19, 21, 23, 25, and 27 post subcutaneous injection; then, plasma was separated by refrigerated centrifuge, and ACTY116 was analysed using a LC-MS/MS method.

Formulations (F17, F18, F19, and F20 in Table 6) were used to evaluate the impact of different types of PLGA on in vivo pharmacokinetics in rats. Eighteen rats were randomly allocated to 3 groups (6 rats/group). Each group of rats received ACTY116 pLAI formulated with a different PLGA type at a single SC dose of 14 mg/kg. The blood samples were collected from the retrobulbar venous plexus at hours 1, 2, and 4 and on days 1, 3, 5, 7, 9, 11, 13, 15, 17, 19, 21, 23, 25, 27, 29, 31, 33, and 35 post subcutaneous injection; then, plasma was separated by refrigerated centrifuge, and ACTY116 was analysed with a LC-MS/MS method.

3. Results

3.1. Stability Evaluation of Different Dosage Forms

The microscope observation of ACTY116 microspheres are displayed in Figure 4a,b. Particle size distribution (Figure 4c) of the microspheres was tested, and the results showed that D (10) was 5.12 µm, D (50) was 16.6 µm, D (90) was 38.3 µm, and D (4,3) was 21.9 µm. Figure 4c depicts the results of three measurements, represented by curves of three different colors. The repeatability of the three measurements is good, the curves almost completely overlap. Encapsulation efficiency was 29.8%.

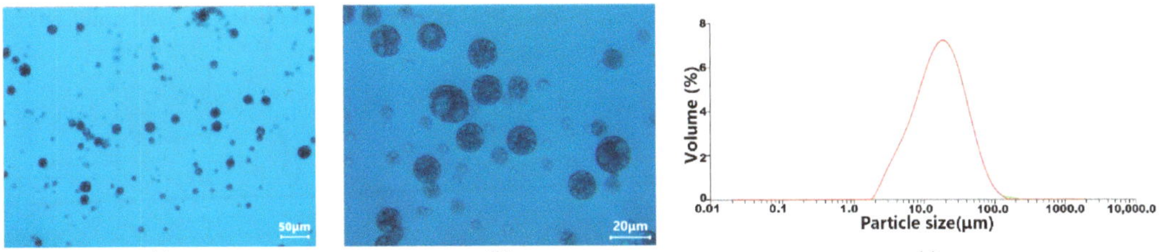

(**a**) (**b**) (**c**)

Figure 4. The polarizing microscope observation of ACTY116 microspheres: (**a**) 20×, (**b**) 80×; (**c**) particle size distribution.

3.1.1. Chemical Stability Evaluation of Different Dosage Forms

Stability data in Table 7 showed that the assay of ACTY116 in microsphere (F2) decreased dramatically to 86.78% after preparation. However, the assay of ACTY116 in solution (F1) and pLAI (F3) were kept constant after preparation.

Table 7. ACTY116 assay change during preparation and short-term stability under 40 °C (n = 4).

	Before Preparation	After Preparation	5 Days @ 40 °C	10 Days @ 40 °C
Solution (F1)	100%	99.43 ± 1.6%	86.75 ± 2.3%	67.39 ± 2.1%
Microsphere (F2)	100%	86.78 ± 2.4%	79.54 ± 3.1%	58.46 ± 2.8%
pLAI in situ depot gel (F3)	100%	99.56 ± 0.8%	99.12 ± 1.7%	98.23 ± 1.3%

Short-term stability under 40 °C showed that the assay in solution (F1) decreased to 86.75% after 5 days and 67.39% after 10 days while the assay in microspheres (F2) decreased to 79.54% after 5 days and 58.46% after 10 days. Surprisingly, the assay was kept at 99.12% after 5 days and 98.23% after 10 days for ACTY116 pLAI in situ depot gel (F3). Data suggested that peptide ACTY116 appears to be much more stable in the pLAI in situ depot gel formulation than that in a solution or microspheres.

Stability comparison results of different dosage forms suggested that neither solution nor the microspheres were stable enough for further development, and non-aqueous in situ depot gel formulations have the potential to maintain the chemical stability of ACTY116; thus, formulation optimization of ACTY116 pLAI in situ depot gel was further conducted.

3.1.2. Secondary Structure of ACTY116 Determined by Circular Dichroism

A secondary structure of a peptide is commonly evaluated by circular dichroism (CD) [38,39]. The circular dichroism (CD) spectrum reveals a prominent negative absorption peak at 208 nm for ACTY116, indicative of its typical α-helical characteristics. Before preparation, the CD spectrum of ACTY116 in solution (Figure 5a) displayed a prominent negative band at 208 nm with a very strong intensity. However, following preparation, the characteristic band at 208 nm gradually diminished. Moreover, after storage at 40 °C for 5 and 10 days, the CD signals decreased further. The CD spectra of ACTY116 in microspheres (Figure 5b) showed a similar pattern after preparation and storage under 40 °C. Because organic solvent evaporation under 50 °C for 4 h was conducted, the process may cause the secondary structure change of peptide ACTY116 during preparation. When stored under 40 °C, the peptide could be aggregated, which may lead to the change of the peptide secondary structure. However, as can be seen (Figure 5c), the CD spectra of ACTY116 in pLAI in situ depot gel have no change in all samples. The CD spectra indicated that the secondary structure of ACTY116 in solution and microspheres had been altered after preparation and storage in high-temperature conditions for several days; however, the characteristic band at 208 nm remained unchanged for samples from different conditions in pLAI in situ gel. Thus, the secondary structure of ACTY116 can be well protected using the pLAI in situ gel formulation approach.

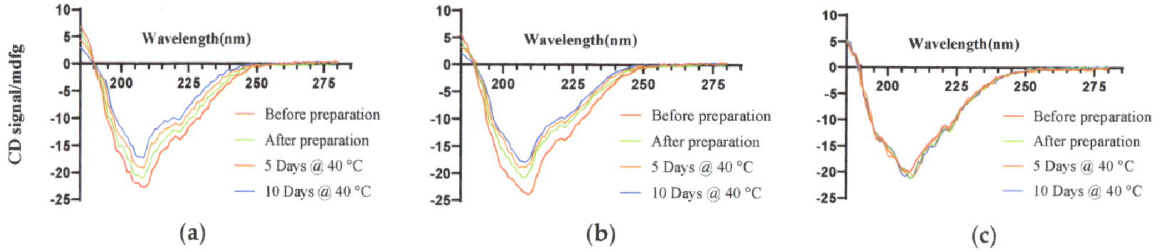

Figure 5. The CD spectra of different ACTY116 dosage forms: (**a**) ACTY116 solution (F1); (**b**) ACTY116 microspheres (F2); (**c**) ACTY116 pLAI in situ depot gel (F3).

Stability comparison results of different dosage forms suggested that neither solution nor microspheres were stable enough for further development, whereas in situ depot gel formulations have the potential for a better stability; thus, formulation optimization of ACTY116 pLAI in situ depot gels were further conducted.

3.2. *Formulation Optimization of ACTY116 pLAI In Situ Depot Gels*

ACTY116 in situ depot gel formulation variables evaluated in this study include quantity of NMP and PLGA, vial diameter, and residual oxygen in headspace.

NMP was used as a non-aqueous solvent in the formulation, which is critical for dissolving PLGA. We varied the ratio of NMP to ACTY116 to explore the impact of NMP on peptide stability. As shown in Figure 6a, an increase in the ratio of NMP to ACTY116 from 20:1 to 50:1 (F4–F7) did not show a negative impact on the assay value of ACTY116, which means that NMP may not impact ACTY116 stability.

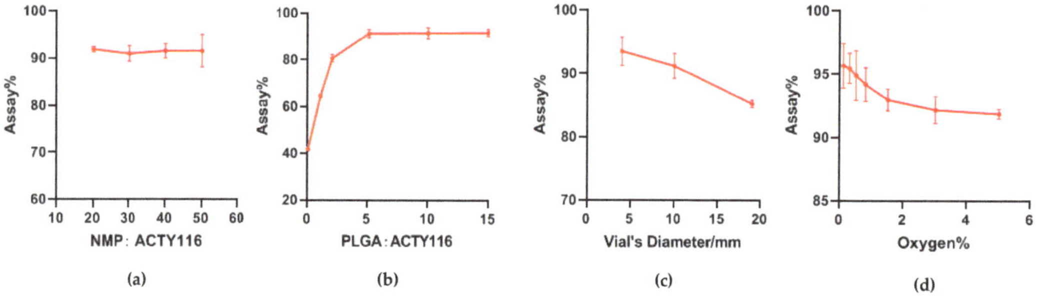

Figure 6. The results of variable evaluation: (**a**) evaluation of impact of NMP quantity on ACTY116 stability in pLAIs (F4–F7); (**b**) evaluation of impact of PLGA quantity on ACTY116 stability in pLAIs (F8–F13); (**c**) evaluation of impact of surface area of liquid–air interface (three sizes of vials with diameters of 4 mm, 10 mm, and 19 mm) on ACTY116 stability in pLAIs; (**d**) evaluation of impact of residual oxygen in the headspace on ACTY116 stability in pLAIs. Data are represented as mean ± SD (n = 4).

PLGA is a controlled-release polymer, which is critical for the long-acting effect of the formulation. The effects on its stability of formulations with different ratios of PLGA (F8–F13) to ACTY116 have been evaluated after terminal sterilization. As shown in Figure 6b, ACTY116 is degraded rapidly without PLGA in the formulation (F8), and only 42% of the assay remained after being treated at 121 °C for 8 min. When the ratio of PLGA to the peptide increased, the assay value of the peptide increased correspondingly after thermal treatment. When the ratio of PLGA to ACTY116 increased 5:1 (F11), the assay of ACTY116 remained above 90% after terminal sterilization. However, increases in the ratios greater than 5:1 did not show further protection of ACTY116 from thermal degradation. Formulation F13 had the highest ratio of PLGA to ACTY116, i.e., 15:1, and the assay of the peptide after terminal sterilization was 91.6%, which is similar to that of F11. The results suggested that PLGA should have a protective function for ACTY116 during terminal sterilization, and a minimal ratio of PLGA to ACTY116 (5:1) is required for maximal protection.

The presence of liquid–air interfaces in peptide/protein pharmaceuticals is known to negatively impact product stability. Vial diameter is a formulation variable because the size has an impact on the surface area of the liquid–air interface. Three sizes of vials with diameters of 4 mm, 10 mm, and 19 mm were filled with the formulation F11 and used in the surface area study. As seen in Figure 6c, the assay value of ACTY116 F11 decreased rapidly with an increase in the vial diameter. When the diameter of the vial was 4 mm, the assay value of ACTY116 was 93.5% after being treated at 121 °C for 8 min while the assay decreased to 85.3% with the vial diameter of 19 mm. Obviously, the vial diameter has a significant impact on degradation of ACTY116, and small diameters reduced the thermal degradation of the peptide, which may be related to the smaller area of liquid–air interface.

Impact of oxygen levels in the headspace of ACTY116 assay has been studied, and the results are provided in Figure 6d. As can be seen, the higher the oxygen level in the headspace is, the lower the assay value would be. When the headspace oxygen was at about 5%, the assay value of ACTY116 decreased to 91.9% after being treated under 121 °C for 8 min while if the oxygen level was reduced to 0.1%, the assay of ACTY116 was 95.7%, which is significantly higher than that of headspace oxygen at 5%. Thus, the oxygen level in the headspace should be controlled to be as low as possible to stabilise the ACTY116 in the pLAI formulation.

3.3. Stability Study of ACTY116 pLAI In Situ Depot Gel

The results demonstrated the excellent stability of ACTY116 pLAI following terminal sterilization at 121 °C for 8 min, with the assay value of ACTY116 remaining as high as 98.6%. Storage at 25 °C/60% RH for up to 6 months and at 40 °C/75% RH for 3 months did not lead to any noticeable changes in assay values. Moreover, no discernible alterations in appearance, headspace oxygen levels, or viscosity were observed (see Table 8).

Table 8. Stability study results for ACTY116 in situ depot gel formulation F11.

Attribute	Initial	6 Months Under 25 °C/60% RH	3 Months Under 40 °C/75% RH
Assay%	98.6 ± 0.85	98.8 ± 1.32	98.3 ± 1.01
Headspace oxygen%	0.07 ± 0.02	0.05 ± 0.03	0.04 ± 0.01
Viscosity (cP)	115 ± 1.50	116 ± 1.83	113 ± 1.83
Appearance observed by polarizing microscope	Uniform shiny ACTY116 crystals in the suspension	Uniform shiny ACTY116 crystals in the suspension	Uniform shiny ACTY116 crystals in the suspension

The polarised microscope observation (30×) of ACTY116 pLAI in situ depot gel is presented in Figure 7; shiny particles were observed in the microscopic image. Since ACTY116 was the sole component exhibiting doubly refracting (optically anisotropic) properties in the pLAI formulation, resulting in interference effects under the polarised light microscope, the shiny particles seen in Figure 7 were identified as ACTY116 peptide crystals. The stability study indicated that the ACTY116 crystals observed through the polarizing microscope in the pLAI formulation remained unchanged throughout the study period.

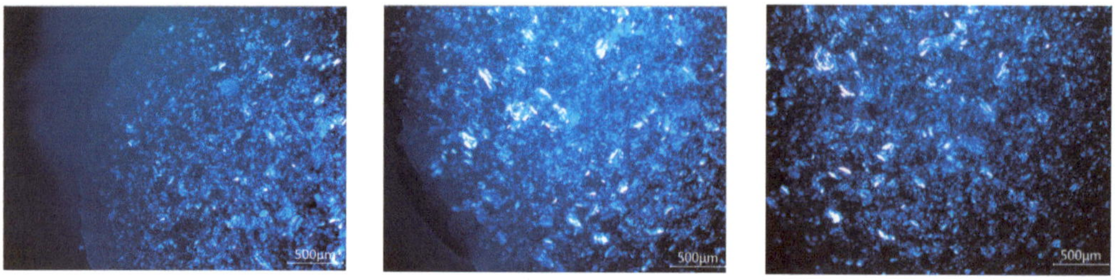

(a) (b) (c)

Figure 7. Polarised microscopic observation of ACTY116 in situ depot gel: (**a**) month 0; (**b**) long-term stability: month 6; 25 °C/60% RH; (**c**) accelerated stability: month 3; 40 °C/75% RH.

In summary, stability data for ACTY116 pLAI in situ depot gel formulation indicated that the formulation is stable and suitable for further in vivo pharmacodynamics and pharmacokinetics studies.

3.4. Conformational Stability Evaluation by Computer Molecular Dynamics (MDs) Simulations

The initial structure of ACTY116 with an alpha helix conformation was established by SYBYL-X 1.3. An ensemble with 12 ACTY116 units was constructed and solvated with water (Figure 8a). After conducting 100 ns of MD simulations, eight units of ACTY116 experienced a conformational change from the middle of the helix when the system was heated to 373.15 K (Figure 8b). To investigate the conformational dynamics of ACTY116, the root mean square fluctuation (RMSF) value during 100 ns of MD simulations were analysed (Figure 8c), in which eleven units of ACTY116 became looser, and the results showed that Lys1-Lys2 and Asn27-Val29 exhibited an obvious change in the displacement of amino acids at C- and N-terminals. The sequences Lys1-Asn6 and Lys24-Val29 were presented in a loop, and seven units of ACTY116 in the middle area (Phe11-Asp16) experienced a secondary structure change. Most fluctuations were observed in Lys1-Asn6, which may be due to the temperature increase that makes the thermodynamic trajectory of amino acids larger. Interestingly, when ACTY116 was complexed with PLGA and solvated into NMP (Figure 8d), only three units of ACTY116 had a slight change in their terminal while others still maintained the same secondary structure (Figure 8e) during 100 ns of MDs simulations. To investigate the conformational dynamics of ACTY116 in PLGA and the NMP system, RMSF values during 100 ns of MDs simulations were analysed (Figure 8f), three units of ACTY116 became looser, and the sequences Lys1-Thr4 and Leu23-Val29 were presented in a loop, while other ACTY116 units maintained a rigid structure during the 100 ns MDs simulation.

Figure 8g indicates that the ensemble with 12 units reached equilibrium from the RMSD value. The average structure was extracted from the latest 20 ns while the system reached equilibrium. ACTY116 complexed with PLGA became more rigid due to the steric hinderance, which has a much lower RMSD value compared to ACTY116 solution. There were some shifts in Lys1-Thr4 and Lys24-Val29 of the ACTY116 secondary structure from alpha-helix to random coil in the water system. Figure 8h indicates that the average hydrogen bonds formed between ACTY116 and different solvent systems during 100 ns MD simulations, and 20 hydrogen bonds were formed between ACTY116 and NMP or PLGA, which shows a higher hydrogen bond value compared to the water system when heated to 373.15 K. In the PLGA and NMP systems, amino acids (such as Lys2, Asn6, Lys15, Asn22, Tyr26, and Leu28) formed hydrogen bonds. That is the reason nine units of ACTY116 remain a rigid structure under 373.15 K for 100 ns MDs simulations, and the hydrogen bonds were kept steady during the whole 100 ns under 373.15 K. However, hydrogen bonds in the water system showed an increasing trend during 100 ns under 373.15 K, which means the secondary structure of ACTY116 changed under high temperature, more amino acids were exposed to water, and more hydrogen bonds were formed between ACTTY116 and water. Figure 8i shows the visualisation of peptide ACTY116 in which it was surrounded by PLGA during the 100 ns MDs simulations.

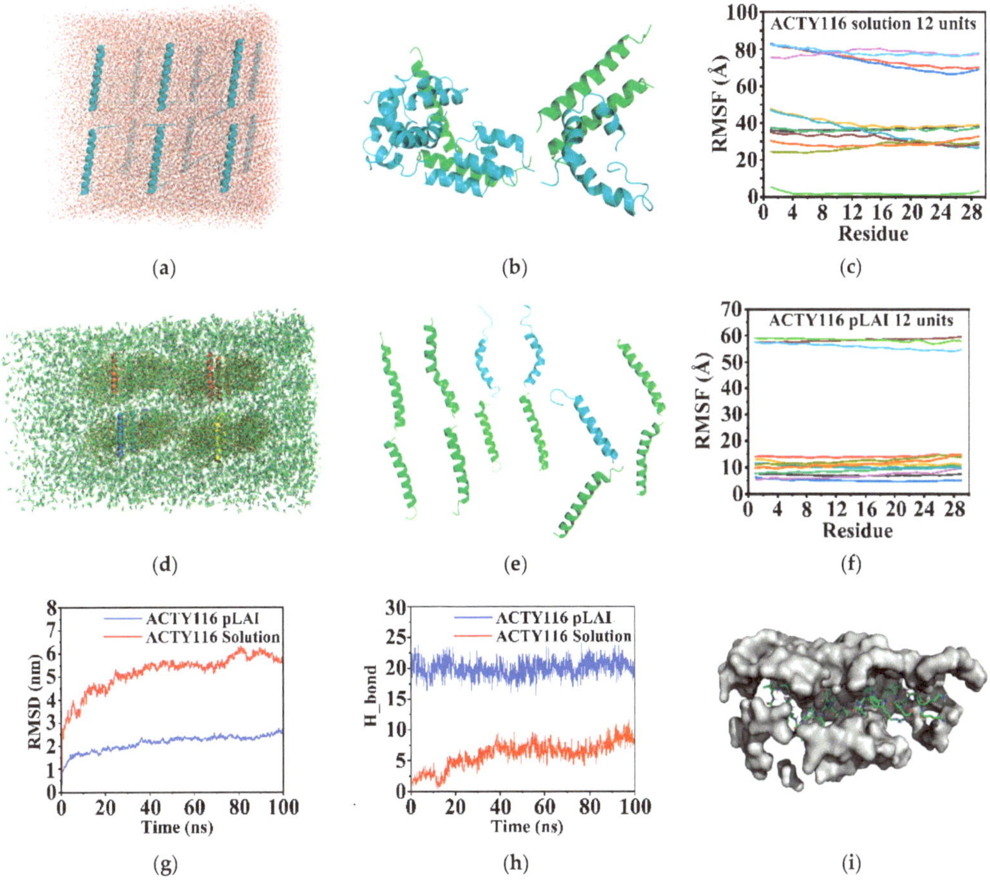

(a) (b) (c)

(d) (e) (f)

(g) (h) (i)

Figure 8. (**a**) Ensemble of ACTY116 initial state solvated in water; (**b**) MDs simulations under 373.15 K for 100 ns in water; (**c**) root mean square fluctuation (RMSF) value of ACTY116 solvated into water under 373.15 K; (**d**) ensemble of ACTY116 initial state complex of ACTY116 and PLGA solvated into NMP; (**e**) MDs simulations under 373.15 K for 100 ns in PLGA and NMP system; (**f**) root mean square fluctuation (RMSF) value of ACTY116 solvated into PLGA and NMP system under 373.15 K; (**g**) root mean square fluctuation (RMSF) value of ACTY116 solvated into water under 373.15 K for 100 ns; (**h**) RMSF value of ACTY116 solvated into PLGA and NMP system under 373.15 K for 100 ns; (**i**) visualisation of ACTY116 unit complexed with PLGA (gray part) around 10 Å distance.

3.5. Pharmacological Effect of ACTY116 Solution and pLAI In Situ Depot Gels on Cardiac Hypertrophy Induced by NE in Mice

Cardiac hypertrophy in mice can be induced by subcutaneous injection of NE for 2 weeks. Pharmacological results showed that many symptoms related to cardiac hypertrophy can be observed in mice, including significant changes in anatomy of the heart and level of BNP, NT-proBNP, and β-MHC. As seen in Figure 9a, NE-treated mice had larger hearts visually than those of mice in the control group. Figure 9b shows that the heart sizes (heart weight (mg)/body weight (g) (HW/BW)) in the ACTY116-solution group appeared similar to those in NE-treated mice. When ACTY116 pLAI in situ depot gel was injected, both dose regimes (i.e., 7 mg/kg once a week for two weeks or 14 mg/kg once every two weeks) showed smaller heart sizes than for the NE-treated group and the ACTY116-solution group by visual observation. The heart weight in the control group was 5.5 mg/g mice while it was increased to 7.2 mg/g body weight after being treated with NE, bid, for 2 weeks, which is a significant increase compared to the control group ($p < 0.0001$). However, if NE-treated mice were given ACTY116 solution at the same time, bid, for 14 days, the heart weight tended to decrease compared with the NE-treated group. At the end of the 14-day treatment, the heart weight for the ACTY116-solution group was 6.6 mg/g body weight, which is significantly lighter than that of the NE-induced group ($p < 0.01$). The results suggested that the ACTY116 solution showed certain pharmacological effect on mice with cardiac hypertrophy. When NE-treated mice were injected with the ACTY116 pLAI formulation at 7 mg/kg, once a week for 2 weeks, the heart weight of mice at day 15 was 6.0 mg/g body weight, which is significantly different in comparison to NE-treated mice ($p < 0.0001$). Another group of NE-treated mice were injected with ACTY116 pLAI formulation at 14 mg/kg, single dose, and the heart weight of the mice at day 15 was 5.9 mg/g body weight. The change in heart weight of mice at the 14 mg/kg dose level was significantly different from that of the NE-treated group. Similar results were obtained for the heart weight (mg)/tibial length (mm) (HW/TL) (Figure 9c) from the above studies. The results indicated that the ACTY116 pLAI formulation has a long-acting effect, and the pharmacological action is superior than that of solution.

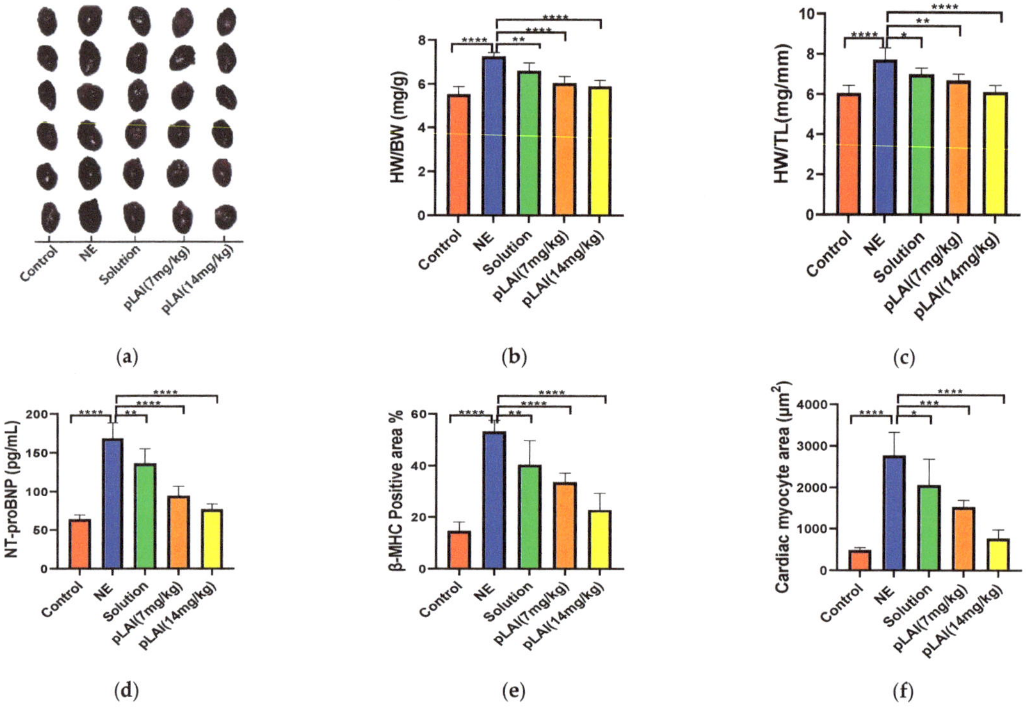

Figure 9. *Cont.*

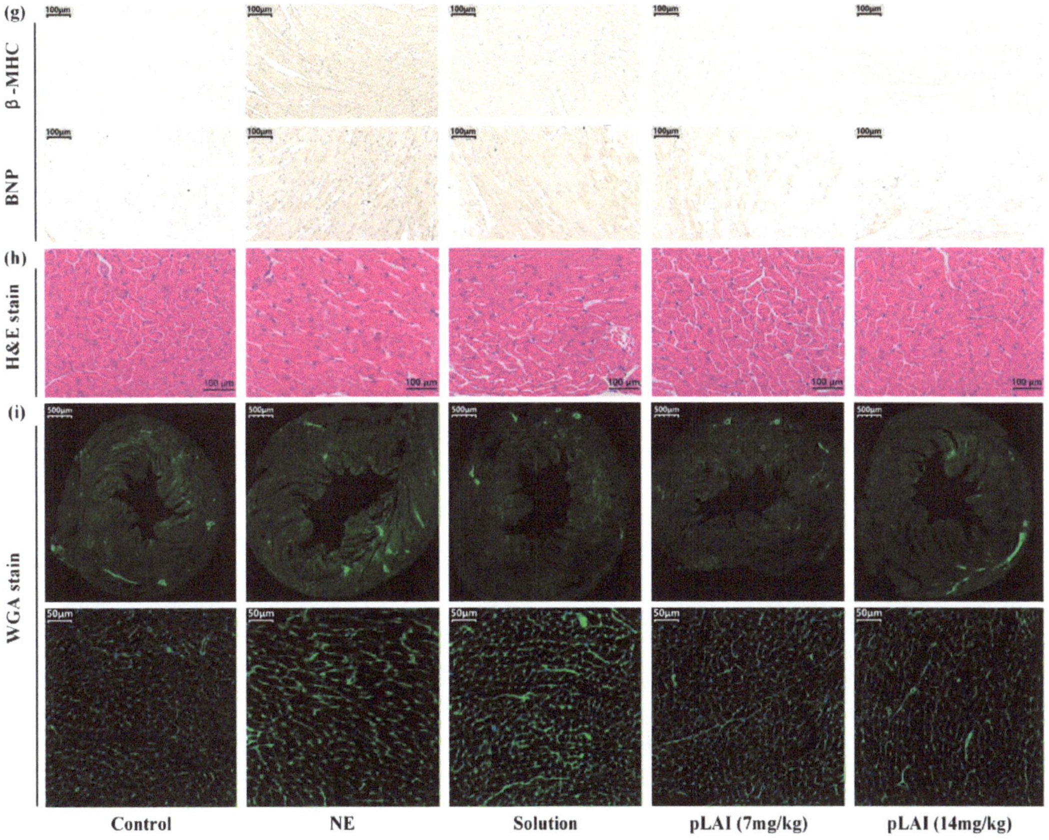

Figure 9. Evaluation of pharmacological activity on ACTY116 solution and pLAI formulations: (**a**) heart sizes; (**b**) heart weight to body weight (HW/BW) ratios; (**c**) heart weight to tibial length (HW/TL) ratios; (**d**) serum levels of NT-proBNP; (**e**) quantitative analysis of β-MHC expression; (**f**) quantitative analysis of myocyte cross-sectional areas in heart tissue sections with HE staining; (**g**) representative images of β-MHC (upper) and BNP (lower) expression (positive expression is brownish yellow); (**h**) representative images of H&E staining of heart tissues; (**i**) representative images of WGA staining of heart tissues. $n = 6$ in each group, * $p < 0.05$, ** $p < 0.01$, *** $p < 0.001$, **** $p < 0.0001$.

A biomarker, i.e., NT-proBNP, in serum is another indicator for cardiac hypertrophy. Two weeks after treatment, the level of NT-proBNT very significantly increased in the NE-treated group (168.43 pg/mL) compared to the control (63.96 pg/mL) group ($p < 0.0001$). Three ACTY116-treated groups showed a significant decrease in serum NT-proBNP (Figure 9d). The serum level of NT-proBNP after the 2-week treatment was 136.12 pg/mL for ACTY116 solution ($p < 0.01$), 94.61 pg/mL for 7 mg/kg once a week for 2 weeks ($p < 0.0001$), and 76.39 pg/mL for 14 mg/kg, single dose ($p < 0.0001$). Similarly, treatment with ACTY116 pLAI obviously decreased β-MHC and BNP expression. The darker the brownish yellow colour, the higher the β-MHC and BNP expression. Results showed that the level of β-MHC expression (Figure 9e) significantly increased in the NE-treated group compared with the control group; the average β-MHC-area of NE-treated group was 53.2%, and 14.6% for the control group ($p < 0.0001$). Three ACTY116-treated groups showed a significant decrease in β-MHC expression. The average β-MHC-positive area was 40.3% for ACTY116 solution ($p < 0.01$) after 2-week treatment, 33.6% for 7 mg/kg once a week for 2 weeks ($p < 0.0001$), and 22.8% for 14 mg/kg, single dose ($p < 0.0001$). Results of BNP expression showed a similar trend, which further proves the pharmacological activity of ACTY116; ACTY116 pLAI in situ depot gel has long-acting effect for cardiac hypertrophy. Representative images of β-MHC (upper) and BNP (lower) expression are shown in Figure 9g.

To investigate the effects of ACTY116 on pathological changes of the heart tissue, H&E (Figure 9h) staining and WGA (Figure 9i) staining were performed, and the quantitative analysis of myocyte cross-sectional areas in heart tissue sections were calculated by software ImageJ (Figure 9f). Compared to the control group, NE markedly increased the cross-sectional area of cardiomyocytes; the mean area increased from 482.7 μm^2 to 2768.2 μm^2. However, treatment with ACTY116 pLAI could significantly decrease the cardiomyocyte cross-sectional area, compared to the NE group: 1530.6 μm^2 for 7 mg/kg once a week for 2 weeks ($p < 0.001$) and 773.1 μm^2 for 14 mg/kg, single dose ($p < 0.0001$). The pharmacological activity is dose-dependent, in which a higher dose (14 mg/kg) showed stronger pharmacological activity than a lower dose (7 mg/kg).

The pharmacodynamics study confirmed the successful establishment of a cardiac hypertrophy mouse model induced by NE. Moreover, the pLAI formulation exhibited superior pharmacological efficacy compared to the ACTY116 solution, allowing for a reduction in injection frequency from twice daily to once weekly or even biweekly.

3.6. *Effect of PLGA Copolymer on In Vitro Drug Release from pLAI In Situ Depot Gels*

Impact of quantity of PLGA on in vitro drug release was studied on formulations with PLGA:ACTY116 ratios of 3:1 (F14), 4:1 (F15), and 5:1 (F16), respectively. When PLGA:ACTY116 ratio was 3:1 (F14), the accumulated drug release was 83.6% at 24 h, and complete release was found at 96 h (Figure 10a). When the ratio of PLGA:ACTY116 increased to 4:1 (F15) and 5:1 (F16), the drug release decreased accordingly, and complete release was 120 h for F15 and 168 h for F16, respectively. Hence, increase in PLGA quantity may significantly decrease the in vitro release rate for ACTY116.

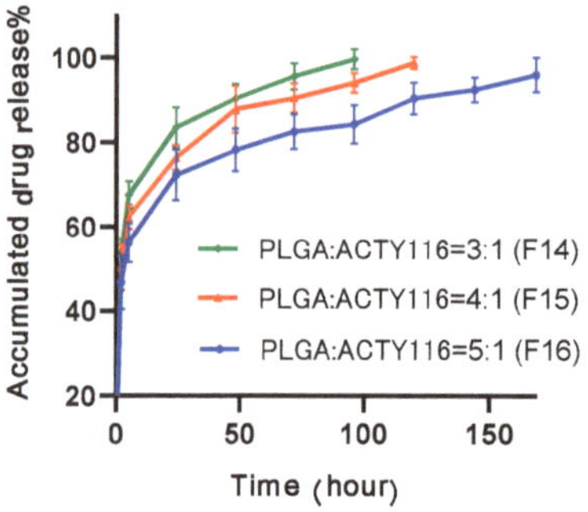

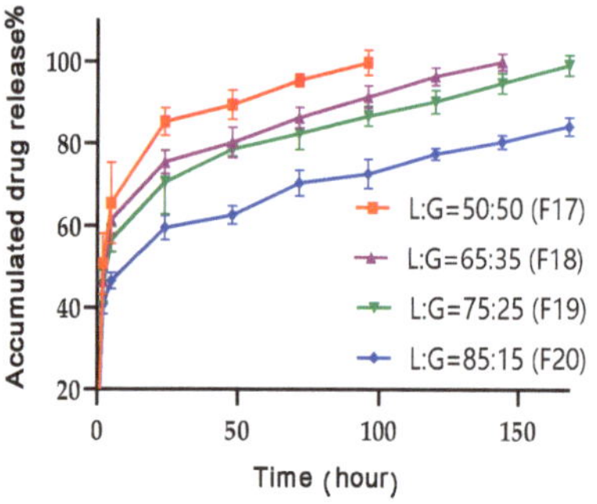

Figure 10. Effect of PLGA copolymer on in vitro drug release from pLAI in situ depot gels: (**a**) impact of PLGA quantity on ACTY116 in vitro release; (**b**) impact of type of PLGA on ACTY116 in vitro release.

Three types of PLGAs have been formulated with ACTY116 and NMP, including a lactide:glycolide (L:G) ratios of 50:50, 65:35, 75:25, and 85:15, respectively. As shown in Figure 10b, when the L:G ratio was 50:50, the accumulated drug release from F16 was 85.4% at 24 h and 95.5% at 72 h. When the L:G ratio was increased to 65:35 (F18), the drug release rate was slowed down. The accumulated drug release was 75.5% at 24 h and 86.4% at 72 h, respectively. By increasing the L:G ratio to 75:25 (F19), the accumulated drug release was only 70.6% at 24 h and 82.4% at 72 h, respectively. Further increasing the L:G ratio to 85:15 (F20) led to the slowest drug release rate in vitro. The results indicated that PLGA should be effective to control the drug release rate, and changes in L:G ratios can be used to formulate the ACTY116 pLAI in situ depot gel with different drug release rates.

Therefore, both quantities of PLGA and different types of PLGAs in formulation can change the release rate of ACTY116 from an in situ depot gel, so a pLAI formulation with an ideal release rate can be designed with varying quantities and types of PLGAs in the formulation.

3.7. Pharmacokinetics of ACTY116 Solution and pLAI Formulations in Rats

The ACTY116 solution (F1) and pLAI formulations with different quantities and types of PLGA were subcutaneously administrated in rats to study pharmacokinetic behaviour. The pharmacokinetic parameters in Table 9 show that ACTY116 pLAI formulations could significantly decrease drug clearance (Cl) from 2167.2 to less than 559.1 mL/h/kg compared to the solution, the half-life and the mean residence time (MRT) was extended from less than 1 h up to hundreds of hours, and the area under curve (AUC) was increased about 100 times, which means the pLAI formulations could reach the long-acting goal.

Table 9. PK parameters of ACTY116 solution and ACTY116 pLAI formulations with different PLGA quantities.

PK Parameters	Solution (F1)	F14	F15	F16
C_{max} (ng/mL)	377.4 ± 20.3	1014.3 ± 388.3	709.5 ± 305.9	587.8 ± 289.9
AUC_{last} (h·ng/mL)	226.9 ± 29.6	29,749.6 ± 12,223.4	28,072.2 ± 3732.3	21,015.0 ± 6374.0
AUC_{INF_obs} (h·ng/mL)	234.1 ± 31.7	31,191.6 ± 116,423.0	31,790.4 ± 2771.5	26,369.1 ± 6491.9
HL_Lambda_z (h)	0.351 ± 0.021	34.1 ± 11.9	103.6 ± 27.1	224.4 ± 114.9
MRT_{last} (h)	0.796 ± 0.024	47.1 ± 10.8	124.6 ± 15.5	161.7 ± 23.0
C_{last} (ng/mL)	14.1 ± 4.0	25.2 ± 15.0	23.3 ± 8.7	16.4 ± 6.4
T_{last} (h)	2 ± 0	168.0 ± 30.4	416.0 ± 36.1	584.0 ± 24.8
Cl_F_obs (mL/h/kg)	2167.2 ± 276.2	507.5 ± 203.8	443.1 ± 37.9	559.1 ± 138.6

The effect of PLGA quantity (formulations are listed in Table 5) on pharmacokinetics was studied. As displayed in Table 9, an increase in the PLGA:ACTY116 ratio resulted in a decrease in Cmax from 1014.3 ng/mL (F14) to 587.8 ng/mL (F16), while extending the half-life from 34.1 h (F14) to 224.4 h (F16) and the MRT from 47.1 h (F14) to 161.7 h (F16). The pharmacokinetic parameters indicated that different PLGA:ACTY116 ratios have an impact on in vivo release of ACTY116 and thus pharmacokinetic profiles in rats. Longer MRTs and half-lives were obtained with a higher PLGA:ACTY116 ratio (Figure 11).

The effect of different types of PLGA on pharmacokinetics was also studied. As displayed in Table 10, an increase in the L:G ratio resulted in a decrease in C_{max} from 806.1 ng/mL (F17) to 552.8 ng/mL (F20), the half-life was extended from 111.4 h (F17) to more than 340 h (F19 and F20), and MRT was extended from 132.1 h (F17) to around 230 h (F19 and F20). The results indicated that different L:G ratios have an impact on in vivo release of ACTY116 and thus the pharmacokinetic profiles in rats. As the ratio of lactide increases (i.e., higher L:G ratio), the polymer degradation slows down due to the presence of a hydrophobic methyl group, and with the increase in lactide portion, the drug release was slower and the half-life and residence time were longer (Figure 11).

Table 10. Pharmacokinetic parameters of ACTY116 pLAI formulations with different PLGA types.

PK Parameters	F17	F18	F19	F20
C_{max} (ng/mL)	806.1 ± 295.0	736.6 ± 289.6	687.4 ± 246.2	552.8 ± 32.3
AUC_{last} (h·ng/mL)	27,601.0 ± 3464.0	21,177.7 ± 3186.0	20,035.8 ± 3527.0	23,157.4 ± 5337.8
AUC_{INF_obs} (h·ng/mL)	32,014.5 ± 5181.5	25,304.8 ± 3693.4	35,578.9 ± 11,920.6	31,563.1 ± 6039.8
HL_Lambda_z (h)	111.4 ± 42.4	156.7 ± 91.5	348.7 ± 121.6	340.9 ± 149.6
MRT_{last} (h)	132.1 ± 15.4	170.3 ± 12.4	232.8 ± 34.9	229.5 ± 34.0
C_{last} (ng/mL)	24.0 ± 16.2	16.0 ± 5.0	28.4 ± 12.8	17.1 ± 7.3
T_{last} (h)	392.0 ± 24.8	496.0 ± 36.1	632.0 ± 39.2	760.0 ± 24.8
Cl_F_obs (mL/h/kg)	445.4 ± 60.1	562.3 ± 74.9	445.9 ± 202.1	456.1 ± 80.1

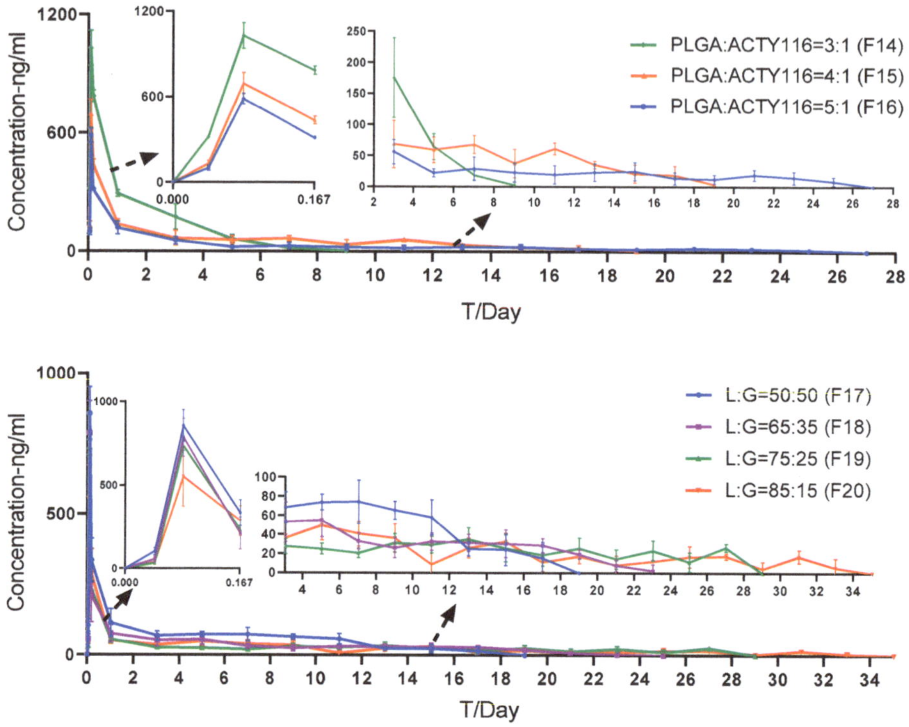

Figure 11. Evaluation of different doses on ACTY116 the in vivo PK profile.

4. Discussion

The U.S. FDA (United States Food and Drug Administration) has approved around 20 long-acting injectables based on PLA/PLGA, primarily in microsphere form. While these products offer improved patient compliance and therapeutic benefits, their complex formulations and intricate processing contribute to high costs; moreover, the high drug load in microspheres makes any unforeseen changes in drug release characteristics risky, potentially leading to adverse effects. Microsphere products are sensitive to manufacturing changes, which may affect their physicochemical attributes, during in vitro and in vivo performance. Manufacturing challenges arise due to the proprietary process, resulting in difficulties achieving consistent high-quality products [39–42]. Peptide molecules often exhibit poor chemical stability, and the production process for microspheres complicates matters further: the peptide is dissolved in water and subjected to vigorous emulsification through high-shear mixing, and following the formation of a double emulsion, the organic solvent necessitates removal at elevated temperatures. Unfortunately, these harsh manufacturing processes serve to accelerate both peptide hydrolysis and oxidation [43,44]. In the early stages of formulation development, we compared two pLAI formulations: microspheres and in situ depot gel. Due to issues such as the complicated preparation process, low encapsulation efficiency, and the fact that ACTY116 showed poor stability in microspheres, we excluded microspheres as a pLAI formulation for ACTY116, and we concentrated on proceeding with the in situ depot gel formulation for further process optimization, molecular dynamics simulation, and pharmacological and pharmacokinetic studies in animals.

In pursuit of achieving extended drug release, this study has developed a long-acting injectable formulation utilising biodegradable polymers and an in situ depot gel, and the preparation process is straightforward, avoiding the use of harsh conditions such as high temperatures, high-shear mixing, or homogenization; furthermore, the maintenance of a water-free and oxygen-free environment ensures the chemical stability of peptide ACTY116. The results revealed superior stability of ACTY116 in the PLGA-based in situ depot gel compared to the solution or microspheres. Molecular dynamics (MDs) simulations highlighted increased rigidity of ACTY116 within the pLAI in situ depot gel, providing stability even under elevated temperatures due to enhanced hydrogen bonding, steric hindrance, and shielding effects. The long-acting release behaviour of in situ depot gel formulations was assessed both in vitro and in vivo. Water absorption starts immediately upon exposure of a PLGA matrix to water, or during in vivo administration. The release rate is initially diffusion-controlled, giving way to degradation/erosion at the end of release period. Diffusion occurs through water-filled pores within the PLGA matrix, which commonly exhibits classic tri-phasic release patterns including an initial burst (phase I) and a slow-release phase (lag time) associated with a diffusion-driven release (phase II), followed by a faster release (phase III) attributed to erosion [45]. Increase in PLGA quantity may significantly decrease the diffusion and erosion of the PLGA matrix, and it may lead to the decreased release rate. PLGA polymer composition (type) is another important factor contributing to degradation rate; it impacts the hydrophilicity, glass transition temperature (Tg), and hydration rate of the PLGA polymer. L:G ratio significantly influences solubility and degradation rate, impacting drug release. The glycolide is more hydrophilic due to the absence of the methyl side group rather than lactide, which means that a higher glycolide percentage causes more water uptake, and consequently an overall weight loss of the PLGA matrix occurs, and a faster degradation rate happens [46]. A pLAI formulation with an ideal release rate can be designed with varying the quantity and type of PLGA in the formulation. Pharmacological effects of different dosage forms also indicate that ACTY116 pLAI in situ depot gel could prolong in vivo release and reduce the dosing interval because of the long residence time.

However, there are still unresolved issues in our study. Similar to FDA-approved microsphere LAIs, our pharmacokinetic findings of ACTY116 pLAI in rats indicated a burst release, primarily due to the rapid drug diffusion from the surface of the in situ depot gel following subcutaneous injection [47,48]. Based on our current pharmacological and pharmacokinetic investigations, the burst release has not resulted in noticeable adverse effects. This might be attributed to the wider safety margin of ACTY116 or the limited duration of our observations. Prior to progressing to clinical trials, further assessments such as long-term toxicity studies are essential to evaluate whether the burst release could potentially lead to severe adverse effects. Currently, it appears that in situ depot gel, as a long-acting injectable formulation, is better suited for drugs with a broader safety margin, whereas it may not be suitable for drugs with a narrow therapeutic index.

5. Conclusions

The purpose of this article was to develop a polymeric long-acting injectable formulation of ACTY116 with high chemical and conformational stability to ensure a sustained and effective blood concentration of ACTY116 in vivo. We demonstrated that the ACTY116 pLAI in situ depot gel significantly reduces the frequency of ACTY116 administration, displaying a dose-dependent release duration. This formulation can achieve the desired long-acting effect as required, and it also exhibits superior in vivo therapeutic efficacy against cardiac hypertrophy in mice compared to ACTY116 solution.

Author Contributions: Y.X.: Conceptualization, methodology, software, validation, investigation, data curation, and writing—original draft; Z.L.: Methodology and writing—review and editing; X.L.: Conceptualization, resources, supervision, resources, project administration and funding acquisition; X.Z.: Conceptualization, software, formal analysis, and writing—review and editing; Y.W.: Methodology and software; J.W.: Validation, investigation, data curation, and Visualisation. All authors have read and agreed to the published version of the manuscript.

Funding: This research was funded by National Natural Scientific Foundation of China (No.: 81773742), Science-Technology Research Program of Chongqing Municipal Education Commission (No.: KJQN202212809), Medical Research Project of Science and Health of Chongqing, China (No.: 2024MSXM028), and Innovation Talents in Key Industries Program of Chongqing Talent Program, China (No.: CQYC20220305379).

Institutional Review Board Statement: All animal experiments were approved by Laboratory Animal Welfare and Ethics Committee of Third Military Medical University (Army Medical University, approval no.: AMUWEC20203377; approval date: 19 May 2020), and all of the experiments were performed in accordance with the National Institutes of Health guidelines for the care and use of laboratory animals.

Informed Consent Statement: Not applicable.

Data Availability Statement: The datasets supporting the results reported in this article may be provided to researchers upon reasonable request. Such requests can be made by contacting the corresponding author (Xiaohui Li, lpsh008@aliyun.com).

Conflicts of Interest: The authors declare no conflicts of interest.

References

1. Chen, D.; Rehfeld, J.F.; Watts, A.G.; Rorsman, P.; Gundlach, A.L. History of key regulatory peptide systems and perspectives for future research. *J. Neuroendocrinol.* **2023**, *35*, e13251. [CrossRef] [PubMed]
2. Dagen, M.M. History of insulin. In *Encyclopedia of Life Sciences (eLS)*; John Wiley & Sons, Ltd.: Chichester, UK, 2016; pp. 1–3.
3. Jimmidi, R. Synthesis and applications of peptides and peptidomimetics in drug discovery. *Eur. J. Org. Chem.* **2023**, *26*, e202300028. [CrossRef]
4. Nugrahadi, P.P.; Hinrichs, W.L.; Frijlink, H.W.; Schöneich, C.; Avanti, C. Designing formulation strategies for enhanced stability of therapeutic peptides in aqueous solutions: A review. *Pharmaceutics* **2023**, *15*, 935. [CrossRef] [PubMed]
5. Yang, H.; Liu, Y.; Lu, X.L.; Li, X.H.; Zhang, H.G. Transmembrane transport of the gαq protein carboxyl terminus imitation polypeptide gcip-27. *Eur. J. Pharm. Sci.* **2013**, *49*, 791–799. [CrossRef] [PubMed]
6. Wang, Y.; Lu, X.L.; Yang, H.; Li, X.H.; Zhang, H.G. Effects of polypeptide drug huilixinkang on cardiac hypertrophy and expressions of myosin heavy chain in mice. *Chin. Pharm. J.* **2011**, *46*, 1566–1569.
7. Zhang, H.G.; Li, X.H.; Zhou, J.Z.; Liu, Y.; Jia, Y.; Yuan, Z.B. Gαq-protein carboxyl terminus imitation polypeptide gcip-27 attenuates cardiac hypertrophy in vitro and in vivo. *Clin. Exp. Pharmacol. Physiol.* **2007**, *34*, 1276–1281. [CrossRef] [PubMed]
8. Lu, X.L.; Tong, Y.F.; Liu, Y.; Xu, Y.L.; Yang, H.; Zhang, G.Y.; Li, X.H.; Zhang, H.G. Gαq protein carboxyl terminus imitation polypeptide gcip-27 improves cardiac function in chronic heart failure rats. *PLoS ONE* **2015**, *10*, e0121007. [CrossRef]
9. Muddineti, O.S.; Omri, A. Current trends in plga based long-acting injectable products: The industry perspective. *Expert Opin. Drug Deliv.* **2022**, *19*, 559–576. [CrossRef] [PubMed]
10. Somayaji, M.R.; Das, D.; Przekwas, A. A new level a type ivivc for the rational design of clinical trials toward regulatory approval of generic polymeric long-acting injectables. *Clin. Pharmacokinet.* **2016**, *55*, 1179–1190. [CrossRef]
11. Butreddy, A.; Gaddam, R.P.; Kommineni, N.; Dudhipala, N.; Voshavar, C. Plga/pla-based long-acting injectable depot microspheres in clinical use: Production and characterization overview for protein/peptide delivery. *Int. J. Mol. Sci.* **2021**, *22*, 8884. [CrossRef]
12. Silva, A.T.C.R.; Cardoso, B.C.O.; e Silva, M.E.S.R.; Freitas, R.F.S.; Sousa, R.G. Synthesis, characterization, and study of plga copolymer *in vitro* degradation. *J. Biomater. Nanobiotechnol.* **2015**, *6*, 8–19. [CrossRef]
13. Mir, M.; Ahmed, N.; ur Rehman, A. Recent applications of plga based nanostructures in drug delivery. *Colloids Surf. B Biointerfaces* **2017**, *159*, 217–231. [CrossRef] [PubMed]
14. Lee, B.K.; Yun, Y.; Park, K. PLA micro-and nano-particles. *Adv. Drug Deliv. Rev.* **2016**, *107*, 176–191. [CrossRef]
15. Su, Y.; Zhang, B.; Sun, R.; Liu, W.; Zhu, Q.; Zhang, X.; Wang, R.; Chen, C. PLGA-based biodegradable microspheres in drug delivery: Recent advances in research and application. *Drug Deliv.* **2021**, *28*, 1397–1418. [CrossRef]
16. Vigani, B.; Rossi, S.; Sandri, G.; Bonferoni, M.C.; Caramella, C.M.; Ferrari, F. Recent advances in the development of in situ gelling drug delivery systems for non-parenteral administration routes. *Pharmaceutics* **2020**, *12*, 859. [CrossRef]
17. Ibrahim, T.M.; El-Megrab, N.A.; El-Nahas, H.M. An overview of plga in-situ forming implants based on solvent exchange technique: Effect of formulation components and characterization. *Pharm. Dev. Technol.* **2021**, *26*, 709–728. [CrossRef] [PubMed]
18. Yamamoto, M.; Okada, H.; Ogawa, Y.; Miyagawa, T. Takeda Chemical Industries, Ltd. Polymer, Production and Use Thereof. U.S. Patent US4849228, 18 July 1989.
19. Pandya, A.K.; Vora, L.K.; Umeyor, C.; Surve, D.; Patel, A.; Biswas, S.; Patel, K.; Patravale, V.B. Polymeric in situ forming depots for long-acting drug delivery systems. *Adv. Drug Deliv. Rev.* **2023**, *200*, 115003. [CrossRef] [PubMed]
20. Bashir, R.; Maqbool, M.; Ara, I.; Zehravi, M. An In sight into Novel Drug Delivery System: In Situ Gels. *CellMed* **2021**, *11*, 6.1–6.7. [CrossRef]

21. Shukr, M.H.; Ismail, S.; El-Hossary, G.G.; El-Shazly, A.H. Design and evaluation of mucoadhesive in situ liposomal gel for sustained ocular delivery of travoprost using two steps factorial design. *J. Drug Deliv. Sci. Technol.* **2021**, *61*, 102333. [CrossRef]
22. Li, Z.; Mu, H.; Larsen, S.W.; Jensen, H.; Østergaard, J. Initial leuprolide acetate release from poly (d,l-lactide-*co*-glycolide) in situ forming implants as studied by ultraviolet–visible imaging. *Mol. Pharm.* **2020**, *17*, 4522–4532. [CrossRef]
23. Ibrahim, T.M.; El-Megrab, N.A.; El-Nahas, H.M. Optimization of injectable plga in-situ forming implants of anti-psychotic risperidone via box-behnken design. *J. Drug Deliv. Sci. Technol.* **2020**, *58*, 101803. [CrossRef]
24. Tripos International. Sybyl x. 2007. Available online: https://www.certara.com/sybyl-x-software/ (accessed on 20 May 2023).
25. Case, D.; Cheatham, T., III; Darden, T.; Gohlke, H.; Luo, R.; Merz, K.M., Jr.; Onufriev, A.; Simmerling, C.; Wang, B.; Woods, R. AMBER 14. University of California, San Francisco. 2014. Available online: https://ambermd.org/ (accessed on 20 May 2023).
26. Maier, J.A.; Martinez, C.; Kasavajhala, K.; Wickstrom, L.; Hauser, K.E.; Simmerling, C. ff14sb: Improving the accuracy of protein side chain and backbone parameters from ff99sb. *J. Chem. Theory Comput.* **2015**, *11*, 3696–3713. [CrossRef] [PubMed]
27. DeLano, W. *Use of Pymol as a Communications Tool for Molecular Science*; Abstracts of Papers of the American Chemical Society; American Chemical Society: Washington, DC, USA, 2004; pp. U313–U314.
28. Moser, L.; Faulhaber, J.; Wiesner, R.J.; Ehmke, H. Predominant activation of endothelin-dependent cardiac hypertrophy by norepinephrine in rat left ventricle. *Am. J. Physiol.-Regul. Integr. Comp. Physiol.* **2002**, *282*, R1389–R1394. [CrossRef] [PubMed]
29. Cao, Z.; Jia, Y.; Zhu, B. BNP and NT-proBNP as diagnostic biomarkers for cardiac dysfunction in both clinical and forensic medicine. *Int. J. Mol. Sci.* **2019**, *20*, 1820. [CrossRef] [PubMed]
30. Tang, K.; Zhong, B.; Luo, Q.; Liu, Q.; Chen, X.; Cao, D.; Li, X.; Yang, S. Phillyrin attenuates norepinephrine-induced cardiac hypertrophy and inflammatory response by suppressing p38/ERK1/2 MAPK and AKT/NF-kappaB pathways. *Eur. J. Pharmacol.* **2022**, *927*, 175022. [CrossRef] [PubMed]
31. Ding, J.; Tang, Q.; Luo, B.; Zhang, L.; Lin, L.; Han, L.; Hao, M.; Li, M.; Yu, L.; Li, M. Klotho inhibits angiotensin II-induced cardiac hypertrophy, fibrosis, and dysfunction in mice through suppression of transforming growth factor-β1 signaling pathway. *Eur. J. Pharmacol.* **2019**, *859*, 172549. [CrossRef] [PubMed]
32. Yuan, M.; Zhao, B.; Jia, H.; Zhang, C.; Zuo, X. Sinomenine ameliorates cardiac hypertrophy by activating Nrf2/ARE signaling pathway. *Bioengineered* **2021**, *12*, 12778–12788. [CrossRef]
33. Jin, Y.G.; Zhou, H.; Fan, D.; Che, Y.; Wang, Z.P.; Wang, S.S.; Tang, Q.Z. TMEM173 protects against pressure overload-induced cardiac hypertrophy by modulating autophagy. *J. Cell. Physiol.* **2021**, *236*, 5176–5192. [CrossRef] [PubMed]
34. Li, Y.; Zhou, W.W.; Sun, J.H.; Yang, H.X.; Xu, G.R.; Zhang, Y.; Song, Q.H.; Zhang, C.; Liu, W.Z.; Liu, X.C.; et al. Modified citrus pectin prevents isoproterenol-induced cardiac hypertrophy associated with p38 signalling and TLR4/JAK/STAT3 pathway. *Biomed. Pharmacother.* **2021**, *143*, 112178. [CrossRef]
35. Lin, X.; Yang, H.; Su, L.; Yang, Z.; Tang, X. Effect of size on the *in vitro/in vivo* drug release and degradation of exenatide-loaded plga microspheres. *J. Drug Deliv. Sci. Technol.* **2018**, *45*, 346–356. [CrossRef]
36. Hu, X.; Zhang, J.; Tang, X.; Li, M.; Ma, S.; Liu, C.; Gao, Y.; Zhang, Y.; Liu, Y.; Yu, F.; et al. An accelerated release method of risperidone loaded plga microspheres with good ivivc. *Curr. Drug Deliv.* **2018**, *15*, 87–96. [CrossRef] [PubMed]
37. Wu, C. Formulation and preparation method of long-acting interferon α-2b loaded injectable microspheres. *Acad. J. Second Mil. Med. Univ.* **2006**, *27*, 76–80.
38. Yoneda, J.S.; Cardoso, M.B. Nanoparticle-induced conformational changes in protein corona revealed by circular dichroism spectroscopy. *Nanomedicine* **2023**, *18*, 709–711. [CrossRef] [PubMed]
39. Bao, X.; Si, X.; Ding, X.; Duan, L.; Xiao, C. pH-responsive hydrogels based on the self-assembly of short polypeptides for controlled release of peptide and protein drugs. *J. Polym. Res.* **2019**, *26*, 278. [CrossRef]
40. O'Brien, M.N.; Jiang, W.; Wang, Y.; Loffredo, D.M. Challenges and opportunities in the development of complex generic long-acting injectable drug products. *J. Control. Release* **2021**, *336*, 144–158. [CrossRef] [PubMed]
41. Zhou, J.; Walker, J.; Ackermann, R.; Olsen, K.; Hong, J.K.; Wang, Y.; Schwendeman, S.P. Effect of manufacturing variables and raw materials on the composition-equivalent plga microspheres for 1-month controlled release of leuprolide. *Mol. Pharm.* **2020**, *17*, 1502–1515. [CrossRef] [PubMed]
42. Park, K.; Otte, A.; Sharifi, F.; Garner, J.; Skidmore, S.; Park, H.; Jhon, Y.K.; Qin, B.; Wang, Y. Formulation composition, manufacturing process, and characterization of poly (lactide-*co*-glycolide) microparticles. *J. Control. Release* **2021**, *329*, 1150–1161. [CrossRef] [PubMed]
43. Green, R.; Hopkinson, I.; Jones, R. Unfolding and intermolecular association in globular proteins adsorbed at interfaces. *Langmuir* **1999**, *15*, 5102–5110. [CrossRef]
44. Yan de Weert, M.; Hennink, W.E.; Jiskoot, W. Protein instability in poly (lactic-co-glycolic acid) microparticles. *Pharm. Res.* **2000**, *17*, 1159–1167. [CrossRef]
45. Allahyari, M.; Mohit, E. Peptide/protein vaccine delivery system based on PLGA particles. *Hum. Vaccines Immunother.* **2016**, *12*, 806–828. [CrossRef]
46. Saini, V.; Jain, V.; Sudheesh, M.S.; Jaganathan, K.S.; Murthy, P.K.; Kohli, D.V. Comparison of humoral and cell-mediated im-mune responses to cationic PLGA microspheres containing recombinant hepatitis B antigen. *Int. J. Pharm.* **2011**, *408*, 50–57. [CrossRef] [PubMed]

47. Schutzman, R.; Shi, N.Q.; Olsen, K.F.; Ackermann, R.; Tang, J.; Liu, Y.Y.; Hong, J.K.Y.; Wang, Y.; Qin, B.; Schwendeman, A.; et al. Mechanistic evaluation of the initial burst release of leuprolide from spray-dried PLGA microspheres. *J. Control. Release* **2023**, *361*, 297–313. [CrossRef] [PubMed]
48. Abdeltawab, H.; Svirskis, D.; Sharma, M. Formulation strategies to modulate drug release from poloxamer based in situ gelling systems. *Expert Opin. Drug Deliv.* **2020**, *17*, 495–509. [CrossRef] [PubMed]

pharmaceutics

Article

The Development of a Stable Peptide-Loaded Long-Acting Injection Formulation through a Comprehensive Understanding of Peptide Degradation Mechanisms: A QbD-Based Approach

Yingxin Xiong [1], Jiawei Wang [2], Xing Zhou [2,*] and Xiaohui Li [1,3,*]

1 Institute of Materia Medica and Department of Pharmaceutics, College of Pharmacy, Army Medical University, Chongqing 400038, China; yx.xiong@gmail.com
2 Chongqing School of Pharmacy and Bioengineering, Chongqing University of Technology, Chongqing 400054, China; wangjiawei0423@gmail.com
3 Engineering Research Center for Pharmacodynamics Evaluation, College of Pharmacy, Army Medical University, Chongqing 400038, China
* Correspondence: diszhou@cqut.edu.cn (X.Z.); lpsh008@aliyun.com (X.L.)

Abstract: Quality by design (QbD) serves as a systematic approach to pharmaceutical development, beginning with predefined objectives and emphasizing an understanding of the product based on sound science and risk management. The purpose of this study is to utilize the QbD concept to develop a stable peptide-loaded long-acting injection formulation. An in-depth comprehension of peptide degradation mechanisms was achieved through forced degradation investigations, elucidating (acid) hydrolysis and oxidation as the primary degradation pathways for the peptide ACTY116. The quality built into the product was focused on risk assessment, for which the critical material attributes (CMAs) and critical process parameters (CPPs) associated with the critical quality attributes (CQAs) of each formulation were identified, leading to the development of the corresponding control strategies. CQAs for three LAI (long-acting injectable) formulations were enhanced by taking the right control strategies. The LAI formulation exhibiting the highest stability for ACTY116 was chosen for subsequent pharmacokinetic investigations in rats. The objective of addressing peptide chemical instability and in vivo long-acting release was achieved. For other molecules with susceptible functionalities like amide bonds, amino groups, and hydroxyl groups, the utilization of PLGA-based in situ gel as an LAI formulation for stabilizing molecules provides valuable insights.

Keywords: quality by design (QbD); control strategy; peptide; stability; degradation mechanisms; long-acting injection

Citation: Xiong, Y.; Wang, J.; Zhou, X.; Li, X. The Development of a Stable Peptide-Loaded Long-Acting Injection Formulation through a Comprehensive Understanding of Peptide Degradation Mechanisms: A QbD-Based Approach. *Pharmaceutics* **2024**, *16*, 266. https://doi.org/10.3390/pharmaceutics16020266

Academic Editor: Juan Torrado

Received: 26 December 2023
Revised: 7 February 2024
Accepted: 7 February 2024
Published: 13 February 2024

1. Introduction

In recent years, the field of peptide therapeutics has undergone substantial advancements. These therapeutic peptides offer several advantages over biologics, including reduced immunogenicity and enhanced cost-effectiveness. Moreover, they exhibit superior safety, selectivity, efficacy, and specificity when compared to small-molecule drugs. One such peptide, ACTY116 (the structure is shown in Figure 1), comprising 29 amino acids ($C_{157}H_{256}N_{40}O_{45}$, with a molecular weight of 3424 g/mol), was designed in our laboratory as a competitive ligand for the binding sites on Gαq (the activated α subunit of the heterotrimeric G protein) in cardiomyocytes. Extensive investigations have been undertaken concerning the structural design of the peptide and the antihypertrophic evaluation of both GCIP (Gαq protein carboxyl terminus imitation peptide) and ACTY116 (an analog of GCIP with specific structural modification) [1–3]. These studies have shown that ACTY116 holds considerable promise as a potential drug candidate for advancing into clinical development. Despite these findings, the formulation design required for its clinical application has yet to be explored.

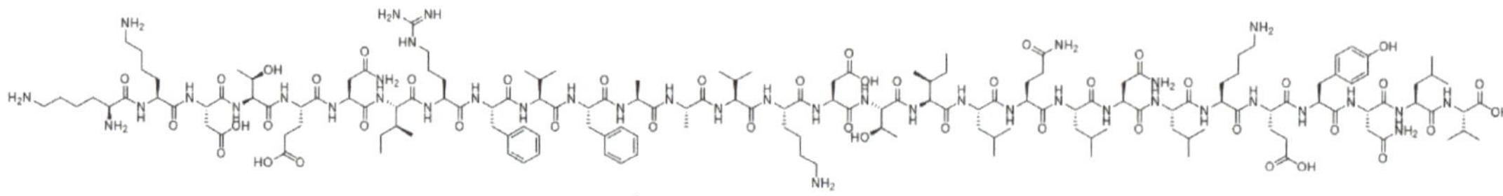

(**a**)

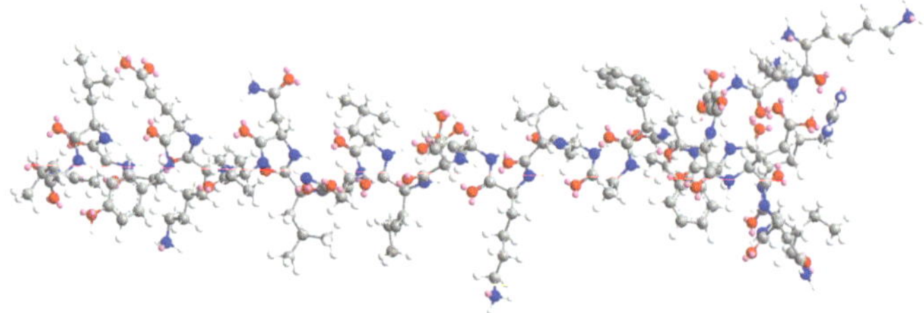

(**b**)

Figure 1. The structure of peptide ACTY116: (**a**) 2D, (**b**) 3D.

Similar to other peptides, ACTY116 presents a set of challenges and limitations that require careful consideration for their successful translation into clinically viable therapeutic products. Peptides typically exhibit a short half-life due to rapid renal filtration and enzymatic degradation. As a result, maintaining a therapeutic level often demands frequent injections or continuous infusions, potentially leading to issues of patient compliance and escalating treatment expenses. Additionally, ACTY116 is susceptible to oxidation and hydrolysis due to the presence of numerous amide bonds, phenolic hydroxyl groups, and amino groups. This chemical instability could compromise both its effectiveness and safety [4–7]. Simultaneously addressing peptide chemical instability and achieving long-acting release presents a substantial challenge.

To address the challenge of limited drug half-life, the utilization of long-acting injectables (LAIs) has emerged as a viable strategy, providing extended drug release through various approaches: (1) chemical modification [8]: modifying drug molecules (such as semaglutide) can enhance stability and prolong drug release [9,10]; (2) active pharmaceutical ingredients (APIs) with low solubility, like Invega Hafyera [11,12], form suspensions for gradual release. The hydrophilic nature of ACTY116 makes it unsuitable for this approach; (3) nonbiodegradable implants (such as Viadur) deliver the drug over months or even years but pose challenges to patient compliance due to the necessity of surgical removal [13]; (4) the formation of drug depots or reservoirs using a biodegradable matrix: The drug is typically formulated as a solution or suspension that undergoes slow release from the depot, extending the availability of the drug. The drug-loaded biodegradable microspheres or in situ gels are administered via injection, and over time, the polymer breaks down into biocompatible byproducts, eliminating the need for device removal [14–19].

Biodegradable microspheres and in situ gels were chosen as LAI approaches for investigating ACTY116, with PLGA and soybean phospholipid selected as the long-acting matrix materials. PLGA (poly(D,L-lactide-co-glycolide)) has achieved success in various US and EU commercial products, including Lupron Depot (leuprolide acetate), Trelstar (triptorelin pamoate), and Risperdal Consta (risperidone) [20–24]. It undergoes biodegradation in vivo, producing biocompatible byproducts like lactic and glycolic acids that can be cleared via the Krebs cycle. The release kinetics of the active pharmaceutical ingredient (API) from PLGA primarily depend on drug diffusion and polymer erosion/degradation process [25]. Soybean phospholipid, comprising a glycerol backbone, two fatty acid chains, a phosphate group, and a choline head group, possesses amphiphilic properties. These properties make it a versatile emulsifier and stabilizer of oil–water interfaces. When employed as a long-acting matrix within in situ gels, soybean phospholipid forms a cross-linked gel network upon administration. This network acts as a barrier, hindering rapid drug release. As the phospholipid matrix gradually degrades over time, the drug is released in a controlled manner, resulting in an extended-release profile [26–29].

The objective of this study was to develop a stable peptide-loaded long-acting injection by following QbD principles (Figure 2). We conducted our study by adhering to the ICH guidelines (Q8, Q9, and Q10) and incorporating recommendations from a highly cited review article titled "Understanding Pharmaceutical Quality by Design" on how to carry out pharmaceutical product development based on the QbD concept [30]. A quality target product profile (QTPP) was established, and ACTY116-loaded LAI formulations were designed based on a comprehensive understanding of ACTY116 degradation mechanisms. The quality built into the product focused on risk assessment, identifying critical material attributes (CMAs) and critical process parameters (CPPs) associated with the critical quality attributes (CQAs) of each formulation, leading to the development of corresponding control strategies. CQAs for different LAI formulations were enhanced by taking the right control strategies. The LAI formulation exhibiting the highest stability for ACTY116 was chosen for further pharmacokinetic investigations in rats. The results were compared with the target product profile to assess the achievement of stability and in vivo long-acting pharmacokinetic behavior objectives.

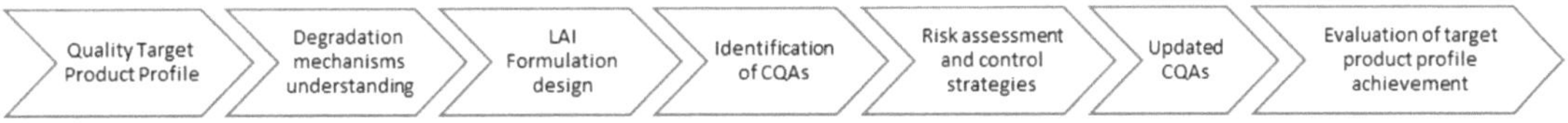

Figure 2. Schematic illustration of long-acting injection development based on quality by design (QbD).

2. Materials and Methods

2.1. Materials

ACTY116 was synthesized by a contract research organization (HLXK, Beijing, China), Poly (D,L-lactide-co-glycolide) (PLGA, with a ratio of lactide to glycolide at 50:50, MW:7000–17,000, acid-terminated) was purchased from Evonik (Darmstadt, Germany), N-methylpyrrolidone (NMP) and dichloromethane (DCM) were purchased from Chengdu Kelong Chemical Co., Ltd. (Chengdu, China), mannitol was purchased from Roquette (Lestrem, France), phospholipid was purchased from Lipoid (Ludwigshafen, Germany), medium chain triglycerides (MCTs) were purchased from Shinsun pharma (Tieling, China), and p-anisidine was purchased from Sinopharm (Shanghai, China).

2.2. Equipment and Instruments

The instruments used in this study included a high-performance liquid chromatograph (e2695-2998, Waters, Milford, MA, USA), a digital mixer (RW20, IKA, Staufen, Germany), a lyophilizer (D-37520, Christ, Osterode, Germany), a polarizing microscope (BK-POL, Aote Optical Instrument, Chongqing, China), a thermostatic oscillator (SHA-C, GY2016-SW, Changzhou Guoyu, Changzhou, China), a digital rotary viscometer (NDJ-8S, Fangrui, Shanghai, China), laser-diffraction particle size analyzers (Mastersizer 3000, Malvern, Worcestershire, UK), a moisture analyzer (Metrohm, Herisau, Switzerland), heat and accelerated stability chambers (Yongsheng, Chongqing, China), a UV spectrophotometer (UV 2450, Shimadzu, Kyoto, Japan), an ultra-high-performance liquid chromatograph (e2695-2998, Waters, Milford, MA, USA), an LC-MS/MS system (6460, Agilent, Santa Clara, CA, USA), and a refrigerated centrifuge (Legend Micro 17R, Thermo, Waltham, MA, USA).

2.3. Degradation Mechanism Studies of ACTY116

2.3.1. Method for ACTY116 Impurity Analysis

The analytical method should be capable of capturing all the potential degradation impurities formed during the stability study. High-performance liquid chromatography

(HPLC) was used as the stability-indicating method for ACTY116 impurity analysis; the detailed information is described below:

- Chromatographic column: XSelect CSH C18, 150 × 4.6 mm, 5 μm;
- Wavelength: 210 nm;
- Column temperature: 40 °C;
- Flow rate: 1 mL/min;
- Injection volume: 25 μL;
- Mobile phase:
    - A: Using phosphate buffer pH 6.5 (containing 20 mM sodium perchlorate);
    - B: Using acetonitrile–water (*v*/*v*) = 80:20.

Gradient elution is shown in Table 1:

Table 1. Gradient elution process.

Time/Min	0	5	6	20	23	28	30	40
A%	90	90	75	50	10	10	90	90
B%	10	10	25	50	90	90	10	10

2.3.2. Forced Degradation Studies

In order to comprehend the chemical properties of ACTY116, a set of stress conditions was utilized to expedite its chemical degradation. This approach enabled the comprehensive assessment of its intrinsic stability and the delineation of degradation pathways [31–33]. The specific studies are outlined as follows:

a. Thermal stress: A measured quantity of ACTY116 was placed into a lidded glass vial and subjected to thermal stress at 60 °C for a duration of 5 days in a heat chamber. Subsequent to the stress period, 1 mg of ACTY116 was precisely weighed and dissolved in 1 mL of purified water for HPLC analysis.

b. Photolytic stress: A measured quantity of ACTY116 was placed into a lidded glass vial and exposed to light under 4500 Lux for a duration of 5 days; then, 1 mg of ACTY116 was precisely weighed and dissolved in 1 mL of purified water for HPLC analysis.

c. Oxidative stress: A measured quantity of ACTY116 (2 mg) was placed into a glass vial and dissolved in 2 mL of 3% H_2O_2. The solution was then subjected to incubation in an oil bath at 100 °C for a duration of 2 h, followed by cooling to room temperature prior to subsequent HPLC analysis.

d. Hydrolytic stress: A measured quantity of ACTY116 (2 mg) was placed into a glass vial and dissolved in 2 mL of purified water. The solution was then subjected to incubation in an oil bath at 100 °C for a duration of 2 h, followed by cooling to room temperature prior to HPLC analysis.

e. Acidic hydrolytic stress: A measured quantity of ACTY116 (2 mg) was placed into a glass vial and dissolved in 2 mL of 1M HCl. The solution was then subjected to incubation in an oil bath at 100 °C for a duration of 2 h, followed by cooling to room temperature prior to HPLC analysis.

2.4. LAI Formulation Design

Three different LAI formulations were designed in this study, and the ingredients in each formulation are presented in Table 2.

Table 2. Formulation ingredients.

	Microsphere	Phospholipid-Based In Situ Gel	PLGA-Based In Situ Gel
Ingredients	ACTY116 PLGA DCM PVA Mannitol	ACTY116 Soybean phospholipid MCT	ACTY116 PLGA NMP

2.4.1. Preparation of Microspheres

The double emulsion-solvent extraction/evaporation method (Figure 3b) was adopted due to the high hydrophilicity of ACTY116. ACTY116 (2 mg) was weighed into a glass vial and dissolved in 200 μL of water for injection (WFI) as the water phase (W_1 phase), and 300 mg of PLGA (with a ratio of lactide to glycolide at 50:50, MW:7000–17,000, acid-terminated, Figure 3a) was dissolved in 2 mL of DCM as the oil phase. A hydrophilic drug solution (W_1 phase) was emulsified in an organic polymer solution (O phase) under 15,000 rpm high-shear mixing to form the primary water-in-oil (W_1/O) emulsion. The obtained W_1/O emulsion was subsequently added to 200 mL of 1% PVA solution (W_2 phase) under 25,000 rpm high-shear mixing to form a double emulsion ($W_1/O/W_2$). The evaporation of DCM was performed under 50 ± 1 °C, 100 rpm continuous shaking for 4 h. The microsphere suspension was centrifuged at 5000 rpm for 2 min (4 °C) and then dispersed with 10 mL of WFI for washing the unencapsulated ACTY116. The washing step was repeated for 5 cycles. Finally, the microspheres were dispersed in a 10% mannitol solution, filled into vials, and lyophilized (F1) with the process shown below (Table 3).

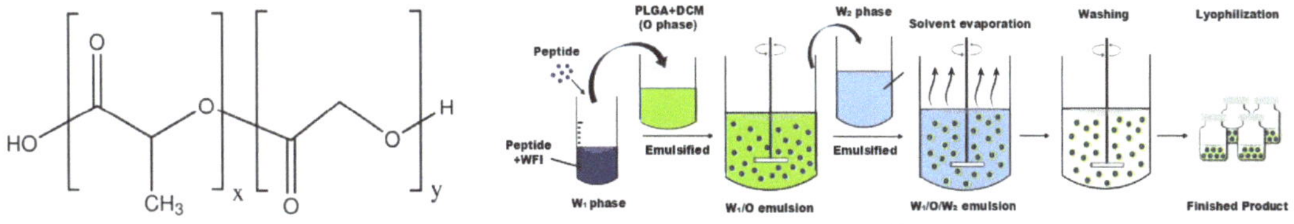

(a) (b)

Figure 3. (**a**) PLGA structure; (**b**) schematic illustration of double emulsion-solvent extraction/evaporation technique for microsphere preparation.

Table 3. Lyophilization process for ACTY116 microspheres.

Temperature/°C	**−40**	**−40**	**−20**	**−20**	**0**	**25**	**25**
Duration/min	30	180	120	270	180	120	600
Pressure/Pa	—	—	10–16	10–16	10–16	10–16	10–16

2.4.2. Preparation of Phospholipid-Based In Situ Gel

Soybean phospholipid (Figure 4a) was selected as the matrix for the in situ gel formulation (F2). Briefly, 1.5 g of soybean phospholipid was dissolved in 3.0 g of medium chain triglycerides (MCTs) under stirring at 80 °C. The mixture was subsequently cooled to room temperature, and then 50 mg of ACTY116 was introduced and stirred for approximately 10 min until the formation of a visible suspension. This resulting suspension was then filled into vials for subsequent use. The preparation method is illustrated in Figure 4b.

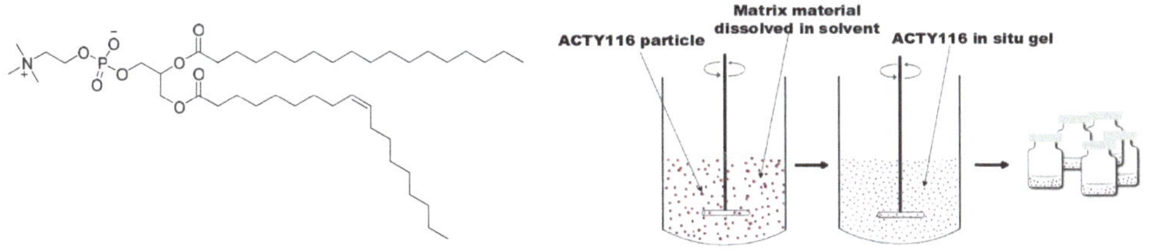

(a) (b)

Figure 4. (**a**) Phospholipid structure; (**b**) schematic illustration of in situ gel preparation.

2.4.3. Preparation of PLGA-Based In Situ Gel

PLGA (with a ratio of lactide to glycolide at 50:50, MW:7000–17,000, acid-terminated) was selected as the polymer to serve as the foundation for the long-acting matrix. The process involved the initial dissolution of 660 mg of PLGA into 1280 mg of NMP; subsequently, 56 mg of ACTY116 was introduced into the solution and stirred for approximately 10 min until the formation of a visibly apparent suspension. This resulting suspension was then transferred into vials for subsequent use (F3).

2.4.4. Characterization of Different Formulations

Polarized microscopic examination was performed by dispersing ACTY116 microspheres in 10 mL of purified water, forming a suspension that was then dropped onto a glass slide. The observation process involved the following parameters: an exposure time of 350 ms, a polarization angle of 4°, and a magnification factor of 30×. The same set of parameter settings was used to examine the in situ gel suspensions after they were applied to glass slides [34,35].

Particle size determination: Particle sizes were determined by employing laser diffraction particle size analyzers. The lyophilized microsphere cake was reconstituted with 2 mL of purified water to form a suspension, which was subsequently dispersed in 250 mL of purified water. Instrument settings included a background measurement duration of 10 s, a sample measurement duration of 30 s, an obscuration range set between 5.0% and 10.0%, and a stirrer speed of 1000 rpm. Similarly, 1 mL of phospholipid-based in situ gel was dispersed in 250 mL of MCT, and 1 mL of PLGA-based in situ gel was dispersed in 250 mL of NMP, with particle size determined using the same parameters.

Encapsulation efficiency (EE): Briefly, 40 mg of microspheres was added to a 5 mL centrifuge tube. Subsequently, 4 mL of purified water was added, and the mixture was shaken to ensure the uniform dispersion of the microspheres. After centrifugation at 10,000 rpm for 5 min, the supernatant was collected to measure unencapsulated peptides. The microspheres settled at the bottom were transferred to a 25 mL volumetric flask using DMSO, the centrifuge tube was rinsed with DMSO five times, and the rinses were pooled in the same volumetric flask. The mixture was then diluted to volume and thoroughly mixed, and the encapsulated peptide (ACTY116) was quantified using HPLC. Encapsulation efficiency was calculated using the following expression:

$$\text{Encapsulation efficiency (EE)}\% = \frac{\text{Encapsulated peptide}}{\text{Unencapsulated peptide} + \text{Encapsulated peptide}} \times 100\% \quad (1)$$

In situ gel viscosity was assessed by using a digital rotary viscometer. The suspension was put in the rotor, after which the instrument was started with a parameter configuration of 3.0 rpm for a duration of 2 min [36]. Then, the viscosity result displayed on the screen after the measurement was recorded.

2.5. *Identification of CQAs*

2.5.1. Impurity Profiles (CQA1) for Different Formulations

Considering the chemical instability of the peptide ACTY116, impurity profiles were identified as critical quality attributes (CQA1). In order to assess the impurity profiles of ACTY116 across different formulations, total impurities were analyzed following storage in a stability chamber (40 °C, 75% RH) for 10 and 20 days.

2.5.2. Other Critical Quality Attributes (CQA2) for Different Formulations

This study primarily focused on addressing the issue of peptide instability, and therefore the in vitro release was not included as a CQA in this study even though it is important to LAI formulations.

Given that (acid) hydrolysis and oxidation were degradation paths of ACTY116, water content, acid value, iodine value, peroxide value, and AV were also considered critical quality attributes (CQA2) for different formulations in this study.

Water content measurement: The sample was weighed and dissolved in anhydrous methanol, and the water content was determined utilizing a moisture analyzer.

The acid value I_A is the number that expresses, in milligrams, the quantity of potassium hydroxide required to neutralize the free acids present in 1 g of the samples. The iodine value I_I is the number that expresses, in grams, the quantity of halogen, calculated as iodine, which can be fixed in the prescribed conditions by 100 g of the sample. The testing methods of I_A and I_I follow general monograph 2.5.4 in the European Pharmacopoeia [37]. The peroxide value I_P is defined as the quantity of peroxide contained in 1000 g of the substance and expressed as in milliequivalents of active oxygen. The testing method follows general monograph 2.5.5 in the European Pharmacopoeia. The anisidine value (AV) is used to evaluate the quantity of aldehydes and ketones in pharmaceutical products. It serves as an important indicator of the extent of the oxidative degradation of lipids in products. AV determination is based on the reaction of aldehydes and ketones with anisidine under alkaline conditions. Aldehydes and ketones undergo a Schiff base reaction (nucleophilic addition) with anisidine under acidic catalysis. The carbonyl group reacts with the amino group of anisidine to form an unstable intermediate (aldimine) structure; then, intramolecular dehydration occurs, yielding a stable colored product, imine. The absorption was measured by UV spectrophotometry to evaluate the quantity of aldehydes and ketones in the sample [38,39]. The testing method follows general monograph 2.5.36 in the European Pharmacopoeia.

2.6. Risk Assessment and Control Strategies

A fundamental aspect of pharmaceutical drug development involves identifying and controlling the critical material attributes (CMAs) and critical process parameters (CPPs) that influence critical quality attributes (CQAs). In this study, we identified CMAs for the input materials (excipients) by understanding the degradation mechanisms of ACTY116. Additionally, we recognized certain process parameters that can directly or indirectly impact peptide stability, particularly those related to peptide oxidation or hydrolysis, such as high temperature and oxygen exposure, as CPPs. To ensure quality is embedded into the product, we focused on risk assessment, which involved the identification of CMAs and CPPs associated with the critical quality attributes (CQAs) for each formulation, ultimately leading to the development of corresponding control strategies.

2.7. Updated CQAs for Different Formulations

An assessment of updated CQAs for different formulations was conducted following the implementation of control strategies. The updated impurity profile (CQA1) for each formulation was investigated by following their storage in an accelerated stability chamber (40 °C, 75% RH) for 10 and 20 days. The other updated critical quality attributes (CQA2) for different formulations such as the water content, acid value, iodine value, peroxide value, and AV were also analyzed.

2.8. Pharmacokinetic Study in Rats

2.8.1. LC-MS/MS Method

The plasma concentrations of ACTY116 were analyzed using an LC-MS/MS system, which consisted of an Agilent 1290 Infinity II UHPLC system coupled with an Agilent 6460 triple quadrupole mass spectrometer equipped with an electrospray ionization source (ESI). The Agilent MassHunter workstation qualitative analysis B.08.00 (Agilent Technologies, Santa Clara, CA, USA) software was used. Chromatographic separation was performed on a BEH C18 column (2.1 mm × 75 mm, 1.7 μm, Waters, Milford, CT, USA). The separation conditions were 40 °C by using formic acid (FA)–water (0.1:99.9, *v*/*v*, A) and FA–acetonitrile (CAN) (0.1:99.9, *v*/*v*, B) solutions at a flow rate of 0.4 mL/min. The sample injection volume was 10 μL, and the autosampler was kept at 4 °C. The initial eluent AB (80:20, *v*/*v*) was changed to A-B (40:60, *v*/*v*) in 6 min and subsequently changed to A-B (20:80, *v*/*v*) in the next 0.5 min in a liner gradient and maintained at this ratio for another 1.5 min. Leuprolide acetate was used as the internal standard (IS). MS analysis was carried out in the multiple-reaction monitoring (MRM) mode with the following operation parameters: capillary voltage, 4.5 KV; gas temperature, 350 °C; nebulizer gas pressure, 50 psi; sheath gas, 11 L/min, 300 °C; fragmentor, 120 V for ACTY116 and IS; collision energy (CE), 15 eV for ACTY116 and 35 eV for IS; and precursor-to-product ion transition, m/z: 685.8→118.1 for ACTY116 and m/z: 606.5→249.4 for IS. Pharmacokinetic parameters were calculated using Phoenix 64 (version 8.3.3.33), and the noncompartmental analysis of pharmacokinetic data was conducted with the 'linear-up log-down' method.

2.8.2. PK Study in Rats

SD rats (200–250 g) were purchased from Ensiweier Biotechnology, Chongqing, China. All animals had free access to a standard diet and drinking water and were housed in a room maintained at 22.0 ± 3 °C and with a 12:12 h cyclic lighting schedule. All animal experiments were approved by the Laboratory Animal Welfare and Ethics Committee of Army Medical University (approval no.: AMUWEC20203377), and all of the experiments were performed in accordance with the National Institutes of Health guidelines for the care and use of laboratory animals.

ACTY116 solution was injected subcutaneously in rats for the analysis of pharmacokinetic (PK) behavior as an immediate-release formulation. Six (6) rats received the ACTY116 solution at a dose of 1.0 mg/kg, and blood samples were collected from the retrobulbar venous plexus 10, 20, 40, 60, 90, 120, and 180 min after subcutaneous administration.

The most stable LAI formulation (PLGA-based in situ gel) was chosen for further pharmacokinetic investigations in rats. Six (6) rats received ACTY116 LAI formulation at a dose of 7 mg/kg. The blood samples were collected from the retrobulbar venous plexus 1, 2, and 4 h post-subcutaneous injection, on days 1, 3, 5, 7, 9, 11, 13, 15, and 17 (i.e., blood was collected every two days).

Plasma was separated via refrigerated centrifugation, and ACTY116 was analyzed with the LC-MS/MS method.

2.9. Evaluation of Target Product Profile Achievement

By comparing the results with the target product profile, the achievement of stability and in vivo long-acting pharmacokinetic behavior objectives was evaluated.

3. Results

3.1. Quality Target Product Profile

This study primarily addresses two objectives: firstly, to design and optimize long-acting injectable (LAI) formulations for maintaining peptide stability during storage and in vivo release, and secondly, to ensure that the LAI formulation can achieve long-acting pharmacokinetic (PK) behavior in rats for at least one week.

The in vivo long-acting characteristic was attained through formulation design using a biodegradable matrix. Consequently, the formulation development based on QbD primarily focused on addressing stability issues in this research.

The quality target product profile was established by referencing the total impurities limits specified in the United States Pharmacopeia (USP) for peptide injectable products, such as exenatide injection (≤10.0%) and teriparatide injection (≤7.0%), both stored at 2–8 °C. We established a target product impurity profile for ACTY116-loaded LAI formulation: In the preparation process, the growth of total impurities should not exceed 1.0%; for the finished product, an accelerated stability study should be undertaken at 40 °C, and the total impurities' growth should not exceed 3.5% in 10 days and 7.0% in 20 days.

3.2. Degradation Mechanism Studies on ACTY116

The HPLC chromatograms in Figure 5 depict the impurity profiles resulting from different forced degradation conditions, illustrating variations in impurity levels.

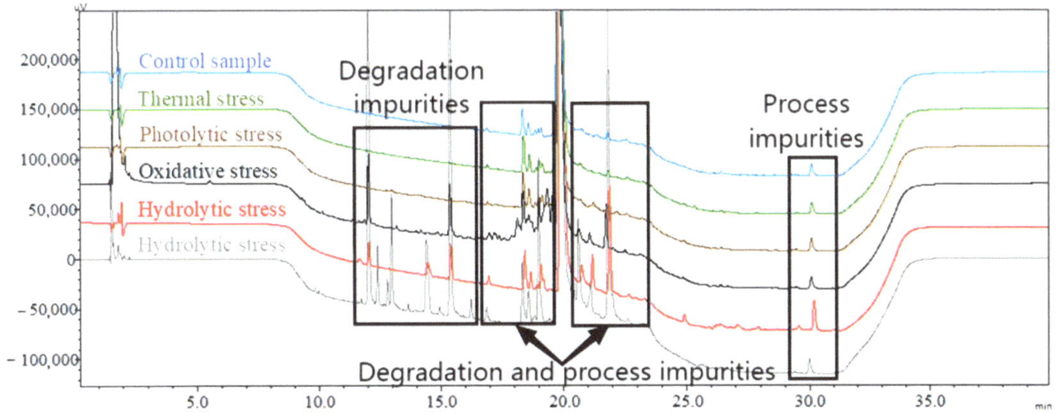

Figure 5. The typical HPLC chromatograms of ACTY116 under various forced degradation conditions; the *X*-axis represents the time, and the *Y*-axis represents the signal intensity: blue—control sample (nonstressed); green—thermal stress; brown—photolytic stress; black—oxidative stress; red—hydrolytic stress; gray—hydrolytic stress under acidic conditions.

The results demonstrated that ACTY116 (with its main peak observed at a retention time of approximately 20 min) remained stable under thermal and photolytic stress conditions, as evidenced by the absence of new degradation impurities compared to the control sample (nonstressed). However, oxidative degradation and (acid) hydrolysis led to a series of new degradation impurities, emphasizing these as the primary degradation pathways for the peptide ACTY116. Notably, hydrolytic stress under acidic conditions generated particularly pronounced degradation impurities, surpassing those observed in hydrolytic and oxidative stress. The total impurities are presented in Table 4.

Table 4. The total impurities under different forced degradation conditions.

Degradation Condition	Control Sample	Thermal Stress	Photolytic Stress	Oxidative Stress	Hydrolytic Stress	Acidic Hydrolytic Stress
Total impurities %	2.2	2.3	2.2	10.1	9.2	34.1

The ACTY116 structure (Figure 1) shows the presence of 32 amide bonds and 1 guanidine group, which account for its susceptibility to hydrolysis. Additionally, the presence of one phenolic hydroxyl group, five amino groups, and two hydroxyl groups contributes to its susceptibility to oxidation. The forced degradation results align with the predicted chemical instability of the peptide structure. The degradation and process impurities are shown on the HPLC chromatogram.

3.3. Characterization of Different LAI Formulations

Figure 6 presents the visual appearance and results of polarizing microscopic observation.

Three formulations are all in the form of suspension, and their particle size, encapsulation efficiency, and viscosity are listed in Table 5.

Table 5. Characterization of different formulations.

	Particle Size (μm)				EE%	Viscosity (cP)
	D(10)	D(50)	D(90)	D(4,3)		
F1	5.12	16.6	38.3	21.9	29.8	NA
F2	6.48	26.6	104	41.6	NA	142
F3	7.11	28.5	107	44.1	NA	115

NA means not applicable.

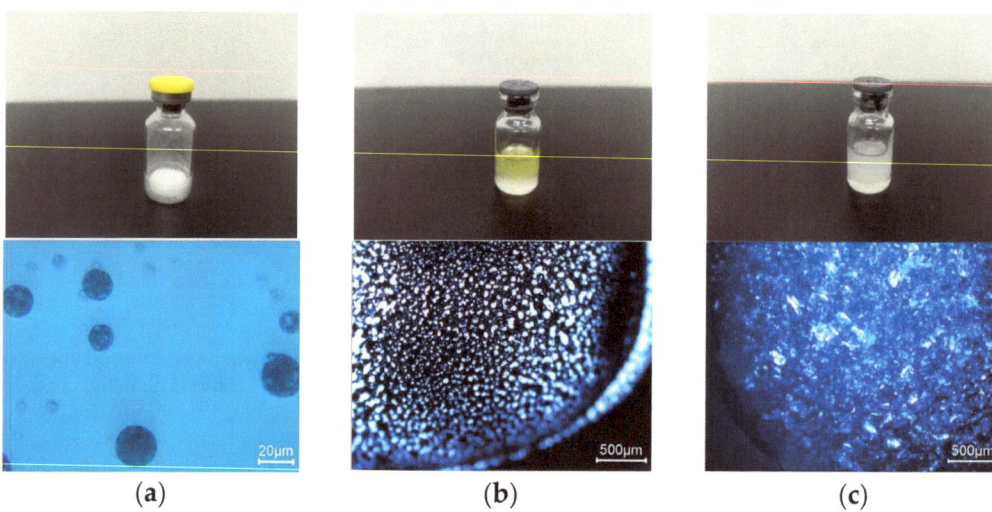

(a) (b) (c)

Figure 6. Visual appearance and polarizing microscope observation of three formulations: (**a**) microspheres (F1); (**b**) phospholipid-based in situ gel (F2); (**c**) PLGA-based in situ gel (F3).

3.4. Initial CQAs

3.4.1. Initial Impurity Profiles (CQA1) for Different Formulations

The chromatograms indicate that the peaks appearing within the retention time range of 24.0 min to 30.0 min are associated with the excipients. In the impurity analysis conducted during the stability study, the subtraction of these impurities was taken into account.

Microspheres (F1): Initial impurity profiles (Figure 7a,b, Table 6) revealed that following the preparation of microspheres, there was a 17.09% increase in total impurities. Throughout the accelerated stability, the levels of total impurities exhibited a consistent trend, namely a 26.39% increase after 10 days, which escalated to 41.22% after 20 days.

Table 6. The initial impurity profiles (CQA1) for different formulations.

	F1	F2	F3
Day 0	17.09 ± 1.18%	1.83 ± 0.87%	0.31 ± 0.08%
Day 10	26.39 ± 4.84%	16.54 ± 0.33%	4.95 ± 0.69%
Day 20	41.22 ± 0.48%	33.90 ± 3.52%	9.85 ± 2.74%

Phospholipid-based in situ gel (F2): Initial impurity profiles (Figure 7c,d, Table 6) demonstrated a time-dependent increase in total impurities within the phospholipid-based in situ gel under 40 °C conditions. Throughout the accelerated stability, the levels of total impurities exhibited a consistent trend, namely a 16.54% increase after 10 days, which escalated to 33.90% after 20 days.

PLGA-based in situ gel (F3): Initial impurity profiles (Figure 7e,f, Table 6) revealed a similar trend of an increase in the total impurities in F3 compared with F1 and F2 but at a noticeably slower pace. The total impurities exhibited a 4.95% increase after 10 days, which escalated to 9.85% after 20 days.

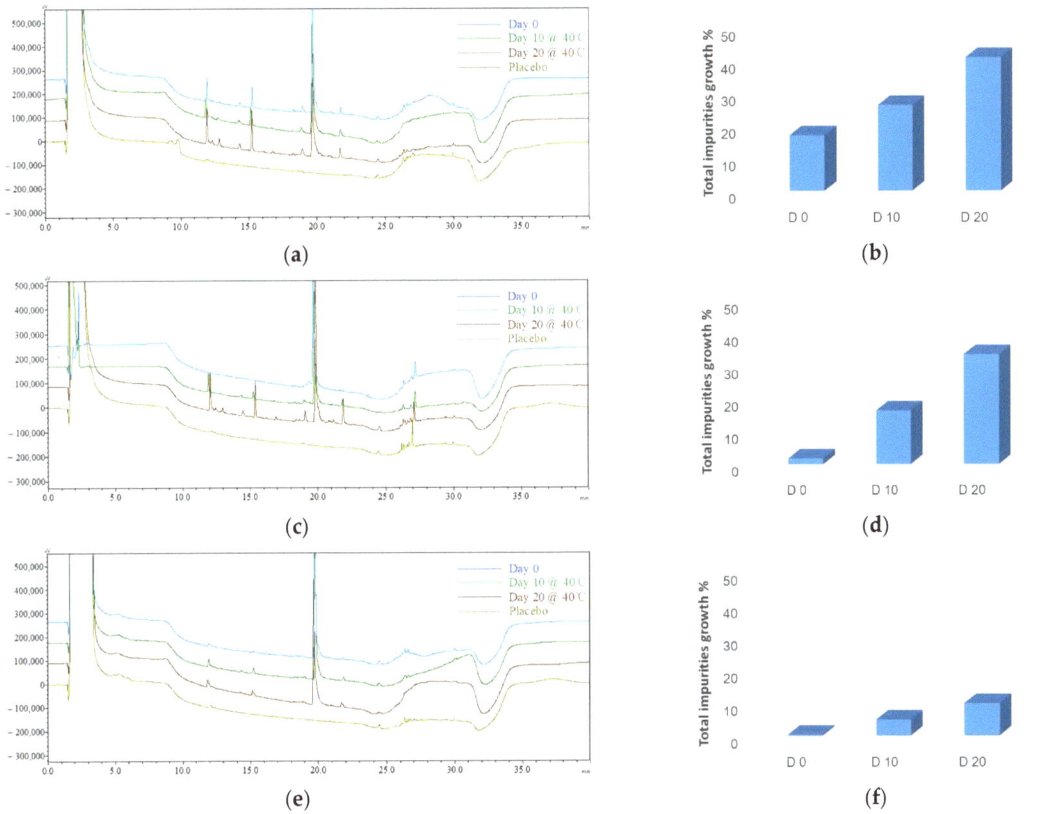

Figure 7. The typical HPLC chromatograms (left: **a**,**c**,**e**; the *X*-axis represents the time, and the *Y*-axis represents the signal intensity) and the impurity profile charts (right: **b**,**d**,**f**) for different formulations. The typical HPLC chromatograms (left: **a**,**c**,**e**): blue—Day 0; green—Day 10 @ 40 °C; brown—Day 20 @ 40 °C; olive—placebo (formulation without ACTY116); (**a**,**b**) microspheres (F1); (**c**,**d**) phospholipid-based in situ gel (F2); (**e**,**f**) PLGA-based in situ gel (F3).

3.4.2. Initial CQA2 for Different Formulations

The other critical quality attributes (CQA2) for different formulations are presented in Table 7. Among the formulations, microspheres (F1) had the highest level of water content, while phospholipid-based in situ gel (F2) had the highest levels of I_A, I_I, I_P, and AV.

Table 7. CQA2 for different formulations.

	Water%	I_A	I_I	I_P	AV
Microspheres (F1)	2.37	0	0	0.2	0
Phospholipid-based in situ gel (F2)	0.6	2.9	37.2	2.6	2.1
PLGA-based in situ gel (F3)	0.03	0	0	0	0

3.5. Risk Assessment and Control Strategies

3.5.1. Critical Material Attributes (CMAs) for Excipients

The CQAs were significantly influenced by the contributions of critical excipients. By examining the CMAs of the excipients, the objective was to identify CMAs that demonstrated a robust relationship with CQAs, enabling the formulation of effective control strategies. In microspheres (F1), PVA and mannitol did not come into direct contact with the inner aqueous phase of the peptide in $W_1/O/W_2$ (ACTY116 was in W_1, and PVA and mannitol were in W_2); therefore, they were not included in the investigation. CMAs for the essential excipients are presented in Table 8.

Table 8. The CMAs of the critical excipients.

		Water%	I_A	I_I	I_P	AV
F1	PLGA	0.01	0	0	0	0
	DCM	0.06	0	0	0	0
F2	Soybean phospholipid	1.4	8.3	105.3	2.8	0.2
	MCT	0.1	0.2	0.9	1.4	0.6
F3	PLGA	0.01	0	0	0	0
	NMP	0.03	0	0	0	0

For Excipients in F1 and F3, the water content, acid value, iodine value, peroxide value, and AV in the excipients were found to be sufficiently low.

CQA2 analysis results in Table 7 reveal that I_A, I_I, I_P, and AV values of the F2 formulation exceed those of the other two formulations. Data in Table 8 demonstrate that soybean phospholipid has the highest levels of water content, I_A, I_I, and I_P, while MCT has the highest AV. These two excipients were critical ingredients in F2, which can explain the high CQAs of F2. Consequently, the control strategy for this formulation encompassed the selection of excipients with superior CMAs (Table 9), and the updated phospholipid-based in situ gel was designated as F5.

Table 9. Excipients with different CMAs in F2 and F5.

		Water%	I_A	I_I	I_P	AV
Soybean phospholipid	F2	1.4	8.3	105.3	2.8	0.2
	F5	1.1	1.6	93.7	1.3	0.1
MCT	F2	0.1	0.2	0.9	1.4	0.6
	F5	0.1	0.1	0.8	0.3	0.2

3.5.2. CPP Control Strategies

For microspheres (F1), process parameters related to peptide oxidation or hydrolysis, such as high temperature and oxygen exposure, were identified as CPPs. The control strategies focused on lowering the DCM evaporation temperature from 50 °C to 40 °C while ensuring compliance with residual solvent regulations; extending the secondary drying phase of the lyophilization process from 10 h to 20 h to reduce water content; and replacing the air in the vial headspace with nitrogen to maintain the oxygen level at $\leq$0.1%. The updated microsphere formulation was designated as F4.

For the in situ gel formulations (F2 and F3), an uncomplicated preparation process was employed without harsh conditions such as high temperatures. The most effective strategy was headspace oxygen level control. The control strategy for phospholipid-based in situ gel encompassed CPP control through the replacement of air in the vial headspace with nitrogen to maintain the oxygen level at $\leq$0.1%, coupled with the selection of excipients with superior CMAs. The updated phospholipid-based in situ gel was designated as F5. The control strategy for PLGA-based in situ gel was the replacement of air in the vial headspace with nitrogen to maintain the oxygen level at ≤0.1%. The updated PLGA-based in situ gel was designated as F6.

The control strategies for the three LAI formulations are summarized in Table 10.

Table 10. Updated CQAs for LAI formulations with control strategies.

		Microsphere F4	Phospholipid-Based In Situ Gel F5	PLGA-Based In Situ Gel F6
CQA1 (impurity profiles)	Day 0	9.42 ± 1.31%	1.62 ± 0.79%	0.00%
	Day 10	18.85 ± 1.06%	10.75 ± 0.81%	2.48 ± 0.42%
	Day 20	27.43 ± 3.33%	17.95 ± 1.67%	4.17 ± 0.42%
CQA2	Water%	1.45	0.4	0.01
	I_A	0	0.6	0
	I_I	0	35.5	0
	I_P	0	0.7	0
	AV	0	0.6	0
Control strategies	CMAs	-	Selection of excipients with superior CMAs	-
	CPPs	• Lowering the evaporation temperature to 40 °C • Extending the secondary drying process to 1200 min • Oxygen headspace ≤ 0.1%	Oxygen in headspace ≤ 0.1%	Oxygen in headspace ≤ 0.1%

3.6. *Updated CQAs for Different Formulations*

The updated impurity profiles (CQA1) for all three formulations demonstrated improvement following the implementation of the control strategies (Figure 8, Table 10). After the completion of microsphere (F4) preparation, a 9.42% increase in total impurities was observed. Subsequently, during the 10-day accelerated storage, total impurities exhibited an 18.85% increase, which further escalated to a 27.43% increase after 20 days. In the case of phospholipid-based in situ gel (F5), there was a 1.62% increase in total impurities following preparation, and during the 10-day accelerated storage, the total impurities displayed a growth of 10.75%, which further increased to 17.95% after 20 days. Surprisingly, for PLGA-based in situ gel (F6), there was no observable increase in total impurities after preparation, and the accelerated stability resulted in a notably sluggish rate of increase under 40 °C conditions: the total impurities increased by 2.48% after 10 days and increased by 4.17% after 20 days.

The introduction of a comprehensive set of control strategies resulted in notable enhancements of ACTY116 stability in all three formulations. The updated CQAs for LAI formulations with control strategies are listed in Table 10, and the impurity profile charts of the three formulations before and after the implementation of the control strategies are visually represented in Figure 9. Remarkably, owing to the exceptional CMAs of excipients within the PLGA-based in situ gel, the absence of moisture and high temperature during the preparation process, coupled with the CPP control over low levels of headspace oxygen, contributed to the most favorable impurity profile observed in F6.

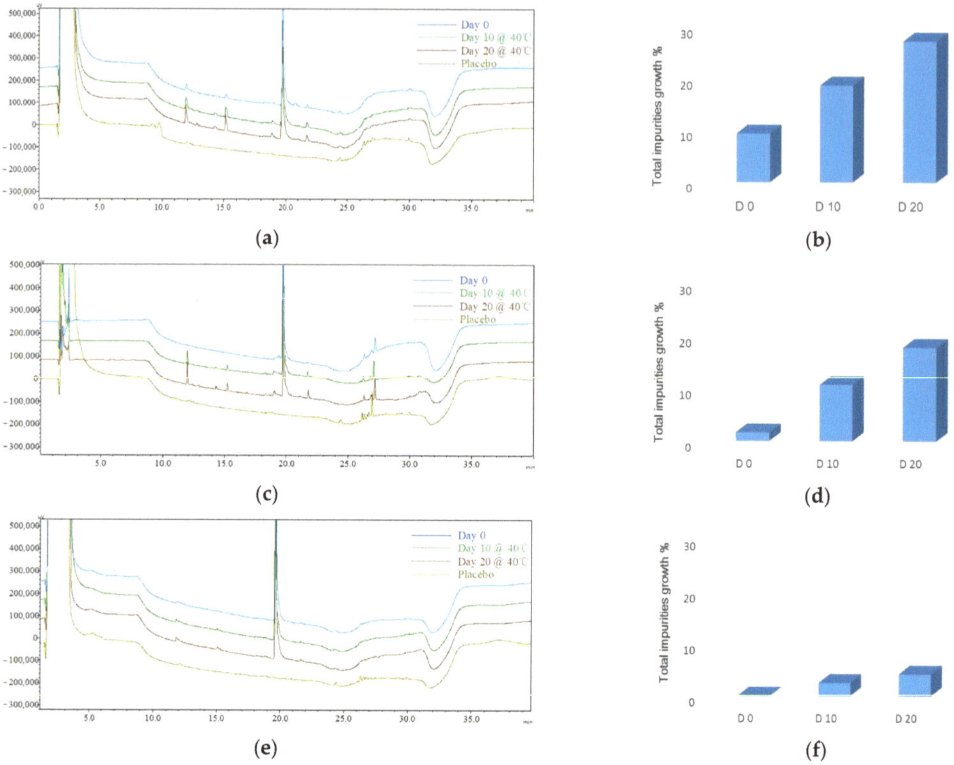

Figure 8. The typical HPLC chromatograms (left: **a**,**c**,**e**; the *X*-axis represents the time, and the *Y*-axis represents the signal intensity) and the impurity profile charts (right: **b**,**d**,**f**) of the updated impurity profile for different formulations. The typical chromatograms (left: **a**,**c**,**e**): blue—Day 0; green—Day 10 @ 40 °C, brown—Day 20 @ 40 °C; olive—placebo (formulation without ACTY116); (**a**,**b**) microspheres (F4); (**c**,**d**) phospholipid-based in situ gel (F5); (**e**,**f**) PLGA-based in situ gel (F6).

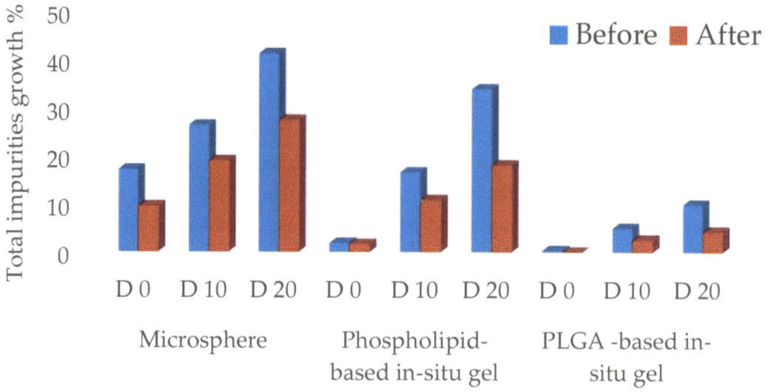

Figure 9. The impurity profile chart of three formulations before and after implementation of control strategies.

3.7. Pharmacokinetic Studies in Rats

PLGA-based in situ gel (F6) was chosen as the LAI formulation for further pharmacokinetic investigations in rats. Pharmacokinetic parameters (Table 11) and profiles (Figure 10) showed that ACTY116 LAI formulation could significantly extend both the half-life and the mean residence time (MRT) from less than 1 h to over 100 h.

Table 11. PK parameters of ACTY116 solution and ACTY116 LAI formulation.

PK Parameters	C_{max} (ng/mL)	AUC_{last} (h·ng/mL)	T_{max} (h)	HL_Lambda_z (h)	MRT_{last} (h)	T_{last} (h)
ACTY116 Solution	377.4 ± 20.3	240.5 ± 29.1	0.67	0.351 ± 0.021	0.796 ± 0.024	2 ± 0
ACTY116 LAI formulation	489.8 ± 44.3	14,385.6 ± 1063.2	1.99	100.4 ± 50.4	117.5 ± 7.2	312 ± 19.2

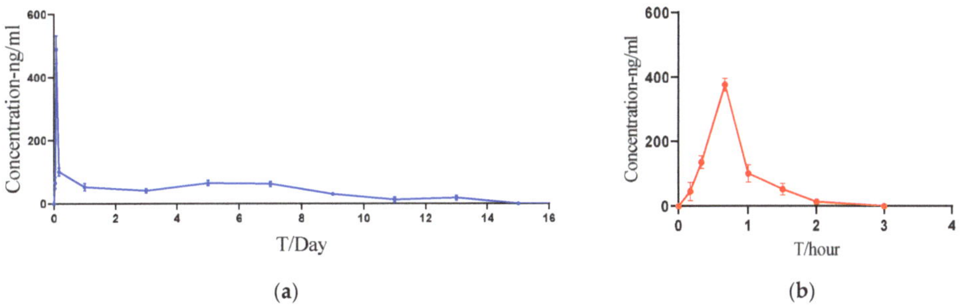

Figure 10. ACTY116 PK profiles: (**a**) ACTY116 LAI formulation (F6); (**b**) ACTY116 solution.

3.8. Evaluation of Target Product Profile Achievement

Applying the QbD concept to the formulation design, control strategies were devised and implemented after identifying CQAs, CMAs, and CPPs for each formulation. These strategies resulted in notable CQA improvements for all formulations. When compared to the target product impurity profile, only F6 successfully met the goal (Table 12).

Table 12. Assessment of target product impurity profile achievement.

	The Total Impurities' Growth		
	During Preparation	10 Days @ 40 °C	20 Days @ 40 °C
Target product impurity profile	≤1.0%	≤3.5%	≤7.0%
Microspheres (F4)	9.42 ± 1.31%	18.85 ± 1.06%	27.43 ± 3.33%
Phospholipid-based in situ gel (F5)	1.62 ± 0.79%	10.75 ± 0.81%	17.95 ± 1.67%
PLGA-based in situ gel (F6)	0	2.48 ± 0.42%	4.17 ± 0.42%

PLGA-based in situ gel exhibited prolonged ACTY116 release and extended residence time compared to the corresponding solution in the PK study. T_{last} values in Table 11 showed that after 2 h following the administration of the solution, ACTY116 was undetectable in the blood, while the LAI formulation maintained a measurable concentration for about 13 days (312 ± 19.2 h). This indicated that the LAI formulation achieved the long-acting goal for at least one week in rats.

4. Discussion

The purpose of this study was to utilize the QbD concept to develop a stable ACTY116-loaded long-acting injection. Simultaneously addressing peptide chemical instability and achieving long-acting release presents a substantial challenge, which is the novelty of this research. We chose biodegradable microspheres and in situ gels as the dosage forms for long-acting drug delivery. For hydrophilic peptides, the preparation of PLGA microspheres was challenging, and encapsulation efficiency was low. As demonstrated by the results of microsphere formulations F1 and F4 in this study, the preparation method not only involved a complex process but also led to peptide degradation under high temperatures. In situ gel formation with an uncomplicated preparation process was designed, and a nonaqueous solvent was selected to overcome these challenges. The principle guiding the choice of this nonaqueous solvent is that the sustained-release matrix can dissolve in the solvent, while the peptide cannot. This results in the formation of a peptide suspension in the solvent. Upon administration, the solvent diffuses into surrounding tissues, forming a solid or semisolid drug delivery depot comprising the peptide and sustained-release matrix. This transformed depot exhibits prolonged residence at the injection site, facilitating sustained drug release [40,41].

We conducted our study by following QbD principles. An in-depth comprehension of peptide degradation mechanisms was achieved through forced degradation investigations, elucidating (acid) hydrolysis and oxidation as the primary pathways for the peptide ACTY116 degradation. The quality built into the product was focused on risk assessment, for which the critical material attributes (CMAs) and critical process parameters (CPPs) associated with the critical quality attributes (CQAs) of each formulation were identified, leading to the development of corresponding control strategies. Following the implementation of a series of control strategies, the CQAs for all three formulations improved, and the PLGA-based in situ gel (F6) achieved the target product impurity profile; thus, it was selected as the LAI formulation for subsequent pharmacokinetic studies. PK profiles showed that the ACTY116 LAI formulation could significantly extend the half-life from less than 1 h to over 100 h. The LAI formulation studies and in vivo pharmacokinetic findings presented in this article establish a robust foundation for the use of ACTY116 in more in-depth preclinical investigations and provide a basis for potential future clinical studies.

The number of novel therapeutic peptide approvals by the US Food and Drug Administration (USFDA) is increasing in the market. About 140 peptide drugs are currently in clinical trials, with more than 500 peptides in preclinical trials [42,43]. Significant research efforts are being made to address drawbacks such as poor stability and short half-life. To this end, structural modifications and novel delivery tactics have been developed to boost their ability to reach their targets as fully functional species. The field is being revolutionized with the inclusion of modern strategies such as synthetic nanochaperone [44] and halloysite nanotubes [45]. In conclusion, the field is in need of novel ideas that can help introduce these peptides to the market.

5. Conclusions

The ACTY116 structure has 32 amide bonds and 1 guanidine group, which account for its susceptibility to hydrolysis. Additionally, the presence of one phenolic hydroxyl group, five amino groups, and two hydroxyl groups makes it susceptible to oxidation. Therefore, maintaining its stability is a significant challenge. According to the QbD principle, PLGA-based in situ gel as an LAI formulation was designed, and an uncomplicated preparation process was employed, which avoided the need for harsh conditions like high temperatures, high shear mixing, or homogenization. Furthermore, the maintenance of a water- and oxygen-free environment ensures the chemical stability of peptide ACTY116. For other molecules with susceptible functionalities like amide bonds, amino groups, hydroxyl groups, etc., the utilization of PLGA-based in situ gel as a long-acting injectable formulation for stabilizing the API provides valuable insights.

Author Contributions: Conceptualization, Y.X., X.L. and X.Z.; methodology, Y.X., X.L. and X.Z.; software, Y.X. and X.Z.; validation, Y.X. and J.W.; formal analysis, X.Z.; investigation, Y.X. and J.W.; resources, X.L.; data curation, Y.X. and J.W.; writing—original draft preparation, Y.X.; writing—review and editing, X.Z.; visualization, J.W.; supervision, X.L.; project administration, Y.X.; funding acquisition, X.L. All authors have read and agreed to the published version of the manuscript.

Funding: This research was funded by the National Natural Scientific Foundation of China (No.: 81773742) and the Science Technology Research Program of Chongqing Municipal Education Commission (No.: KJQN202212809), Talent Plan Project of Chongqing (No.: CQYC20220305379).

Institutional Review Board Statement: Not applicable.

Informed Consent Statement: Not applicable.

Data Availability Statement: Data are contained within the article.

Conflicts of Interest: The authors declare no conflicts of interest.

References

1. Yang, H.; Liu, Y.; Lu, X.L.; Li, X.H.; Zhang, H.G. Transmembrane transport of the gαq protein carboxyl terminus imitation polypeptide gcip-27. *Eur. J. Pharm. Sci.* **2013**, *49*, 791–799. [CrossRef]
2. Wang, Y.; Lu, X.L.; Yang, H.; Li, X.H.; Zhang, H.G. Effects of polypeptide drug huilixinkang on cardiac hypertrophy and expressions of myosin heavy chain in mice. *Chin. Pharm. J.* **2011**, *46*, 1566–1569.
3. Lu, X.L.; Tong, Y.F.; Liu, Y.; Xu, Y.L.; Yang, H.; Zhang, G.Y.; Li, X.H.; Zhang, H.G. Gαq protein carboxyl terminus imitation polypeptide gcip-27 improves cardiac function in chronic heart failure rats. *PLoS ONE* **2015**, *10*, e0121007.
4. Blessy, M.R.D.P.; Patel, R.D.; Prajapati, P.N.; Agrawal, Y.K. Development of forced degradation and stability indicating studies of drugs—A review. *J. Pharm. Anal.* **2014**, *4*, 159–165. [CrossRef] [PubMed]
5. Naazneen, S.; Sridevi, A. Development of assay method and forced degradation study of valsartan and sacubitril by RP-HPLC in tablet formulation. *Int. J. Appl. Pharm.* **2017**, *9*, 9–15. [CrossRef]
6. Jimmidi, R. Synthesis and applications of peptides and peptidomimetics in drug discovery. *Eur. J. Org. Chem.* **2023**, *26*, e202300028. [CrossRef]
7. Nugrahadi, P.P.; Hinrichs, W.L.; Frijlink, H.W.; Schöneich, C.; Avanti, C. Designing formulation strategies for enhanced stability of therapeutic peptides in aqueous solutions: A review. *Pharmaceutics* **2023**, *15*, 935. [CrossRef] [PubMed]
8. Shi, Y.; Lu, A.; Wang, X.; Belahadj, Z.; Wang, J.; Zhang, Q. A review of existing strategies for designing long-acting parenteral formulations: Focus on underlying mechanisms, and future perspectives. *Acta Pharm. Sin. B.* **2021**, *11*, 2396–2415. [CrossRef] [PubMed]
9. Ahmed, N.R.; Kulkarni, V.V.; Pokhrel, S.; Akram, H.; Abdelgadir, A.; Chatterjee, A.; Khan, S. Comparing the efficacy and safety of obeticholic acid and semaglutide in patients with non-alcoholic fatty liver disease: A systematic review. *Cureus* **2022**, *14*. [CrossRef]
10. Knudsen, L.B.; Lau, J. The discovery and development of liraglutide and semaglutide. *Front. Endocrinol.* **2019**, *10*, 155. [CrossRef]
11. Citrome, L. Paliperidone palmitate—Review of the efficacy, safety and cost of a new second-generation depot antipsychotic medication. *Int. J. Clin. Pract.* **2010**, *64*, 216–239. [CrossRef]
12. Li, G.; Rui-Guo, Z.; Yu-Ting, Q.; Yun-Chun, C.; Hua-Ning, W.; Psychosomatic, D.O. Efficacy and Safety of Paliperidone Palmitate or Long-acting Injectable Risperidone in Patients with Schizophrenia. *Prog. Mod. Biomed.* **2017**, *17*, 688–691.
13. Fowler, J.E., Jr.; Flanagan, M.; Gleason, D.M.; Klimberg, I.W.; Gottesman, J.E.; Sharifi, R. Evaluation of an implant that delivers leuprolide for 1 year for the palliative treatment of prostate cancer. *Urology* **2000**, *55*, 639–642. [CrossRef] [PubMed]
14. Park, K.; Skidmore, S.; Hadar, J.; Garner, J.; Park, H.; Otte, A.; Soh, B.K.; Yoon, G.; Yu, D.; Yun, Y. Injectable, long-acting plga formulations: Analyzing plga and understanding microparticle formation. *J. Control. Release* **2019**, *304*, 125–134. [CrossRef] [PubMed]
15. Lee, W.Y.; Asadujjaman, M.; Jee, J.P. Long acting injectable formulations: The state of the arts and challenges of poly (lactic-co-glycolic acid) microsphere, hydrogel, organogel and liquid crystal. *J. Pharm. Investig.* **2019**, *49*, 459–476. [CrossRef]
16. O'Brien, M.N.; Jiang, W.; Wang, Y.; Loffredo, D.M. Challenges and opportunities in the development of complex generic long-acting injectable drug products. *J. Control. Release* **2021**, *336*, 144–158. [CrossRef]
17. Zhou, J.; Walker, J.; Ackermann, R.; Olsen, K.; Hong, J.K.; Wang, Y.; Schwendeman, S.P. Effect of manufacturing variables and raw materials on the composition-equivalent plga microspheres for 1-month controlled release of leuprolide. *Mol. Pharm.* **2020**, *17*, 1502–1515. [CrossRef]
18. Park, K.; Otte, A.; Sharifi, F.; Garner, J.; Skidmore, S.; Park, H.; Jhon, Y.K.; Qin, B.; Wang, Y. Formulation composition, manufacturing process, and characterization of poly (lactide-co-glycolide) microparticles. *J. Control. Release* **2021**, *329*, 1150–1161. [CrossRef]
19. Nair, H.A.; Begum, N. Development and evaluation of a poloxamer- and chitosan-based in situ gel-forming injectable depot. *Asian J. Pharm. Clin. Res.* **2020**, *13*, 36–41. [CrossRef]
20. Muddineti, O.S.; Omri, A. Current trends in plga based long-acting injectable products: The industry perspective. *Expert Opin. Drug Deliv.* **2022**, *19*, 559–576. [CrossRef]
21. Somayaji, M.R.; Das, D.; Przekwas, A. A new level a type ivivc for the rational design of clinical trials toward regulatory approval of generic polymeric long-acting injectables. *Clin. Pharmacokinet.* **2016**, *55*, 1179–1190. [CrossRef]
22. Butreddy, A.; Gaddam, R.P.; Kommineni, N.; Dudhipala, N.; Voshavar, C. Plga/pla-based long-acting injectable depot microspheres in clinical use: Production and characterization overview for protein/peptide delivery. *Int. J. Mol. Sci.* **2021**, *22*, 8884. [CrossRef]
23. Silva, A.T.C.R.; Cardoso, B.C.O.; e Silva, M.E.S.R.; Freitas, R.F.S.; Sousa, R.G. Synthesis, characterization, and study of plga copolymer in vitro degradation. *J. Biomater. Nanobiotechnol.* **2015**, *6*, 8. [CrossRef]

24. Mir, M.; Ahmed, N.; ur Rehman, A. Recent applications of plga based nanostructures in drug delivery. *Colloids Surf. B Biointerfaces* **2017**, *159*, 217–231. [CrossRef] [PubMed]
25. Lim, Y.W.; Tan, W.S.; Ho, K.L.; Mariatulqabtiah, A.R.; Abu Kasim, N.H.; Abd Rahman, N.; Wong, T.W.; Chee, C.F. Challenges and Complications of Poly(lactic-co-glycolic acid)-Based Long-Acting Drug Product Development. *Pharmaceutics* **2022**, *14*, 614. [CrossRef] [PubMed]
26. Hu, M.; Zhang, Y.; Xiang, N.; Zhong, Y.; Gong, T.; Zhang, Z.R.; Fu, Y. Long-Acting Phospholipid Gel of Exenatide for Long-Term Therapy of Type II Diabetes. *Pharm. Res.* **2016**, *33*, 1318–1326. [CrossRef] [PubMed]
27. Nanxi, X.; Yu, Z.; Xinyi, H.E.; Jinjie, Z.; Xun, S.; Tao, G. Preparation and pharmacokinetic study of Huperzine A phospholipid in situ-gel. *West China J. Pharm. Sci.* **2017**, *32*, 136–146.
28. Li, H.; Liu, T.; Zhu, Y.; Fu, Q.; Wu, W.; Deng, J.; Shi, S. An in situ-forming phospholipid-based phase transition gel prolongs the duration of local anesthesia for ropivacaine with minimal toxicity. *Acta Biomater.* **2017**, *58*, 136–145. [CrossRef] [PubMed]
29. Xu, X.; Dai, Z.; Zhang, Z.; Kou, X.; You, X.; Sun, H.; Zhu, H. Fabrication of oral nanovesicle in-situ gel based on Epigallocatechin gallate phospholipid complex: Application in dental anti-caries. *Eur. J. Pharmacol.* **2021**, *897*, 173951. [CrossRef]
30. Yu, L.X.; Amidon, G.; Khan, M.A.; Hoag, S.W.; Polli, J.; Raju, G.K.; Woodcock, J. Understanding pharmaceutical quality by design. *AAPS J.* **2014**, *16*, 771–783. [CrossRef]
31. Devi, M.S.; Babu, G.R.; Mulukuri, N.S. A new stability indicating RP-HPLC method for the simultaneous estimation of Diloxanide and Ornidazole in bulk and Pharmaceutical Dosage forms. *Res. J. Pharm. Technol.* **2017**, *12*, 4247–4254. [CrossRef]
32. Lakka NSKuppan, C.; Srinivas, K.S.; Yarra, R. Separation and Characterization of New Forced Degradation Products of Dasatinib in Tablet Dosage Formulation Using LC-MS and Stability-Indicating HPLC Methods. *Chromatographia* **2020**, *83*, 947–962. [CrossRef]
33. Rathor, S.; Sherje, A. Forced degradation studies of tizanidine hydrochloride and development of validated stability-indicating RP-HPLC method. *Indian Drugs* **2021**, *58*, 50–55. [CrossRef]
34. Li, Z.; Mu, H.; Larsen, S.W.; Jensen, H.; Østergaard, J. Initial leuprolide acetate release from poly (d, l-lactide-co-glycolide) in situ forming implants as studied by ultraviolet–visible imaging. *Mol. Pharm.* **2020**, *17*, 4522–4532. [CrossRef]
35. Ibrahim, T.M.; El-Megrab, N.A.; El-Nahas, H.M. Optimization of injectable plga in-situ forming implants of anti-psychotic risperidone via box-behnken design. *J. Drug Deliv. Sci. Technol.* **2020**, *58*, 101803. [CrossRef]
36. Shukr, M.H.; Ismail, S.; El-Hossary, G.G.; El-Shazly, A.H. Design and evaluation of mucoadhesive in situ liposomal gel for sustained ocular delivery of travoprost using two steps factorial design. *J. Drug Deliv. Sci. Technol.* **2021**, *61*, 102333. [CrossRef]
37. *European Pharmacopoeia 11.0*; European Directorate for the Quality of Medicines & Healthcare: Strasbourg, France, 2022.
38. Doleschall, F.; KemÉNy, Z.; Recseg, K.; Kővári, K. A new analytical method to monitor lipid peroxidation during bleaching. *Eur. J. Lipid Sci. Technol.* **2002**, *104*, 14–18. [CrossRef]
39. Lai-Lin, Z.; Qing-He, Z.; Jie-Sheng, Z.; Shu-Li, W. Effects of storage conditions on oil-making quality of sesame seeds. *J. Henan Univ. Technol.* **2015**, *36*, 47–51.
40. Vigani, B.; Rossi, S.; Sandri, G.; Bonferoni, M.C.; Caramella, C.M.; Ferrari, F. Recent advances in the development of in situ gelling drug delivery systems for non-parenteral administration routes. *Pharmaceutics* **2020**, *12*, 859. [CrossRef]
41. Ibrahim, T.M.; El-Megrab, N.A.; El-Nahas, H.M. An overview of plga in-situ forming implants based on solvent exchange technique: Effect of formulation components and characterization. *Pharm. Dev. Technol.* **2021**, *26*, 709–728. [CrossRef]
42. Al Shaer, D.; Al Musaimi, O.; Albericio, F.; de la Torre, B.G. 2021 FDA TIDES (Peptides and Oligonucleotides) Harvest. *Pharmaceuticals* **2022**, *15*, 222. [CrossRef] [PubMed]
43. Lau, J.L.; Dunn, M.K. Therapeutic peptides: Historical perspectives, current development trends, and future directions. *Bioorg. Med. Chem.* **2018**, *26*, 2700–2707. [CrossRef] [PubMed]
44. Park, I.S.; Kim, S.; Yim, Y.; Park, G.; Choi, J.; Won, C.; Min, D.H. Multifunctional synthetic nano-chaperone for peptide folding and intracellular delivery. *Nat. Commun.* **2022**, *13*, 4568. [CrossRef] [PubMed]
45. Massaro, M.; Licandro, E.; Cauteruccio, S.; Lazzara, G.; Liotta, L.F.; Notarbartolo, M.; Raymo, F.M.; Sánchez-Espejo, R.; Viseras-Iborra, C.; Riela, S. Nanocarrier based on halloysite and fluorescent probe for intracellular delivery of peptide nucleic acids. *J. Colloid Interface Sci.* **2022**, *620*, 221–233. [CrossRef]

pharmaceutics

MDPI

Article

Nano-Topographically Guided, Biomineralized, 3D-Printed Polycaprolactone Scaffolds with Urine-Derived Stem Cells for Promoting Bone Regeneration

Fei Xing [1], Hui-Yuan Shen [2], Man Zhe [3], Kai Jiang [2], Jun Lei [2], Zhou Xiang [1], Ming Liu [1,*], Jia-Zhuang Xu [2,*] and Zhong-Ming Li [2]

1 Department of Orthopedic Surgery, Orthopedic Research Institute, Laboratory of Stem Cell and Tissue Engineering, State Key Laboratory of Biotherapy, West China Hospital, Sichuan University, Chengdu 610041, China; xingfeihuaxi@163.com (F.X.); xiangzhoui5@hotmail.com (Z.X.)

2 College of Polymer Science and Engineering and State Key Laboratory of Polymer Materials Engineering, Sichuan University, Chengdu 610065, China; shyhuiyuanshen@163.com (H.-Y.S.); jiangkaijkcd@163.com (K.J.); leijun@scu.edu.cn (J.L.); zmli@scu.edu.cn (Z.-M.L.)

3 Animal Experiment Center, West China Hospital, Sichuan University, Chengdu 610041, China; zheman@wchscu.cn

* Correspondence: liuminglm15@163.com (M.L.); jzxu@scu.edu.cn (J.-Z.X.)

Abstract: Currently, biomineralization is widely used as a surface modification approach to obtain ideal material surfaces with complex hierarchical nanostructures, morphologies, unique biological functions, and categorized organizations. The fabrication of biomineralized coating for the surfaces of scaffolds, especially synthetic polymer scaffolds, can alter surface characteristics, provide a favorable microenvironment, release various bioactive substances, regulate the cellular behaviors of osteoblasts, and promote bone regeneration after implantation. However, the biomineralized coating fabricated by immersion in a simulated body fluid has the disadvantages of non-uniformity, instability, and limited capacity to act as an effective reservoir of bioactive ions for bone regeneration. In this study, in order to promote the osteoinductivity of 3D-printed PCL scaffolds, we optimized the surface biomineralization procedure by nano-topographical guidance. Compared with biomineralized coating constructed by the conventional method, the nano-topographically guided biomineralized coating possessed more mineral substances and firmly existed on the surface of scaffolds. Additionally, nano-topographically guided biomineralized coating possessed better protein adsorption and ion release capacities. To this end, the present work also demonstrated that nano-topographically guided biomineralized coating on the surface of 3D-printed PCL scaffolds can regulate the cellular behaviors of USCs, guide the osteogenic differentiation of USCs, and provide a biomimetic microenvironment for bone regeneration.

Keywords: 3D printing; nano-topography; coating; hydroxyapatite; polycaprolactone

Citation: Xing, F.; Shen, H.-Y.; Zhe, M.; Jiang, K.; Lei, J.; Xiang, Z.; Liu, M.; Xu, J.-Z.; Li, Z.-M. Nano-Topographically Guided, Biomineralized, 3D-Printed Polycaprolactone Scaffolds with Urine-Derived Stem Cells for Promoting Bone Regeneration. *Pharmaceutics* **2024**, *16*, 204. https://doi.org/10.3390/pharmaceutics16020204

Academic Editor: Dong Keun Han

Received: 30 November 2023
Revised: 21 January 2024
Accepted: 26 January 2024
Published: 31 January 2024

1. Introduction

In nature, the unique biological functions of various tissues are based on their complex hierarchical nanostructures after long-term evolution and natural selection [1]. Among the various tissues of the human body, dense bone tissue possessing plate-like mineral nanostructures endows bone tissue with excellent mechanical properties that support the various movements of the body in daily life [2]. Bone tissue is a hard and mineralized connective tissue composed of biogenic hierarchical biominerals that exhibit distinct topographies and functions [3]. Biominerals in bone tissue are generated by a biochemical process in body fluids or interstitial fluids, which is called biomineralization [4]. Biominerals inside a living organism consist of various inorganic substances, such as phosphates, carbonates, sulfates, and halides, and emerge as kinds of crystalline, paracrystalline, and amorphous phases [5]. As the hardest substances in vertebrates, the growth and development of bone tissue rely on a self-assembly dynamic biomineralization process. Biomineralization plays a pivotal role in the process of endochondral ossification, facilitating the gradual replacement of cartilage with bone, which is guided by a series of interactive activities of bone tissue and microenvironments. After biomineralization, complex hierarchical nanostructures, morphologies, and unique biological functions are formed in bone tissue [6].

Biomineralization is a complex, multi-level process that deposits inorganic mineralized nanomaterials onto a surface template in a self-assembly manner under mild conditions [7]. The biomineralization process can be adjusted by altering organic templates, inorganic mineralized agents, and external factors, such as pH, time, and temperature [8]. In addition, various nanostructures on the surface of organic templates, such as nanotubes and nanoarrays, can also regulate the biomineralization process. Recently, more and more researchers have utilized biomimetic mineralization as a modification approach to obtain ideal material surfaces with complex nanostructures, unique biological functions, and categorized organizations [9–11]. Most biomimetic mineralization approaches are conducted in aqueous environments with controllable conditions. As a calcium phosphate crystal derivative, hydroxyapatite (HA) is the main inorganic substance existing in natural bone tissue and possesses unique crystallographic nanostructures, hierarchically arranged between the collagen fibrils [12]. In vitro, due to similar components to native bone tissue, HA has been widely used as a calcium–phosphate (CaP)-based bone substitute for bone regeneration. After implantation in vivo, the chemical properties of HA are stable. In addition, under physiological conditions, HA has the ability to regulate various cellular behaviors of osteoblasts, such as proliferation, migration, osteogenic differentiation, and cell adhesion [13]. Due to its excellent bioactivity and biocompatibility, HA has gradually become one of the most prominent biomaterials in the fabrication of various bone substitutes. Nevertheless, the direct application of bulk HA as bone implants is limited due to its weak mechanical properties. Researchers have utilized many approaches to enhance the mechanical properties of bulk HA, such as altering the sintering temperature [14]. Simultaneously, applying HA as an additive material coating onto scaffolds, such as metal implants and polymer implants, has also attracted attention to the practical applications of HA [15–17].

Due to its excellent biocompatibility, high customizability, good tensile strength, high resistance to degradation, and high stability under physiological conditions, synthetic polymers, including polycaprolactone (PCL), polylactic-co-glycolic acid (PLGA), poly(l-lactic acid) (PLLA), poly(lactic acid) (PLA), and poly(glycolic acid) (PGA), have been widely used as bone substitutes [18,19]. However, the surface of the synthetic polymer scaffolds is bioinert and has the disadvantages of low wettability and weak cell adhesion and thus cannot provide favorable microenvironments for osteogenesis in vivo. Therefore, the biomineralization of HA onto surfaces of synthetic polymer scaffolds can form a bioactive surface with higher wettability and better osteoinductivity, which provides a more favorable microenvironment for osteoblast adhesion, proliferation, and differentiation [20,21]. Currently, soaking in a simulated body fluid (SBF) that contains similar ion levels to those of human body fluid is one of the most common biomineralization approaches and has the advantages of being a simple procedure and having high efficiency [22]. However, biomineralized coating fabricated by immersion in simulated body fluid is uneven and unstable. Researchers can alter the ion concentrations of SBF to regulate biomimetic calcium–phosphate coatings during the biomineralization process [23,24]. In addition, the surface properties, such as topography, charge, and hydrophilicity, greatly affect the surface mineralization of HA during SBF soaking. In recent years, many researchers have altered the surface topography of implants, including nanotubes, nanopits, nanofibers, nanocolloids, nanopillars, nanogrooves, nanodots, and random roughness, to regulate bone formation in vivo [25–28]. In addition, the surface roughness of scaffolds can directly regulate cellular behaviors and biomineralization on the surfaces of scaffolds [29–31]. However, few studies focus on biomineralization on the surface of synthetic polymer scaffolds. Moreover, the propagation of HA in the space between collagens fibrils relies on the continuous supplement of calcium and phosphate ions [32]. Achieving the long-term release of bioactive ions from

HA coating plays an important role in continuously regulating bone regeneration in vivo after implantation.

Among various cells in bone tissues, osteoblasts and stem cells are the main source of bone regeneration. Stem cells can differentiate into various cells under various physiochemical or biological activations and directly participate in bone regeneration in vivo [33,34]. As carriers of various stem cells, the surface properties of scaffolds, including physicochemical and biological characteristics, can directly regulate cellular behaviors, such as proliferation, survival, migration, adhesion, and differentiation. Hence, fabricating a favorable surface microenvironment in scaffolds to direct stem cell fate is essential for stem cell delivery in bone repair. HA coating on the surface of scaffolds can provide an osteoinductive microenvironment for stem cells due to its native osteoinductivity. After implantation, the calcium ions and phosphate released from the HA coating can effectively guide stem cells to differentiate into osteoblasts or osteocytes. Recently, the existence of urine-derived stem cells (USCs) in urine has been confirmed by many studies [35]. Compared with other kinds of mesenchymal stem cells (MSCs), USCs possess similar capacities of self-proliferation and multi-potential differentiation [36,37]. Additionally, the isolation procedure of USCs is simple, non-invasive, and cost-effective, which makes it a potential alternative seed cell for stem cell therapy. Therefore, the construction of biomineralized coating on the surface of scaffolds to load and manipulate USCs' cellular fate can be a promising alternative approach.

In the present study, aiming to enhance the surface osteoinductivity of 3D-printed PCL scaffolds, we optimized the surface biomineralization procedure by nano-topographical guidance. The optimized surface biomineralized coating on the surfaces of customized scaffolds achieved the continuous release of calcium and phosphorus ions and regulated various cellular behaviors of USCs, such as osteogenic differentiation. To this end, the in vivo osteogenesis of nano-topographically guided biomineralized 3D-printed PCL scaffolds combined with USCs was also evaluated. This study provided 3D-printed polymer scaffolds with a promising alternative surface biomineralization strategy to regulate stem cell fate for the guidance of subsequent bone regeneration after implantation.

2. Materials and Methods

2.1. The Preparation of 3D-Printed PCL Scaffolds

In this study, a 3D bioprinter (Esun 600C, Shenzhen Guanghua Weiye Industrial Co., Ltd., Shenzhen, China) with a printing mechanism of melt extrusion deposition was used to fabricate 3D-printed PCL scaffolds. The viscosity-averaged molecular weight of the PCL pellets used as the raw materials for the PCL scaffolds was 6 × 104 g/mol. In addition, the melting temperature of the PCL pellets was 60 °C. The residual moisture from the PCL pellets was removed by drying at 37 °C for 24 h. Then, the PCL pellets were fabricated into PCL filaments by a single-screw extruder. Then, the PCL filaments were melted in the high-temperature cavity for subsequent shaping. A nozzle with a diameter of 0.5 mm extruded the melted PCL onto the platform surface, and the printed fibers were arrayed orthogonally. The PCL printing temperature was set at 70 °C. The moving speed of the printer nozzle was set at 0.5 mm/s. To this end, the customized PCL scaffolds were vacuum-dried for subsequent surface biomineralization.

2.2. Nano-Topographically Guided Biomineralization

Nano-topographically guided biomineralization was conducted through immersion in various functionalized solutions. Nano-topographical modification was essential in this procedure of biomineralization, which was carried out via the approach of epitaxial crystallization. Acetic acid (Chengdu Kelong Co., Ltd., Chengdu, China) and distilled water were mixed at a volume ratio of 77%/23%. Then, the nutrition solution for epitaxial crystallization was fabricated by dissolving PCL pellets into the mixed solution at 60 °C for 3 h. The nano-topographical modification was conducted by immersing 3D-printed PCL scaffolds into the nutrition solution for 15 min at 37 °C. Then, the nano-topographical scaffolds were dried at 37 °C for 24 h. The nano-topographical modification was confirmed by scanning electronic microscopy (SEM, Nova NanoSEM450, FEI Co., Ltd., Hillsboro, OR, USA). Furthermore, the thick distribution of the nano-ridge and the periodic distance distribution of the nano-topographical surface were also calculated according to SEM results.

After surface nano-topographical modification, the subsequent biomineralization procedure was carried out by immersing nano-topographical 3D-printed PCL scaffolds in specific biomineralizing solutions, which were supersaturated four-fold concentrations of simulated body fluids (SBFs). The biomineralizing solutions were prepared by sequentially dissolving 15.95 g of NaCl (Shanghai Macklin Co., Ltd., Shanghai, China), 0.7 g of $NaHCO_3$ (Shanghai Macklin Co., Ltd., China), 0.45 g of KCl (Shanghai Macklin Co., Ltd., Shanghai, China), 0.46 g of $K_2HPO_4 \cdot H_2O$ (Shanghai Macklin Co., Ltd., Shanghai, China), 0.56 g of $CaCl_2$ (Shanghai Macklin Co., Ltd., Shanghai, China), 0.61 g of $MgCl_2 \cdot 6H_2O$ (Shanghai Macklin Co., Ltd., Shanghai, China), and 0.14 g of Na_2SO_4 (Shanghai Macklin Co., Ltd., Shanghai, China) into 500 mL of deionized water. Then, the Tris-HCl solution was used as a buffer to adjust the pH value of the biomineralizing solutions to 7.4. The nano-topographically guided biomineralized scaffolds were prepared by immersing nano-topographical scaffolds in biomineralizing solutions at 37 °C for seven days. The biomineralizing solutions were changed every 24 h during the biomineralized coating formation on the surface of the scaffolds. Simultaneously, as a control group, bare 3D-printed PCL scaffolds without nano-topographical modification were also immersed into biomineralized solutions at 37 °C for seven days to form biomineralized scaffolds. After this procedure of biomineralization, biomineralized scaffolds were dried at 37 °C for 24 h. To this end, the bare 3D-printed PCL scaffolds, nano-topographical 3D-printed PCL scaffolds, biomineralized 3D-printed PCL scaffolds, and nano-topographically guided biomineralized 3D-printed PCL scaffolds were named BS, NS, MS, and NMS, respectively. All scaffolds were sterilized by ethylene oxide at a low temperature for subsequent cell and animal experiments.

2.3. Characteristics of Scaffolds

During the processes of nano-topographically guided biomineralization and conventional biomineralization, the surface morphology of BS, NS, MS, and NMS at nano and micro levels was observed by SEM (Nova NanoSEM450, FEI, Charlottesville, VA, USA). In addition, the water contact angle of BS, NS, MS, and NMS was also investigated. During the procedure of biomineralization, the surface chemistry of BS, NS, MS, and NMS was evaluated by Fourier transform infrared spectroscopy (FTIR, Nicolet 6700, Thermal Scientific Co., Ltd., Waltham, MA, USA). In addition, the wavenumber range of FTIR was set at 700–4000 cm^{-1}. The crystallographic structure was evaluated by X-ray diffraction (XRD, Geigerflex Co., Ltd., Rigaku, Japan). In addition, the scan range was set at 5–60°. The surface elements were assessed by X-ray photoelectron spectroscopy (XPS, XSAM800, Shimadzu-Kratos Ltd., Tokyo, Japan). Moreover, the C (1s), O (1s), Ca (2p), and P (2p) core-level spectra of the XPS results were also compared. A universal testing machine (Instron 5976, Thermal Scientific Co., Ltd., Waltham, MA, USA) was used to assess the effects of biomineralized coating on the mechanical properties. Furthermore, stress–strain and force–displacement curves were calculated.

The surface characteristics of the biomineralized coating of MS and NMS were further investigated to compare the approaches of nano-topographically guided biomineralization and conventional biomineralization. Calcium (Ca) and phosphorus (P) were the two main components of the biomineralized coating. The Ca and P ion distribution on the surface of MS and NMS was investigated by elemental energy dispersive spectrum (EDS). The Ca ions are marked green, while the P ions are marked red. The thermal stability of MS and NMS was measured by thermogravimetric analysis (TGA). In addition, the TG–temperature curves of MS and NMS were calculated. The release of Ca and P ions is an important aspect in investigating the characteristics of biomineralized coating. The bioactive ions released from MS and NMS at different time points were evaluated by inductively coupled plasma atomic emission spectroscopy (ICP-AES; Vista AX, Thermal Scientific Co., Ltd., Waltham, MA, USA). The protein adsorption capacity of MS and NMS was investigated by the protein estimation kit (Beyotime, BCA Protein Assay Kit, Shanghai, China). In order to investigate the adhesion of the biomineralized coating of scaffolds, the scaffolds were immersed in PBS and placed on the horizontal shaker. Then, the scaffolds were immersed in an alizarin red solution for 30 min.

2.4. Isolation of USCs

According to our previous studies, the USCs were isolated and obtained by the method of two times centrifugations [35,36]. After obtaining informed consent from all urine donors, 200–250 mL of fresh urine from healthy adults was collected into a sterile glass beaker. Then, the urine was separated into several 50 mL centrifuge tubes. Then, the centrifuged speed of the centrifuge tubes was set at 1700 rpm and the centrifuged time was set to 15 min. Then, the tubes were centrifuged at a centrifuge speed of 1700 rpm for 15 min. The pellets of the solution were resuspended with a specific culture medium for USCs, which is fabricated by mixing embryo fibroblast medium (EFM) (Thermo Fisher Scientific Inc., Fremont, CA, USA) and keratinocyte serum-free medium (KSFM) (Thermo Fisher Scientific Inc., Fremont, CA, USA) at a volume ratio of 1:1. Then, the suspension of USCs was seeded in cell culture plates.

2.5. Cellular Behaviors of USCs Co-Cultured with MS and NMS

In order to investigate the cellular behaviors directed by nano-topographically guided biomineralized coating, the USCs were co-cultured with MS and NMS. The cellular behaviors include proliferation, cell morphology, cell viability, migration, and invasion. Co-culturing USCs with scaffolds was performed in Transwell plates (Corning. Inc., New York, NY, USA). The USCs were seeded onto the lower chamber, while the scaffolds were placed in the upper chamber. Cell Counting Kit-8 (CCK-8, Beyotime Biotech. Inc., Shanghai, China) was applied to quantitatively evaluate the proliferation of USCs co-cultured with MS and NMS at different time points. Briefly, after discarding the medium, the CCK8 working solution was used to incubate the USCs for 1 h. Then, the absorption values of the CCK8 working solution were texted. The cytotoxicity of the nano-topographically guided biomineralized coating was investigated by live/dead staining (Beyotime Biotech. Inc., Shanghai, China) of the USCs co-cultured with MS and NMS on day 1, day 4, and day 7. The live/dead staining solution contained two fluorescent dyes to label live and dead cells separately. The live USCs were stained green and the dead USCs were stained red. After incubation with a working solution for 5 min, the samples were analyzed by fluorescent microscopy. In addition, the cell viability of USCs was also calculated according to the live/dead staining results. Cytoskeleton changes can affect various cellular behaviors. Phalloidin/DAPI staining (Beyotime Biotech. Inc., Shanghai, China) was used to observe the cytoskeleton changes of USCs co-cultured with MS and NMS. Briefly, after discarding the supernatant, the USCs were fixed in PBS containing 4% formaldehyde for 1 h. Then, the USCs were immersed in a 0.1% Triton X-100 solution for 30 min at room temperature. Then, the USCs were treated with a phalloidin staining working solution for 1 h in the dark. After being treated with a DAPI working solution, the cytoskeleton changes were observed by fluorescent microscopy. In addition, the cell area of USCs was calculated according to the cytoskeleton staining results.

The cell migration and invasion of USCs co-cultured with MS and NMS were investigated by the scratch–wound assay and transwell invasion assay. The USCs were seeded onto a microwell plate. When the USCs covered the bottom of the plate, the cell layer was scraped in a straight line using a 1 mm pipette tip. Then, the microscope was used to image the same pot at 0 h, 6 h, 12 h, and 24 h. Different from the above co-culture approach, the USCs were seeded on the top chamber of the transwell plates and the scaffolds were placed on the lower chamber during the transwell invasion assay. After incubation for 24 h, USCs that migrated to the lower surface of the top chamber membrane were fixed with

4% formaldehyde and stained with DAPI. The number of migrated USCs was calculated. In addition, in order to observe cellular behaviors on the surface of MS and NMS, the USCs were also directly seeded onto the surface of MS and NMS. Live/dead staining and phalloidin/DAPI staining were used to investigate the proliferation and cytoskeleton changes of USCs when directly co-cultured on the surface of scaffolds. In addition, the cell viability and cell area of USCs on the biomineralized coating were also calculated.

2.6. The Osteogenesis of USCs Co-Cultured with MS and NMS

The osteogenesis of USCs co-cultured with MS and NMS at different time points was conducted in transwell plates. The USCs were seeded onto the lower chamber while the scaffolds were placed on the top chamber. Alkaline phosphatase (ALP) staining was used to investigate the early osteogenesis of USCs regulated by nano-topographically guided biomineralized coating. Briefly, after co-culturing USCs with scaffolds, the medium was discarded and fixed with 10% formaldehyde for 15 min. Then, the USCs were incubated in an ALP buffer for 15 min. The BCIP/NBT color development substrate solution was used to stain USCs. In addition, the positive areas of ALP staining results were also calculated. Alizarin red staining (ARS) is a common approach for investigating the mineralization of various osteoblasts. On day 14 and day 28, the medium in the transwell plate was discarded. Then, the USCs were immersed in an alizarin red working solution for 30 min. Moreover, the positive area of ARS was assessed to quantitatively analyze the USCs' mineralization regulated by nano-topographically guided biomineralized coating. After co-culturing with MS and NMS for 7 and 21 days, the osteogenesis-related gene expression of the USCs, including collagen type 1 alpha 1 (COL1A1), alkaline phosphatase (ALP), osteocalcin (OCN), and runt-related transcription factor 2 (RUNX2), was investigated by using RT-qPCR. In addition, GAPDH was used as a reference gene. Supplementary Table S1 reports the primer sequences of the target genes. Briefly, the TRIzol solution was applied to extract the total RNA of cells. Then, RNA was reverse-transcribed into cDNA by using the QuantiTect Reverse Transcription Kit. Then, the amplification of the specific transcripts on the real-time fluorescence quantitative instrument was completed on a LightCycler 96 system by utilizing the SYBR Green Mix Kit. The condition was set at 94 °C for 5 min followed by 40 cycles of 94 °C for 15 s, 55 °C for 30 s, and 72 °C for 30 s. The 2-DDCq method was utilized to evaluate the relative levels of osteogenic gene expression. In addition, the USCs were seeded onto the surface of MS and NMS to assess the direct effect of scaffolds on cellular behaviors. In addition, live/dead staining and phalloidin staining were used to investigate the proliferation and cytoskeleton changes of USCs after being seeded onto the surface of scaffolds. The cell viability and cell area of USCs on the surface of MS and NMS were also calculated. Moreover, the osteogenesis-related gene expression of USCs on the surface of MS and NMS, including COL1A1, ALP, OCN, and RUNX2, was evaluated by using RT-qPCR.

2.7. In Vivo Bone Regeneration

All animal procedures were performed in accordance with the Guidelines for Care and Use of Laboratory Animals of West China Hospital, Sichuan University, and experiments were approved by the Animal Ethics Committee of West China Hospital, Sichuan University. The rabbit cranial bone defect models were used as in vivo osteogenesis models to evaluate the bone regeneration mediated by NMS loaded with USCs. Twenty New Zealand white rabbits (body weight: 2.5–3.0 kg; gender: male) were randomly separated into five groups: NMS loaded with USCs (NMS/USCs, n = 4), MS loaded with USCs (MS/USCs, n = 4), NMS (n = 4), MS (n = 4), and a control (n = 4). In groups of NMS/USCs and MS/USCs, the USCs were seeded onto the surface of NMS and MS and then implanted into cranial bone defects. The NMS and MS were implanted in groups of NMS and MS. In the control group, no scaffolds were implanted.

The procedure for the in vivo osteogenesis model was as follows. Briefly, after general anesthesia, the surgeon performed an incision with a longitudinal length of 4 cm. Then, the subcutaneous tissue under the skin was cut layer by layer. After the removal of the periosteum of the cranial, the cranial was fully exposed. After the construction of two circular defects with a diameter of 10 mm, the scaffolds were implanted. The information on animal grouping was reported above. After the implantation of scaffolds, the wounds were closed layer by layer with 4-0 sutures. After surgery, intramuscular penicillin was administered for 3 days at a dose of 100,000 U/day to prevent the occurrence of infection.

All animals were sacrificed by overdose of anesthesia at 8 and 16 weeks after implantation. The micro-computed tomography (Micro-CT, Trifoil Imaging Inc., Chatsworth, CA, USA) was utilized to observe newborn bone formation. In addition, the BV/TV and bone density of new bone were calculated. After imaging evaluation, the cranial samples were fixed with 10% formaldehyde and then immersed in a decalcification solution of EDTA for 8 weeks. Histological staining, including HE and Masson staining, was used to assess the new bone formation in the bone defect site. Moreover, new bone areas in the middle of the bone defect were also calculated according to the histological results.

2.8. Statistical Analysis

All experimental data analyses were performed by SPSS (Version 25). The statistical analysis of significant differences between the study groups was conducted by using the Mann–Whitney U-test or Student's *t*-test. Furthermore, p-values of <0.05 were interpreted as statistically significant.

3. Results and Discussion

3.1. The Fabrication of Nano-Topographically Guided Biomineralized 3D-Printed PCL Scaffolds

Currently, due to their good biocompatibility and abundant resources, various polymer scaffolds have been used as orthopedic implants such as joint prostheses, bone screws, nails, and plates. However, the bioinert and poor osteoinductive surface of polymer implants cannot chemically bind to surrounding bone tissue, resulting in limiting their further application for orthopedic implants [38]. Thus, the formation of a natural bone-like hydroxyapatite coating layer on polymer scaffolds plays an important role in enhancing osteointegration after implantation. In addition, few studies focus on fabricating biomineralized coating on the surface of 3D-printed polymer scaffolds. In our study, we report a simple biomineralization approach for 3D-printed polymer scaffolds via surface nano-topographical modification. Figure 1A shows the fabrication procedure for the 3D-printed PCL scaffolds. The procedures for the nano-topographically guided mineralization and conventional mineralization of the 3D-printed polymer scaffolds are shown in Figure 1B,C. Conventional mineralization was conducted by immersing the scaffolds into mineralized solutions. As shown in Figure 1D, the general views of BS, NS, MS, and NMS exhibited a similar appearance of white mesh. In addition, according to the SEM results, no significant differences were found among BS, NS, MS, or NMS when magnified to the micron level. When magnified to the nanoscale, BS, NS, MS, and NMS possessed totally different surface nano-topographies. The surface of BS was flat and smooth, while the NS exhibited a nano ridge-like surface. Altering surface properties, such as topography, roughness, and grain structure, has proven to be an effective approach to enhance the osteointegration of implants [39,40]. Moreover, our previous study demonstrated that the topography surface of polymer sheets fabricated by surface epitaxial crystallization could provide sufficient crystallization sites to enhance the in vitro biomineralization and osteogenic differentiation of preosteoblasts [41,42]. After conventional biomineralization, some mineralized crystals with irregular shapes could be observed on the MS surface. After nano-topographically guided biomineralization, a large amount of mineralized crystals with clustered shapes formed on the surface of NMS. In terms of section views of the scaffolds, some scattered mineralized crystals could be observed on the MS surface, while there was still a large amount of mineralized crystal formed on the inner fibers. In addition, compared with MS, the mineralized crystals of NMS almost fully covered the PCL fibers.

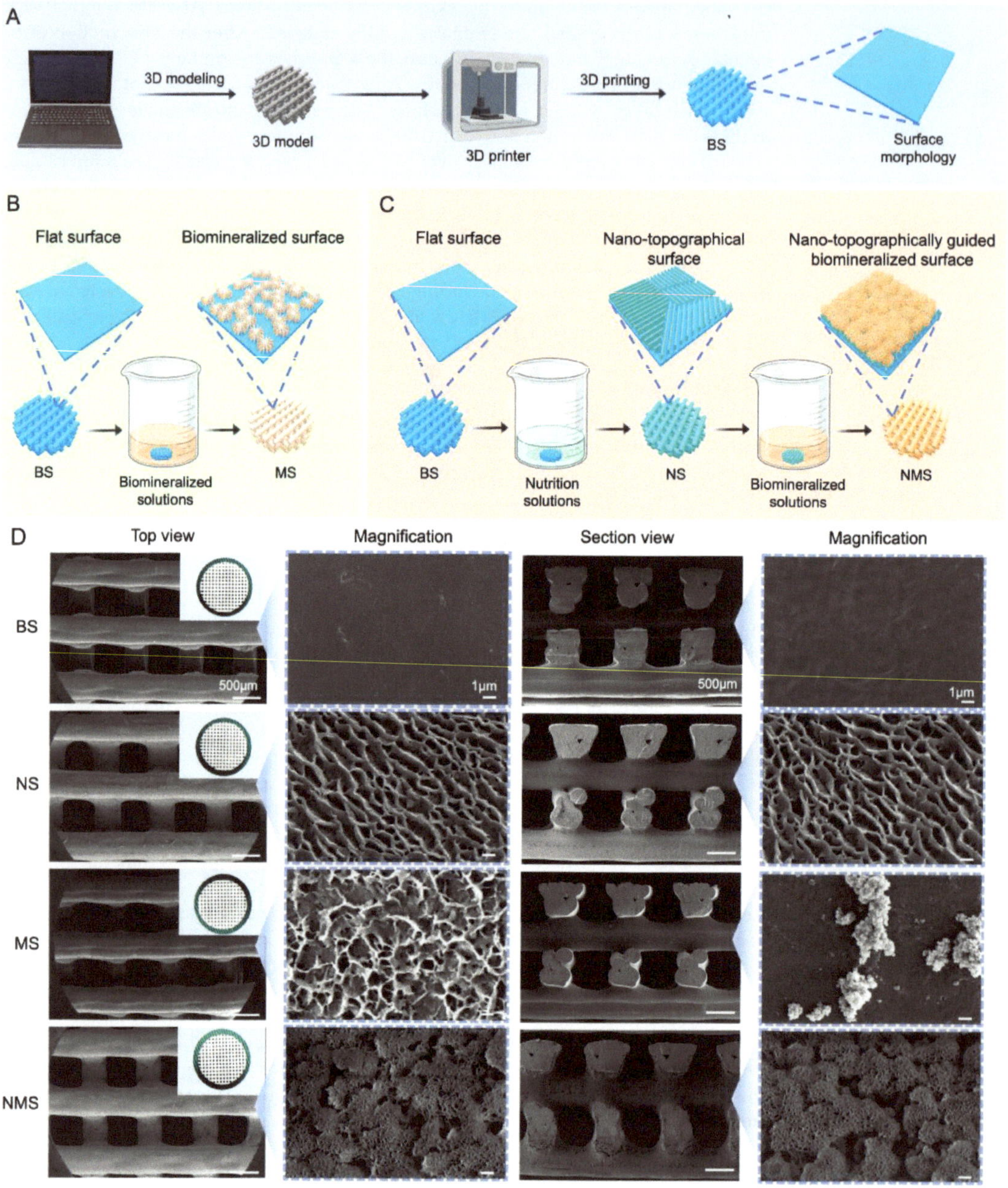

Figure 1. (**A**) The fabrication of 3D-printed PCL scaffolds. (**B**) The procedure for conventional biomineralization. (**C**) The procedure for nano-topographically guided biomineralization. (**D**) General view and SEM results of BS, NS, MS, and NMS, respectively.

3.2. Characteristics of Nano-Topographically Guided Biomineralized 3D-Printed PCL Scaffolds

The thick distribution of the nano-ridge and periodic distance distribution are shown in Figure 2A,B. Based on the SEM results, the average thickness of the nano-ridge on the surface of NS was 92.04 ± 13.69, while the average periodic distance of the nano-ridge on the surface of NS was 725.639 ± 103.93 nm. In addition to adjusting the ion concentrations of the SBF solution, changing the surface properties of scaffolds can also affect the biomineralization process [23,24]. Compared with the flat surface of NS, the nano-ridge increased the surface area as well as the roughness and provided more binding sites for subsequent biomineralization. The water contact angle of the surface of bone substitutes is important in regulating the various cellular behaviors of stem cells. As shown in Figure 2C, the water contact angle of BS, NS, MS, and NMS was 110.21 ± 3.88°, 105.71 ± 4.27°, 79.85 ± 5.12°, and 53.62 ± 5.33°. After biomineralization, the biomineralized coating gave a lower surface water contact angle for MS and NMS due to the deposition of mineralized substances. In addition, the water contact angle of NMS was significantly lower than that of MS, which indicated the greater existence of mineralized substances deposited onto the scaffolds. In the field of bone repair, the surface charge of biological scaffolds plays an important role in regulating various cell behaviors [43,44]. The Zeta potential of BS, NS, MS, and NMS was −49.44 ± 3.75 mV, 58.35 ± 4.04 mV, 43.37 ± 3.15 mV, and −18.71 ± 3.57 mV at a pH of 7.4, respectively. Moreover, as shown in Figure 2D,E, FTIR and XRD were applied to observe the chemical composition and crystal structure of the surface of BS, NS, MS, and NMS. The FTIR results demonstrated that BS and NS shared the same strong peaks at 1750 cm^{-1} and 1084 cm^{-1} (C=O and C-O-C), which indicated that the nano-topographical surface fabricated by epitaxial crystallization possessed a similar composition to that of the base material. After biomineralization, the surface FTIR of NMS and MS showed characteristic peaks of HA at 1046 cm^{-1}, which confirmed the existence of biomineralized coating. In addition, compared with MS, the characteristic peaks of the HA of NMS were more obvious and even covered the characteristic peaks of PCL, which indicated a greater existence of HA on the scaffolds' surface. XRD is a common technique to evaluate the type and content of crystal phases. XRD demonstrated that NS and BS shared a similar XRD curve, which confirmed that nano-topographical modification does not introduce new substances to the scaffold surface. Furthermore, the XRD results also revealed the typical peaks of the HA of NMS and MS. In addition, compared with MS, NMS possessed higher typical peaks of HA at 31.9°, which also demonstrated that more HA had deposited onto the scaffold surface. Figure 2F shows the XPS results of BS, NS, MS, and NMS. Figure 2G,J show the C (1s), O (1s), Ca (2p), and P (2p) core-level spectra of BS, NS, MS, and NMS, which demonstrated the obvious existence of Ca and P substances on the surface of NMS. The two kinds of biomineralized approaches could deposit HA onto the surface of PCL, while nano-graphically guided biomineralization could deposit more mineralized substances onto polymer scaffolds. In addition, Figure 2K,L show that BS, NS, MS, and NMS shared similar stress–strain curves and force–displacement curves. The mechanical properties showed that nano-topographical medication and mineralization did not change the mechanical properties of the scaffolds. The FTIR, XPS, and XRD results demonstrated the existence of biomineralized coating on the surface of MS and NMS, which is consistent with the above SEM results.

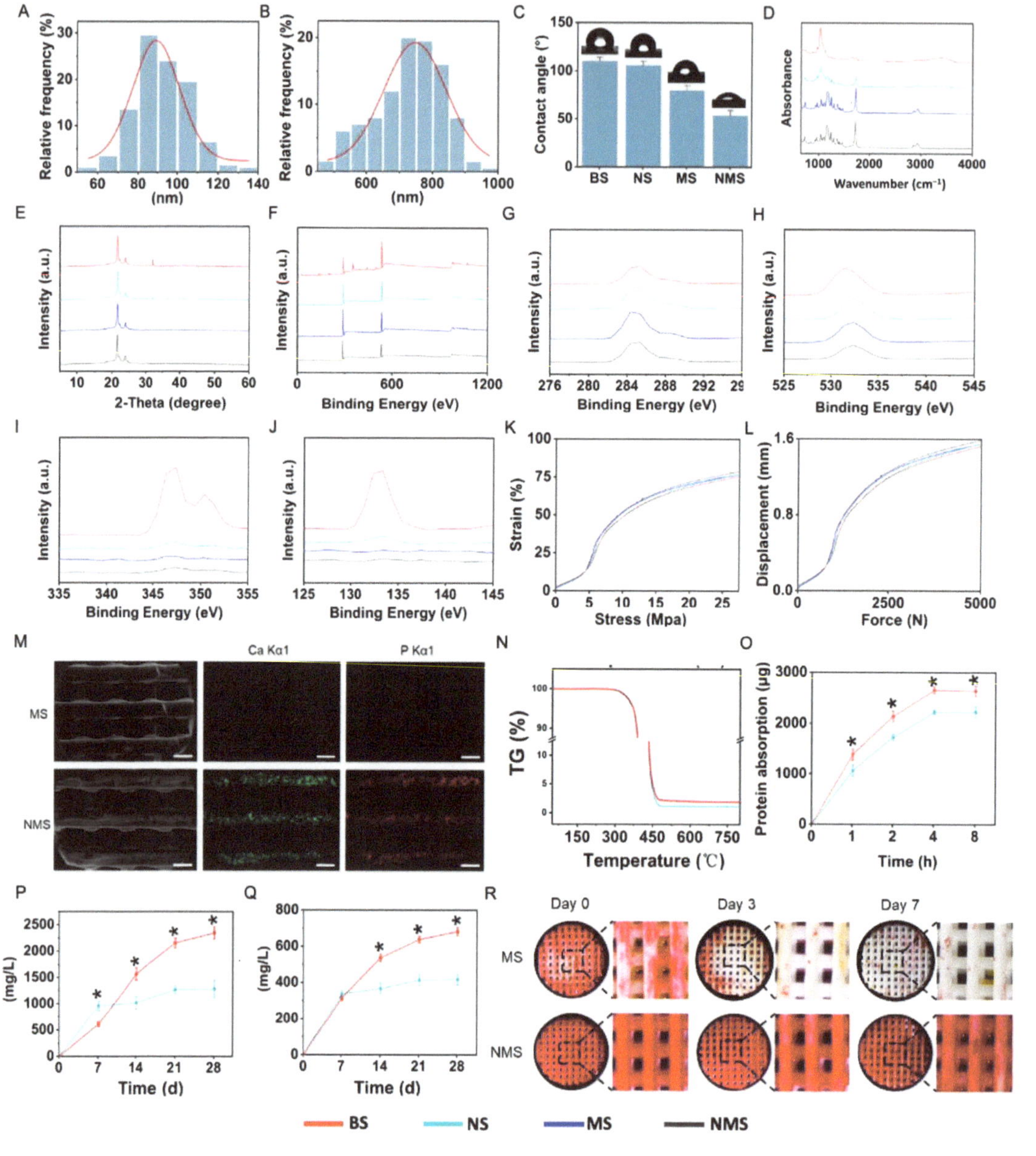

Figure 2. (**A**) The thick distribution of the nano-ridge on the surface of NS. (**B**) The periodic distance distribution on the surface of NS. (**C**) The water contact angle. (**D**) The FTIR results of the scaffolds. (**E**) The XRD results of the scaffolds. (**F**) The XPS results of the scaffolds. (**G–J**) The C (1s), O (1s), Ca (2p), and P (2p) core-level spectra of BS, NS, MS, and NMS. (**K**) The stress–strain curves of the scaffolds. (**L**) The force–displacement curves of the scaffolds. (**M**) The SEM-EDS elemental mapping of the scaffolds. Scale bar = 500 μm (**N**) The TG curve of the scaffolds. (**O**) The Ca ions released from the scaffolds. (**P**) The P ions released from the scaffolds. (**Q**) The protein absorption of the scaffolds. (**R**) The ARS results of the scaffolds. * $p < 0.05$.

In natural bone tissue, as the main inorganic component, HA can regulate various osteoblasts and reinforce the collagen fibrils as the basic building blocks. Fabricating biomineralized coating on polymer scaffolds plays an important role in structural and functional bionics, leading to scaffolds that are close to natural bone in composition and structure. The surface nano-topography of scaffolds can effectively affect the biomineralized coating. Thus, the development of biomineralization based on surface topology can enable the regulation of the procedure of biomineralization without introducing new chemical components into scaffolds. In our study, two kinds of biomineralization coating were further compared. The SEM-EDS elemental mapping of NMS and MS is shown in Figure 2M. The green and red dots represent the existence of Ca and P ions, respectively. The Ca and P ions were evenly distributed on the biomineralized coating of MS and NMS. Compared with MS, more Ca and P ions were deposited on the surface of the scaffolds, which indicated that a nano-topographical surface can effectively enhance biomineralization. Thermogravimetric (TG) analysis is an analytical technique used to investigate the weight change of biomaterials, such as polymers, under controlled temperatures. Figure 3N shows the TG curves of MS and NMS. With the temperature heated up to over 300 °C, the weight of MS and NMS decreased dramatically. With the temperature heated up to over 500 °C, the weight of MS and NMS remained stable. Due to the native TG differences between polymer and biomineralized coating, most of the remaining substances, when heated up to over 500 °C, were inorganic biomineralization substances. The TG results show that the remaining substance weight of NMS was higher than that of MS, which indicated that the method of nano-topographically guided biomineralization can deposit more inorganic biomineralization substances than conventional mineralization. Protein adsorption occurring on the surface of scaffolds is an essential mediator of various biological responses. In addition, the interaction between the scaffold and cells in the human body after implantation is achieved by protein adsorption [45]. As shown in Figure 2O, the protein adsorption of NMS was higher than that of MS. The higher protein adsorption capacity of the nano-topographically guided biomineralized coating might enhance the polymer scaffolds' surface bioactivity for bone regeneration. The osteoinductivity of biomineralized coating is achieved by releasing bioactive Ca and P ions, which are involved in various complex biological processes, such as bone regeneration and bone remodeling. In addition, the Ca and P ions released from biomineralized coating on the surface of scaffolds can directly take part in directing the fate of stem cells. Figure 2P,Q show the Ca and P ions released from MS and NMS, respectively. At day 7, the level of Ca and P ions released from MS was higher than that from NMS, which could be attributed to the adhesion of the biomineralized coating to the scaffold. After day 7, the Ca and P ion levels of the NMS group continued to rise, and the level at day 28 was almost four times the level at day 7. As for the MS group, the Ca and P ion levels increased in a small range. The Ca and P ion levels of NMS were significantly higher than those of MS on day 14, day 21, and day 28. The long-term efficient release of Ca and P ions from biomineralized coating is conducive to the long-term regulation of stem cells' biological activities and in vivo bone regeneration. The whole period of bone regeneration goes on for several months [46] and, thus, an ideal biomineralized coating needs to possess a high adhesion capacity to scaffolds, which can continuously regulate the process of osteogenesis after implantation. Figure 3F shows the ALP staining of MS and NMS after horizontal shaking in PBS. After shaking, the biomineralized coating on the surface of MS gradually fell off. By day 7, the biomineralized coating on the surface of the MS almost completely fell off. The biomineralized coating constructed by nano-topographical guidance could stably exist on the surface of NMS after shaking.

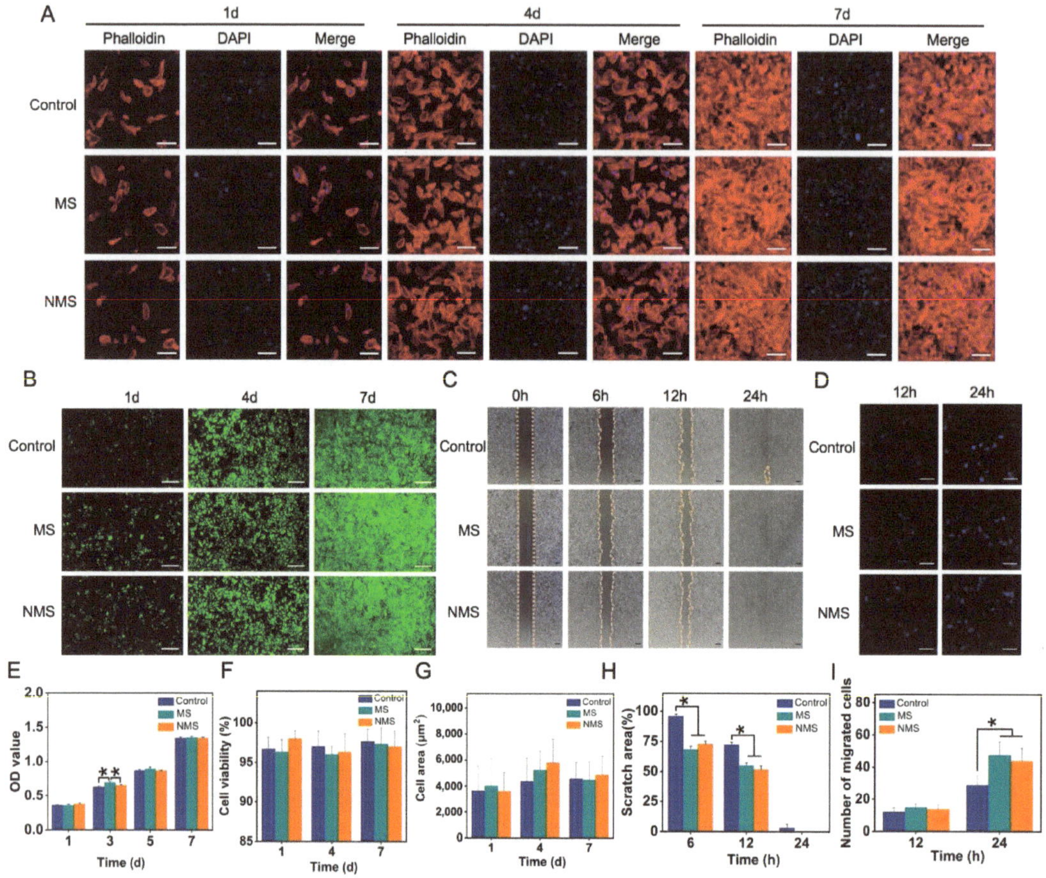

Figure 3. (**A**) Phalloidin/DAPI staining of USCs co-cultured with scaffolds. (**B**) Live/dead staining of USCs co-cultured with scaffolds. (**C**) The scratch–wound assay of USCs co-cultured with scaffolds. (**D**) The number of migrated cells. (**E**) The CCK-8 results of USCs when co-cultured with scaffolds. (**F**) The cell viability of USCs co-cultured with scaffolds. (**G**) The cell area of USCs co-cultured with scaffolds. (**H**) The cell viability of USCs co-cultured with scaffolds. (**I**) The number of migrated cells. * represent $p < 0.05$.

3.3. Cellular Behaviors of USCs Co-Cultured with MS and NMS

USCs were co-cultured with MS and NMS in transwell plates to investigate the cellular behaviors affected by scaffolds. The biomineralized coating on the surface of 3D-printed PCL scaffolds is able to promote bone regeneration by regulating cellular behaviors and the fate of stem cells. Among these cellular behaviors, as the basic functions of stem cells, the cell proliferation ability has been widely used to investigate the cytocompatibility and cytotoxicity of scaffolds. Maintaining normal cell morphology is essential for maintaining the biological viability of stem cells. Figure 3A shows the cytoskeleton staining of USCs co-cultured with scaffolds. Compared with the control group, USCs co-cultured with MS and NMS possessed normal cell morphology. In addition, no significant differences were found in terms of the cell area calculated according to the control, MS, and NMS. (Figure 3G) The CCK-8 results of the USCs co-cultured with MS and NMS at different time points are shown in Figure 3E. On day 3, the OD value of MS was significantly higher than those of the control and NMS. Furthermore, no significant differences were found between the groups control, MS, and NMS, which indicated the good cytocompatibility of MS and NMS. In order to investigate the visible cell proliferation of USCs co-cultured with scaffolds, live/dead staining was also conducted. With the extension of the culture time, each group of cells exhibited a stable cell proliferation capacity. Compared with the control group, the USCs co-cultured with MS and NMS showed a similar cell proliferation capacity (Figure 3B). In addition, the cell viability of USCs when co-cultured with scaffolds was calculated according to the live/dead staining results (Figure 4F). No significant differences were observed among the groups control, MS, and NMS, which also demonstrated the good cytocompatibility of MS and NMS. Cellular morphology changes contribute to various cellular functions such as cell division, signaling, and differentiation [47,48]. Cell migration is an important process involving many biological activities, such as tissue regeneration, development, inflammation, and differentiation [49]. In order to investigate the cell migration and invasion of USCs co-cultured with MS and NMS, scratch–wound and transwell invasion assays were performed. As shown in Figure 3C, the scratch–wound assay results demonstrated that the MS and NMS could enhance the migration of USCs compared with the control group. Additionally, the scratch area of MS and NMS, calculated according to the scratch–wound assay results, was significantly lower than that of the control group at 6 h and 12 h (Figure 3H). The transwell invasion assay results are shown in Figure 3D. No significant differences in cell numbers were found among the groups MS, NMS, and control at 12 h. The invasion cell numbers of MS and NMS were significantly higher than those of the control group at 24 h, which demonstrated that MS and NMS could effectively enhance the invasion of USCs (Figure 3I).

3.4. The Osteogenesis of USCs Co-Cultured with MS and NMS

Ideal biomineralized coating on the surface of scaffolds can mimic the microenvironment of natural bone tissue, provide appropriate biochemical and physical signals, guide the osteogenic differentiation of stem cells, and enhance the deposition and mineralization of bone matrix after implantation [50]. Alkaline phosphatase (ALP) is highly expressed in the cells of mineralized tissue and plays an important role in hard tissue formation. In addition, ALP has been considered to be an initial marker during the process of osteogenic differentiation. Figure 4A shows the ALP staining results of USCs co-cultured with scaffolds. The positive area of ALP staining is calculated in Figure 4B. The ALP-positive areas of MS and NMS were significantly higher than that of the control group on day 5 and day 10. In addition, the ALP-positive area of NMS was significantly higher than that of MS on day 10. Alizarin red staining (ARS) was used to evaluate calcium-rich deposits by cells in the culture. As shown in Figure 4C, the ARS results show that more calcium nodules were found in the NMS group than in other groups. The positive area of the ARS results is also calculated in Figure 4D. The ARS-positive area of the NMS group was higher than that of the groups MS and control on day 14 and day 28. In addition, the ARS-positive area of the MS group was higher than that of the control group. Figure 4E shows the osteogenic-related gene expression of USCs co-cultured with scaffolds. As a member of the RUNX family of transcription factors, RUNX2 regulates the process of osteogenic differentiation. The RUNX2 expression of the NMS group was significantly higher than that of the groups MS and control on day 7 and day 21. ALP is produced mainly by bones and the liver. In addition, ALP can take part in hydrolyzing inorganic pyrophosphate and provide inorganic phosphate to modulate the process of biomineralization in bone tissues. The ALP expression of groups NMS and MS was significantly higher than that of the control group. As an early maker of osteogenesis, COL1A1 plays a crucial role in the formation of collagen fiber and the strengthening of bone tissue. The COL1A1 expression of the NMS group was significantly higher than that of the groups MS and control on day 7 and day 21. As a late maker of osteogenesis, osteocalcin is produced by osteoblasts or stem cells. In addition, OCN is a non-collagen protein and plays a vital role in regulating the processes of mineral deposition and bone remodeling. The OCN expression of groups of NMS and MS was significantly higher than that of the control group on day 7 and day 21. Additionally, the OCN expression of the NMS group was significantly higher than that of MS on day 21. Compared with biomineralized coating fabricated by the conventional method, the biomineralized coating fabricated by nano-topographical guidance showed a better regulation capacity in guiding the osteogenic differentiation of USCs.

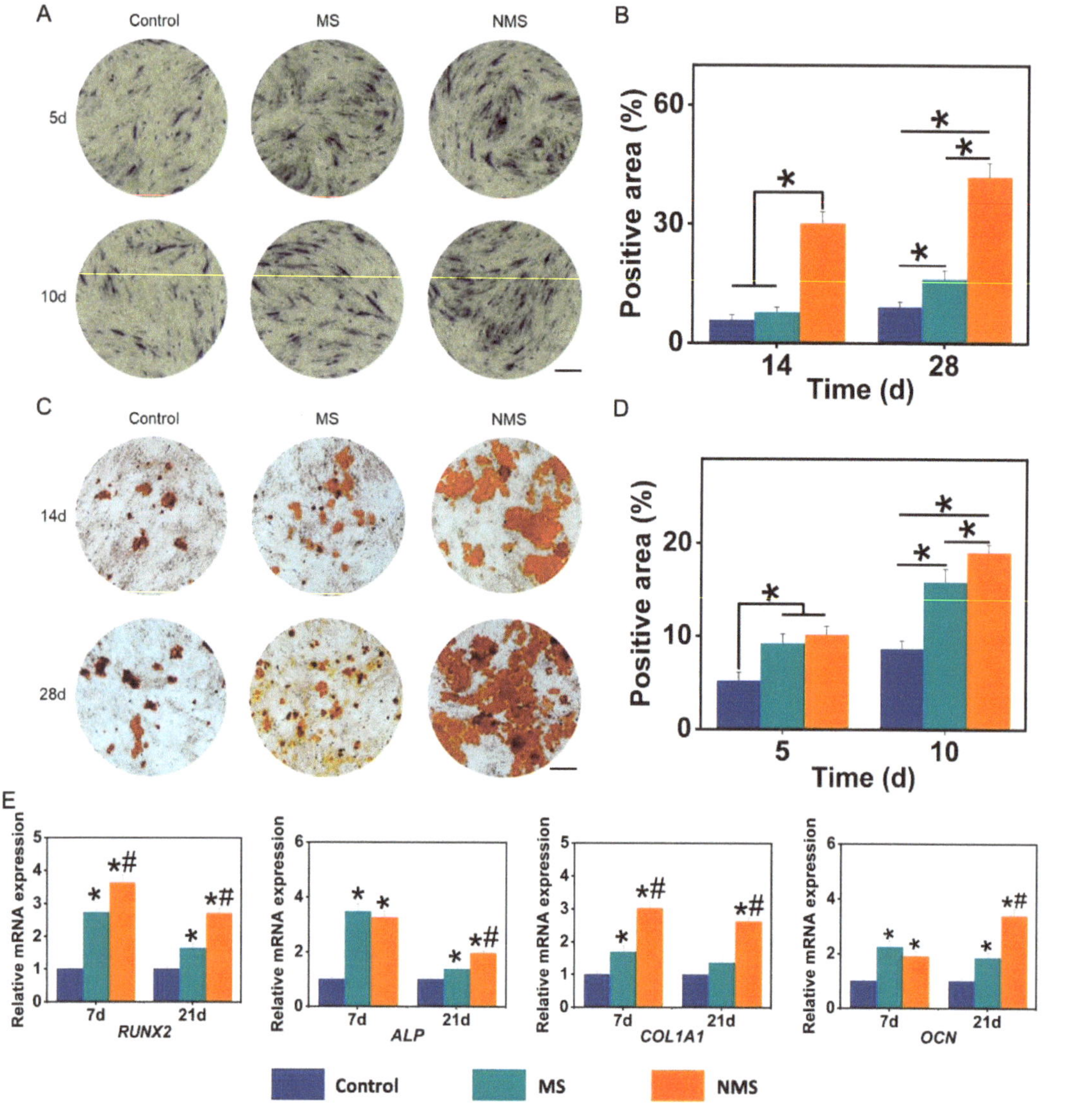

Figure 4. (**A**) ALP staining of USCs co-cultured with scaffolds. (**B**) The positive area of the ALP staining results. * $p < 0.05$. (**C**) ARS staining of USCs co-cultured with scaffolds. (**D**) The positive area of the ARS staining results. * $p < 0.05$. (**E**) The osteogenic-related gene expression of USCs co-cultured with scaffolds. * $p < 0.05$, compared with control, # $p < 0.05$, compared with MS.

In our study, USCs were also seeded onto the scaffolds to evaluate the direct effect of two mineralized scaffolds on cellular behaviors. The proliferation and cellular morphology changes of stem cells on the surface of scaffolds play a very important role in osteogenesis in vitro and in vivo. As shown in Figure 5A, the USCs on the surface of MS and NMS exhibited a stable proliferation ability. With the expansion of the culture time, the number of USCs on the scaffolds gradually increased. Compared with the MS group, more USCs could be observed on the surface of NMS. On day 7, USCs on the surface of NMS could fuse together and cover the scaffold fiber. However, as shown in Figure 5B, no significant differences were found in terms of cell viability between the groups MS and NMS. Figure 5C shows the results of the phalloidin staining of USCs seeded onto scaffolds on day 7. The USCs on the surface of MS were scattered while the USCs on the surface of NMS merged. In addition, as shown in Figure 5D, the cell area of the NMS group was significantly higher than that of the MS group on day 4. Figure 5D shows the osteogenesis-related gene expression of USCs on the surface of MS and NMS. The COL1A1, ALP, and RUNX2 expression of the NMS group was significantly higher than that of the MS group, which confirmed the direct contribution to osteogenesis in vitro.

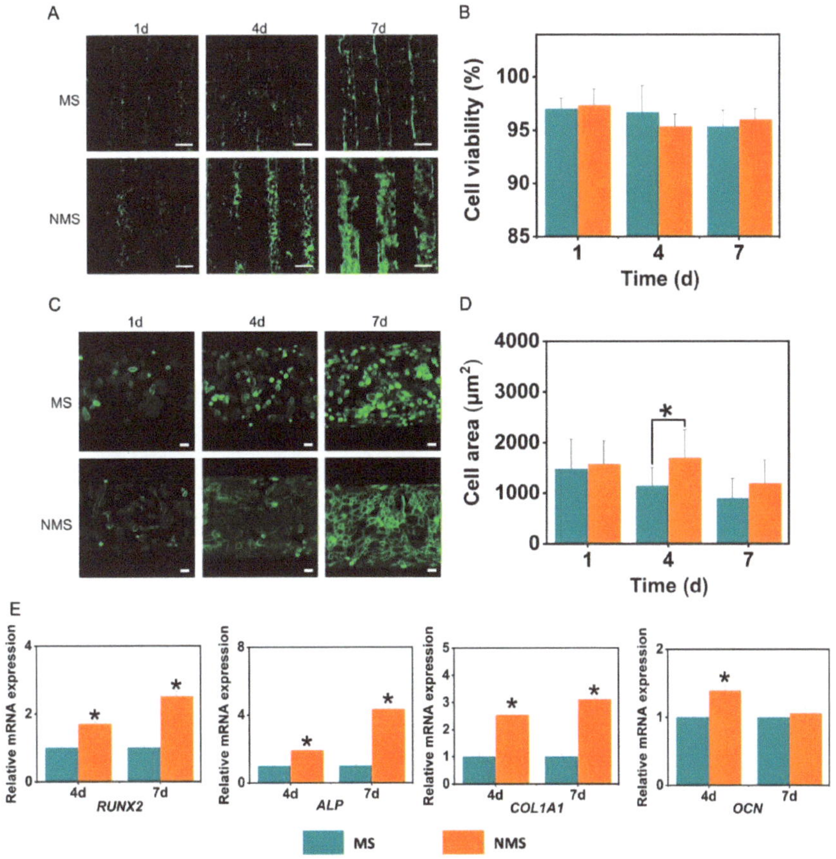

Figure 5. (**A**) Live/dead staining of USCs seeded onto scaffolds. (**B**) The cell viability of USCs seeded onto scaffolds. Scale bar = 500 μm. (**C**) Phalloidin staining of USCs seeded onto scaffolds. Scale bar = 50 μm. (**D**) The cell area of USCs seeded onto scaffolds. * $p < 0.05$, compared with MS. (**E**) The osteogenic-related gene expression of USCs seeded onto scaffolds. * $p < 0.05$, compared with MS.

3.5. In Vivo Bone Regeneration

Micro-CT was utilized to observe newborn bone formation in the bone defects after implantation. Figure 6A shows the micro-CT results of scaffolds implanted into bone defects. At 8 weeks after implantation, no obvious newborn bone formation was found in the control group. In the MS group, a small amount of newborn bone formation was found at the edge of bone defects. In the NMS group, more newborn bone formation was found at the edge of bone defects. In the MS/USCs group, a small amount of newborn bone formation was found in the central area of bone defects. In the NMS/USCs group, newborn bone formation could be found at the edge and central area of bone defects. At 16 weeks after implantation, only a small amount of newborn bone formation was found at the edge of bone defects in the control group. In the MS group, the newborn bone formation covered part of the bone defects. Compared with the MS group, more newborn bone formation was found in the NMS group. In the MS/USCs group, newborn bone formation occurred inside the scaffolds. In the NMS/USCs group, a large amount of newborn bone fused together in the bone defects. As shown in Figure 6B, BV/TV was also calculated to quantitatively investigate the bone formation occurring at the site of bone defects. The BV/TV of each scaffold group was significantly higher than that of the control group at 8 weeks and 16 weeks after implantation. The BV/TV of the NMS group was significantly higher than that of the MS group. The BV/TV of the NMS/USCs group was significantly higher than that of the other groups. No significant differences were found between the NMS group and the MS/USCs group. Moreover, newborn bone density in the bone defects was also calculated according to the micro-CT results. As shown in Figure 6C, the results show that all groups shared similar newborn bone density, which confirmed the homogeneity of the newborn bone tissue.

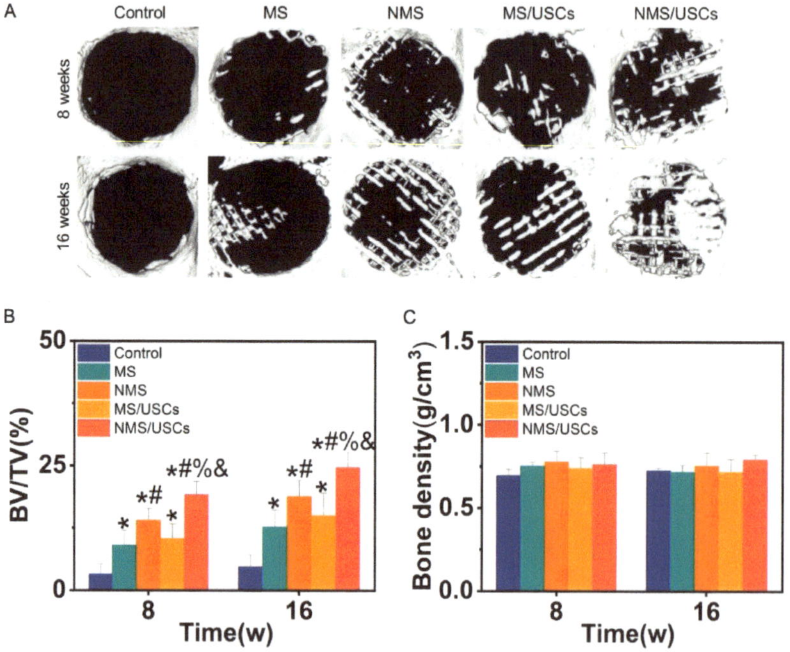

Figure 6. (**A**) Micro-CT results of scaffolds implanted into bone defects. (**B**) The BV/TV of each group after implantation. (**C**) The bone density of newborn bone formation in bone defects. * $p < 0.05$, compared with control, # $p < 0.05$, compared with MS, % $p < 0.05$, compared with NMS, & $p < 0.05$, compared with MS/USCs.

After implantation, the biomineralized coating on the surface of polymer scaffolds is able to provide the proper microenvironment for bone regeneration by continuously releasing Ca and P ions [51]. The crystals of calcium and phosphorus compounds in the biomineralized coating can serve as a template for bone matrix formations. In addition, various proteins can adhere to the surface of scaffolds and mediate and regulate the process of bone formation. The HE staining results of the central area of the bone defects at 8 and 16 weeks after implantation are shown in Figure 7. At 8 weeks after implantation, no obvious newborn bone formation was found on the bone defects of the control group. In the MS group, only a small amount of newborn bone formation was found at the edge of the bone defects. In addition, some of the fibrous tissue was distributed around the scaffold fiber. Compared with the MS group, more newborn bone formation was distributed inside the NMS scaffolds. Furthermore, newborn bone formation mainly occurred around scaffold fibers. In the MS/USCs group, many fibrous tissues were found inside the scaffolds and no obvious newborn formation occurred in bone defects. In the NMS/USCs group, newborn bone formation occurred inside the scaffolds. Compared with the NMS group, more newborn bone formation was distributed in the central area of bone defects. At 16 weeks after implantation, only a small amount of newborn bone formation occurred at the edge of bone defects. Compared with the MS groups, more newborn bone formation occurred along the scaffold fiber in NMS. In the MS/USCs group, few newborn bone formations were found inside the scaffolds. Compared with the other groups, a large amount of newborn bone formation was found in the NMS/USCs group. In addition, the newborn bone formed along the scaffold fibers and almost filled the inside of the scaffolds.

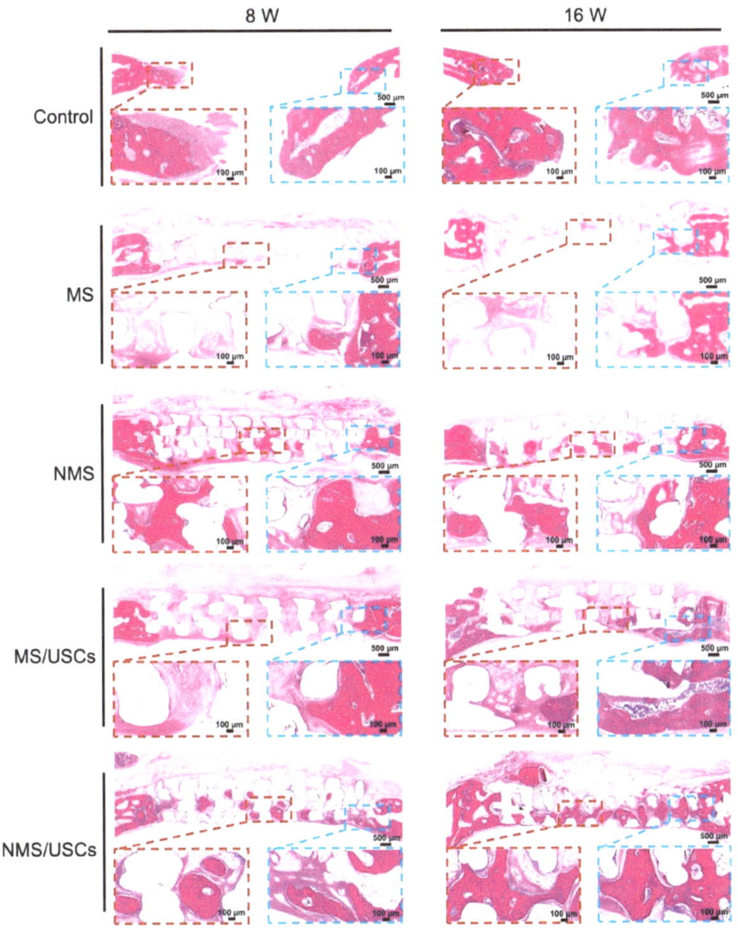

Figure 7. The HE staining of the bone defects after implantation.

The Masson staining results of the central area of bone defects at 8 and 16 weeks after implantation are shown in Figure 8. The blue area represents the mineralized bone of newborn bone formation and the red area represents the osteoid, unmineralized bone tissue [52]. The Masson staining results of all groups were consistent with the HE staining results. According to the Masson staining results, the newborn bone tissue of all groups was calculated to quantitatively investigate the bone regeneration in the central areas of bone defects (Figure 9). The new bone area of each scaffold group was significantly higher than that of the control group at 8 and 16 weeks after implantation. The new bone area of the NMS group was significantly higher than that of the MS group at 8 and 16 weeks after implantation. Interestingly, the new bone area of the NMS group was significantly higher than that of the MS/USCs group at 16 weeks after implantation, which demonstrated that effective biomineralized coating is better than stem cells combined with weak biomineralized coating for the long-term regulation of osteogenesis in vivo. In addition, the new bone area of the NMS/USCs group was significantly higher than that of the other groups at 8 and 16 weeks after implantation, which demonstrated that nano-topographically guided biomineralized coating combined with USCs can exert a good synergistic effect on the induction of osteogenesis in vivo.

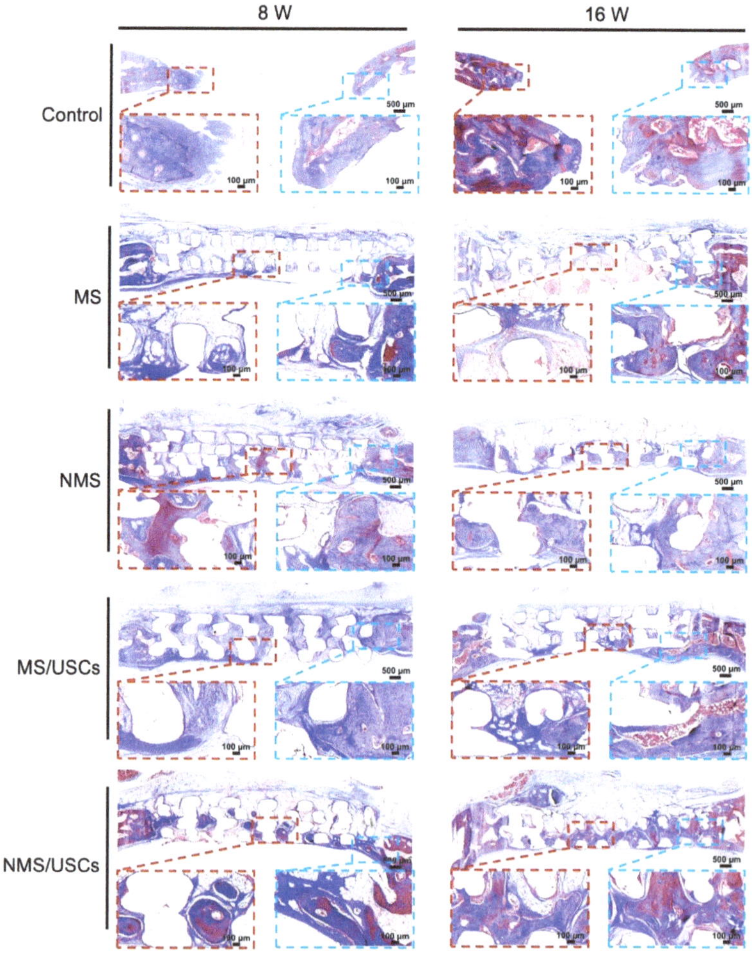

Figure 8. Masson staining of the bone defects after implantation.

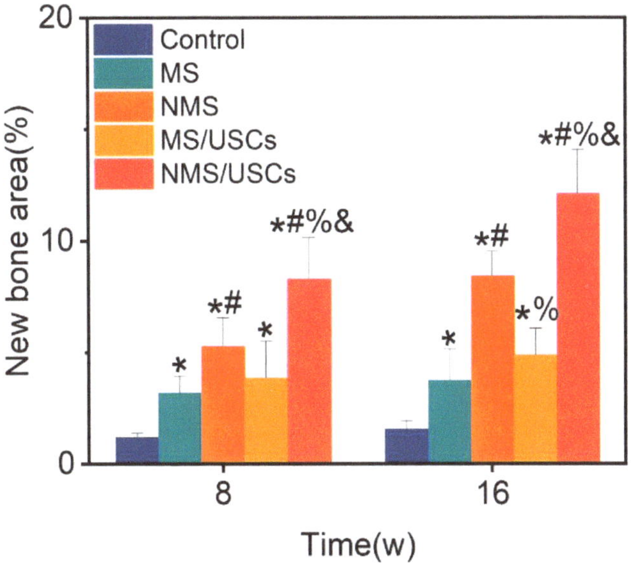

Figure 9. The new bone area of Masson staining results. * $p < 0.05$, compared with control, # $p < 0.05$, compared with MS, % $p < 0.05$, compared with NMS, & $p < 0.05$, compared with MS/USCs.

4. Conclusions

In the current study, we fabricated a biomineralized coating on the surface of 3D-printed PCL scaffolds by nano-topographically guided modifications for bone regeneration. Compared with biomineralized coating constructed by the conventional method, the nano-topographically guided biomineralized coating possessed more mineral substances and more firmly existed on the surface of the scaffolds. In addition, nano-topographically guided biomineralized coating possessed a better protein adsorption capacity and Ca–P ion release capacity. Regarding the cellular behaviors of USCs co-cultured with scaffolds, the nano-topographically guided biomineralized coating could maintain the proliferation capacity of USCs and enhance the migration and invasion of USCs. Regarding the in vitro osteogenesis of USCs co-cultured with scaffolds, compared with biomineralized coating constructed by the conventional method, the nano-topographically guided biomineralized coating could better promote the in vitro mineralization of USCs and the expression of osteogenesis-related genes. After being implanted into bone defect models, compared with conventional biomineralized scaffolds, nano-topographically guided biomineralized scaffolds exhibited a better ability to induce bone regeneration. In addition, the combination of nano-topographically guided biomineralized scaffolds with USCs exhibited a good synergistic effect on the induction of osteogenesis in vivo. The present work demonstrated that nano-topographically guided biomineralized coating on the surface of 3D-printed PCL scaffolds can achieve the long-term release of Ca and P ions, regulate the cellular behaviors of USCs, guide the osteogenic differentiation of USCs, and provide a biomimetic microenvironment for in vivo bone regeneration after implantation. Overall, our study provides 3D-printed polymer scaffolds with a promising alternative surface biomineralization strategy to regulate stem cell fate for the guidance of subsequent bone regeneration after implantation.

Supplementary Materials: The following supporting information can be downloaded at https://www.mdpi.com/article/10.3390/pharmaceutics16020204/s1: Table S1: Primers for real-time polymerase chain reaction.

Author Contributions: Conceptualization, M.L. and J.-Z.X.; methodology, F.X., H.-Y.S., M.Z., K.J. and J.L.; investigation, H.-Y.S.; writing—original draft preparation, F.X.; writing—review and editing, Z.X. and Z.-M.L.; supervision, M.L. and J.-Z.X.; project administration, Z.X. and Z.-M.L. All authors have read and agreed to the published version of the manuscript.

Funding: This work was supported by the National Natural Science Foundation of China (52273142, 52022061, 82202705), the Project of the Science and Technology Department of Sichuan Province (nos. 2023YFS0162, 2023NSFSC1944, 2023NSFSC1738), the Sino–German Center for Research Promotion (GZ1219), and State Key Laboratory of Polymer Materials Engineering (no. sklpme2022-2-05).

Institutional Review Board Statement: This study was approved by the institutional ethical review board of our institution (West China Hospital, Sichuan University, Chengdu, China). The Research Ethics Board for both human urine samples and animal protocols was approved by the Ethics Committee of West China Hospital, Sichuan University, Chengdu, China (Protocol code 20220303068HX). Written informed consent was obtained from all participants. This study was performed under the Guide for the Care and Use of Laboratory Animals of the National Institutes of Health. This study was conducted in accordance with the Declaration of Helsinki.

Informed Consent Statement: Informed consent was obtained from all subjects involved in the study.

Data Availability Statement: Data are contained within the article and Supplementary Materials.

Conflicts of Interest: The authors declare no conflicts of interest.

References

1. Li, Q.; Wang, Y.; Zhang, G.; Su, R.; Qi, W. Biomimetic mineralization based on self-assembling peptides. *Chem. Soc. Rev.* **2023**, *52*, 1549–1590. [CrossRef] [PubMed]
2. Lv, Z.; Hu, T.; Bian, Y.; Wang, G.; Wu, Z.; Li, H.; Liu, X.; Yang, S.; Tan, C.; Liang, R.; et al. A MgFe-LDH Nanosheet-Incorporated Smart Thermo-Responsive Hydrogel with Controllable Growth Factor Releasing Capability for Bone Regeneration. *Adv. Mater.* **2023**, *35*, 2206545. [CrossRef] [PubMed]
3. Kaushik, N.; Nhat Nguyen, L.; Kim, J.H.; Choi, E.H.; Kumar Kaushik, N. Strategies for Using Polydopamine to Induce Biomineralization of Hydroxyapatite on Implant Materials for Bone Tissue Engineering. *Int. J. Mol. Sci.* **2020**, *21*, 6544. [CrossRef] [PubMed]
4. Hao, J.-X.; Shen, M.-J.; Wang, C.-Y.; Wei, J.-H.; Wan, Q.-Q.; Zhu, Y.-F.; Ye, T.; Luo, M.-L.; Qin, W.-P.; Li, Y.-T.; et al. Regulation of biomineralization by proteoglycans: From mechanisms to application. *Carbohydr. Polym.* **2022**, *294*, 119773. [CrossRef]
5. Wang, L.-N.; Meng, Y.-F.; Feng, Y.; Wang, H.-C.; Mao, L.-B.; Yu, S.-H.; Wang, Z.-L. Amorphous Precursor-Mediated Calcium Phosphate Coatings with Tunable Microstructures for Customized Bone Implants. *Adv. Healthc. Mater.* **2022**, *11*, 2201248. [CrossRef]
6. Jiang, Y.; Tan, S.; Hu, J.; Chen, X.; Chen, F.; Yao, Q.; Zhou, Z.; Wang, X.; Zhou, Z.; Fan, Y.; et al. Amorphous calcium magnesium phosphate nanocomposites with superior osteogenic activity for bone regeneration. *Regen Biomater.* **2021**, *8*, rbab068. [CrossRef]
7. Kovacs, C.S.; Chaussain, C.; Osdoby, P.; Brandi, M.L.; Clarke, B.; Thakker, R.V. The role of biomineralization in disorders of skeletal development and tooth formation. *Nat. Rev. Endocrinol.* **2021**, *17*, 336–349. [CrossRef] [PubMed]
8. Arnold, A.; Dennison, E.; Kovacs, C.S.; Mannstadt, M.; Rizzoli, R.; Brandi, M.L.; Clarke, B.; Thakker, R.V. Hormonal regulation of biomineralization. *Nat. Rev. Endocrinol.* **2021**, *17*, 261–275. [CrossRef] [PubMed]
9. Liao, Z.; Zhang, L.; Lan, W.; Du, J.; Hu, Y.; Wei, Y.; Hang, R.; Chen, W.; Huang, D. In situ titanium phosphate formation on a titanium implant as ultrahigh bonding with nano-hydroxyapatite coating for rapid osseointegration. *Biomater. Sci.* **2023**, *11*, 2230–2242. [CrossRef] [PubMed]
10. Pang, Y.; Li, D.; Zhou, J.; Liu, X.; Li, M.; Zhang, Y.; Zhang, D.; Zhang, X.; Cai, Q. In vitro and in vivo evaluation of biomimetic hydroxyapatite/whitlockite inorganic scaffolds for bone tissue regeneration. *Biomed. Mater.* **2022**, *17*, 065020. [CrossRef]
11. Ling, L.; Cai, S.; Zuo, Y.; Tian, M.; Meng, T.; Tian, H.; Bao, X.; Xu, G. Copper-doped zeolitic imidazolate frameworks-8/hydroxyapatite composite coating endows magnesium alloy with excellent corrosion resistance, antibacterial ability and biocompatibility. *Colloids Surf. B Biointerfaces* **2022**, *219*, 112810. [CrossRef]
12. Chen, J.; Wen, J.; Fu, Y.; Li, X.; Huang, J.; Guan, X.; Zhou, Y. A bifunctional bortezomib-loaded porous nano-hydroxyapatite/alginate scaffold for simultaneous tumor inhibition and bone regeneration. *J. Nanobiotechnol.* **2023**, *21*, 174. [CrossRef]
13. Wang, F.; Wang, Q.; Zhao, Y.; Tian, Z.; Chang, S.; Tong, H.; Liu, N.; Bai, S.; Li, X.; Fan, J. Adipose-derived stem cells with miR-150-5p inhibition laden in hydroxyapatite/tricalcium phosphate ceramic powders promote osteogenesis via regulating Notch3 and activating FAK/ERK and RhoA. *Acta Biomater.* **2023**, *155*, 644–653. [CrossRef]
14. Zhang, B.; Xing, F.; Chen, L.; Zhou, C.; Gui, X.; Su, Z.; Fan, S.; Zhou, Z.; Jiang, Q.; Zhao, L.; et al. DLP fabrication of customized porous bioceramics with osteoinduction ability for remote isolation bone regeneration. *Biomater. Adv.* **2023**, *145*, 213261. [CrossRef]
15. Akiyama, N.; Patel, K.D.; Jang, E.J.; Shannon, M.R.; Patel, R.; Patel, M.; Perriman, A.W. Tubular nanomaterials for bone tissue engineering. *J. Mater. Chem. B* **2023**, *11*, 6225–6248. [CrossRef]
16. Zhao, Y.; Chen, H.; Ran, K.; Zhang, Y.; Pan, H.; Shangguan, J.; Tong, M.; Yang, J.; Yao, Q.; Xu, H. Porous hydroxyapatite scaffold orchestrated with bioactive coatings for rapid bone repair. *Biomater. Adv.* **2023**, *144*, 213202. [CrossRef] [PubMed]

17. Wang, L.; Xu, C.; Meng, K.; Xia, Y.; Zhang, Y.; Lian, J.; Wang, X.; Zhao, B. Biomimetic Hydroxyapatite Composite Coatings with a Variable Morphology Mediated by Silk Fibroin and Its Derived Peptides Enhance the Bioactivity on Titanium. *ACS Biomater. Sci. Eng.* **2023**, *9*, 165–181. [CrossRef] [PubMed]
18. Murab, S.; Herold, S.; Hawk, T.; Snyder, A.; Espinal, E.; Whitlock, P. Advances in additive manufacturing of polycaprolactone based scaffolds for bone regeneration. *J. Mater. Chem. B* **2023**, *11*, 7250–7279. [CrossRef] [PubMed]
19. Li, G.; Li, Y.; Zhang, X.; Gao, P.; Xia, X.; Xiao, S.; Wen, J.; Guo, T.; Yang, W.; Li, J. Strontium and simvastatin dual loaded hydroxyapatite microsphere reinforced poly(ε-caprolactone) scaffolds promote vascularized bone regeneration. *J. Mater. Chem. B* **2023**, *11*, 1115–1130.
20. Egorov, A.; Riedel, B.; Vinke, J.; Schmal, H.; Thomann, R.; Thomann, Y.; Seidenstuecker, M. The Mineralization of Various 3D-Printed PCL Composites. *J. Funct. Biomater.* **2022**, *13*, 238.
21. Fazeli, N.; Arefian, E.; Irani, S.; Ardeshirylajimi, A.; Seyedjafari, E. 3D-Printed PCL Scaffolds Coated with Nanobioceramics Enhance Osteogenic Differentiation of Stem Cells. *ACS Omega* **2021**, *6*, 35284–35296. [CrossRef]
22. Huang, R.; Hao, Y.; Pan, Y.; Pan, C.; Tang, X.; Huang, L.; Du, C.; Yue, R.; Cui, D. Using a two-step method of surface mechanical attrition treatment and calcium ion implantation to promote the osteogenic activity of mesenchymal stem cells as well as biomineralization on a β-titanium surface. *RSC Adv.* **2022**, *12*, 20037–20053. [CrossRef]
23. Costa, D.O.; Allo, B.A.; Klassen, R.; Hutter, J.L.; Dixon, S.J.; Rizkalla, A.S. Control of Surface Topography in Biomimetic Calcium Phosphate Coatings. *Langmuir* **2012**, *28*, 3871–3880. [CrossRef]
24. Miguel, B.S.; Kriauciunas, R.; Tosatti, S.; Ehrbar, M.; Ghayor, C.; Textor, M.; Weber, F.E. Enhanced osteoblastic activity and bone regeneration using surface-modified porous bioactive glass scaffolds. *J. Biomed. Mater. Res. Part A* **2010**, *94A*, 1023–1033. [CrossRef]
25. Boyan, B.D.; Lotz, E.M.; Schwartz, Z. Roughness and Hydrophilicity as Osteogenic Biomimetic Surface Properties. *Tissue Eng. Part A* **2017**, *23*, 1479–1489. [CrossRef]
26. Dobbenga, S.; Fratila-Apachitei, L.E.; Zadpoor, A.A. Nanopattern-induced osteogenic differentiation of stem cells—A systematic review. *Acta Biomater.* **2016**, *46*, 3–14. [CrossRef]
27. Gandolfi, M.G.; Taddei, P.; Siboni, F.; Perrotti, V.; Iezzi, G.; Piattelli, A.; Prati, C. Micro-Topography and Reactivity of Implant Surfaces: An In Vitro Study in Simulated Body Fluid (SBF). *Microsc. Microanal.* **2015**, *21*, 190–203. [CrossRef] [PubMed]
28. Li, X.; Liu, M.; Chen, F.; Wang, Y.; Wang, M.; Chen, X.; Xiao, Y.; Zhang, X. Design of hydroxyapatite bioceramics with micro-/nano-topographies to regulate the osteogenic activities of bone morphogenetic protein-2 and bone marrow stromal cells. *Nanoscale* **2020**, *12*, 7284–7300. [CrossRef] [PubMed]
29. Park, J.; Lee, S.J.; Jung, T.G.; Lee, J.H.; Kim, W.D.; Lee, J.Y.; Park, S.A. Surface modification of a three-dimensional polycaprolactone scaffold by polydopamine, biomineralization, and BMP-2 immobilization for potential bone tissue applications. *Colloids Surf. B Biointerfaces* **2021**, *199*, 111528.
30. Vannozzi, L.; Gouveia, P.; Pingue, P.; Canale, C.; Ricotti, L. Novel Ultrathin Films Based on a Blend of PEG-b-PCL and PLLA and Doped with ZnO Nanoparticles. *ACS Appl. Mater. Interfaces* **2020**, *12*, 21398–21410. [CrossRef] [PubMed]
31. Alvarez Perez, M.A.; Guarino, V.; Cirillo, V.; Ambrosio, L. In vitro mineralization and bone osteogenesis in poly(ε-caprolactone)/gelatin nanofibers. *J. Biomed. Mater. Res. Part A* **2012**, *100A*, 3008–3019. [CrossRef]
32. Collins, M.T.; Marcucci, G.; Anders, H.-J.; Beltrami, G.; Cauley, J.A.; Ebeling, P.R.; Kumar, R.; Linglart, A.; Sangiorgi, L.; Towler, D.A.; et al. Skeletal and extraskeletal disorders of biomineralization. *Nat. Rev. Endocrinol.* **2022**, *18*, 473–489. [CrossRef] [PubMed]
33. de Morree, A.; Rando, T.A. Regulation of adult stem cell quiescence and its functions in the maintenance of tissue integrity. *Nat. Rev. Mol. Cell Biol.* **2023**, *24*, 334–354. [CrossRef] [PubMed]
34. Zhao, J.; Zhou, Y.-H.; Zhao, Y.-Q.; Gao, Z.-R.; Ouyang, Z.-Y.; Ye, Q.; Liu, Q.; Chen, Y.; Tan, L.; Zhang, S.-H.; et al. Oral cavity-derived stem cells and preclinical models of jaw-bone defects for bone tissue engineering. *Stem Cell Res. Ther.* **2023**, *14*, 39. [CrossRef]
35. Xing, F.; Li, L.; Sun, J.; Liu, G.; Duan, X.; Chen, J.; Liu, M.; Long, Y.; Xiang, Z. Surface mineralized biphasic calcium phosphate ceramics loaded with urine-derived stem cells are effective in bone regeneration. *J. Orthop. Surg. Res.* **2019**, *14*, 419. [CrossRef] [PubMed]
36. Xing, F.; Yin, H.-M.; Zhe, M.; Xie, J.-C.; Duan, X.; Xu, J.-Z.; Xiang, Z.; Li, Z.-M. Nanotopographical 3D-Printed Poly(ε-caprolactone) Scaffolds Enhance Proliferation and Osteogenic Differentiation of Urine-Derived Stem Cells for Bone Regeneration. *Pharmaceutics* **2022**, *14*, 1437. [CrossRef]
37. Carvalho, C.M.F.; Leonel, L.; Cañada, R.R.; Barreto, R.S.N.; Maria, D.A.; Del Sol, M.; Miglino, M.A.; Lobo, S.E. Comparison between placental and skeletal muscle ECM: In vivo implantation. *Connect. Tissue Res.* **2021**, *62*, 629–642. [CrossRef]
38. Dai, W.; Zheng, Y.; Li, B.; Yang, F.; Chen, W.; Li, Y.; Deng, Y.; Bai, D.; Shu, R. A 3D-printed orthopedic implant with dual-effect synergy based on MoS2 and hydroxyapatite nanoparticles for tumor therapy and bone regeneration. *Colloids Surf. B Biointerfaces* **2023**, *228*, 113384. [CrossRef] [PubMed]
39. Huang, R.; Lu, S.; Han, Y. Role of grain size in the regulation of osteoblast response to Ti–25Nb–3Mo–3Zr–2Sn alloy. *Colloids Surf. B Biointerfaces* **2013**, *111*, 232–241. [CrossRef]
40. Wong, P.-C.; Song, S.-M.; Tsai, P.-H.; Nien, Y.-Y.; Jang, J.S.-C.; Cheng, C.-K.; Chen, C.-H. Relationship between the Surface Roughness of Biodegradable Mg-Based Bulk Metallic Glass and the Osteogenetic Ability of MG63 Osteoblast-Like Cells. *Materials* **2020**, *13*, 1188. [CrossRef]

41. Zhu, G.-Y.; Liu, Y.-H.; Liu, W.; Huang, X.-Q.; Zhang, B.; Zheng, Z.-L.; Wei, X.; Xu, J.-Z.; Zhao, Z.-H. Surface Epitaxial Nano-Topography Facilitates Biomineralization to Promote Osteogenic Differentiation and Osteogenesis. *ACS Omega* **2021**, *6*, 21792–21800. [CrossRef] [PubMed]
42. Yin, H.-M.; Liu, W.; Huang, Y.-F.; Ren, Y.; Xu, L.; Xu, J.-Z.; Zhao, B.; Li, Z.-M. Surface Epitaxial Crystallization-Directed Nanotopography for Accelerating Preosteoblast Proliferation and Osteogenic Differentiation. *ACS Appl. Mater. Interfaces* **2019**, *11*, 42956–42963. [CrossRef] [PubMed]
43. Matsuzaki, T.; Terutsuki, D.; Sato, S.; Ikarashi, K.; Sato, K.; Mitsuno, H.; Okumura, R.; Yoshimura, Y.; Usami, S.; Mori, Y.; et al. Low Surface Potential with Glycoconjugates Determines Insect Cell Adhesion at Room Temperature. *J. Phys. Chem. Lett.* **2022**, *13*, 9494–9500. [CrossRef] [PubMed]
44. Bai, Y.; Zheng, X.; Zhong, X.; Cui, Q.; Zhang, S.; Wen, X.; Heng, B.C.; He, S.; Shen, Y.; Zhang, J.; et al. Manipulation of Heterogeneous Surface Electric Potential Promotes Osteogenesis by Strengthening RGD Peptide Binding and Cellular Mechanosensing. *Adv. Mater.* **2023**, *35*, 2209769. [CrossRef]
45. Shen, S.; Gao, Y.; Ouyang, Z.; Jia, B.; Shen, M.; Shi, X. Photothermal-triggered dendrimer nanovaccines boost systemic antitumor immunity. *J. Control. Release* **2023**, *355*, 171–183. [CrossRef]
46. Zhao, T.; Zhang, J.; Gao, X.; Yuan, D.; Gu, Z.; Xu, Y. Electrospun nanofibers for bone regeneration: From biomimetic composition, structure to function. *J. Mater. Chem. B* **2022**, *10*, 6078–6106. [CrossRef] [PubMed]
47. Huang, L.; Peng, Y.; Tao, X.; Ding, X.; Li, R.; Jiang, Y.; Zuo, W. Microtubule Organization Is Essential for Maintaining Cellular Morphology and Function. *Oxid. Med. Cell. Longev.* **2022**, *2022*, 1623181. [CrossRef]
48. Zhang, W.; Taheri-Ledari, R.; Ganjali, F.; Mirmohammadi, S.S.; Qazi, F.S.; Saeidirad, M.; KashtiAray, A.; Zarei-Shokat, S.; Tian, Y.; Maleki, A. Effects of morphology and size of nanoscale drug carriers on cellular uptake and internalization process: A review. *RSC Adv.* **2023**, *13*, 80–114. [CrossRef] [PubMed]
49. Su, Y.; Wang, X.; Yang, Y.; Chen, L.; Xia, W.; Hoi, K.K.; Li, H.; Wang, Q.; Yu, G.; Chen, X.; et al. Astrocyte endfoot formation controls the termination of oligodendrocyte precursor cell perivascular migration during development. *Neuron* **2023**, *111*, 190–201.e8. [CrossRef] [PubMed]
50. Dommeti, V.K.; Roy, S.; Pramanik, S.; Merdji, A.; Ouldyerou, A.; Özcan, M. Design and Development of Tantalum and Strontium Ion Doped Hydroxyapatite Composite Coating on Titanium Substrate: Structural and Human Osteoblast-like Cell Viability Studies. *Materials* **2023**, *16*, 1499. [CrossRef]
51. Zhang, X.; He, J.; Qiao, L.; Wang, Z.; Zheng, Q.; Xiong, C.; Yang, H.; Li, K.; Lu, C.; Li, S.; et al. 3D printed PCLA scaffold with nano-hydroxyapatite coating doped green tea EGCG promotes bone growth and inhibits multidrug-resistant bacteria colonization. *Cell Prolif.* **2022**, *55*, e13289. [CrossRef] [PubMed]
52. Ralis, Z.A.; Watkins, G. Modified Tetrachrome Method for Osteoid and Defectively Mineralized Bone in Paraffin Sections. *Biotech. Histochem.* **1992**, *67*, 339–345. [CrossRef] [PubMed]

pharmaceutics

MDPI

Article

Thermo-Responsive Hydrogels Encapsulating Targeted Core–Shell Nanoparticles as Injectable Drug Delivery Systems

Elif Gulin Ertugral-Samgar [1], Ali Murad Ozmen [1] and Ozgul Gok [1,2,*]

[1] Medical Engineering Program, Graduate School of Natural and Applied Sciences, Acibadem Mehmet Ali Aydinlar University, 34752 Istanbul, Turkey; elif.ertugral@live.acibadem.edu.tr (E.G.E.-S.); alimurad93@gmail.com (A.M.O.)

[2] Department of Biomedical Engineering, Faculty of Engineering and Natural Sciences, Acibadem Mehmet Ali Aydinlar University, 34752 Istanbul, Turkey

* Correspondence: ozgul.gok@acibadem.edu.tr; Tel.: +90-216-5004188

Abstract: As therapeutic agents that allow for minimally invasive administration, injectable biomaterials stand out as effective tools with tunable properties. Furthermore, hydrogels with responsive features present potential platforms for delivering therapeutics to desired sites in the body. Herein, temperature-responsive hydrogel scaffolds with embedded targeted nanoparticles were utilized to achieve controlled drug delivery via local drug administration. Poly(N-isopropylacrylamide) (pNIPAM) hydrogels, prepared with an ethylene-glycol-based cross-linker, demonstrated thermo-sensitive gelation ability upon injection into environments at body temperature. This hydrogel network was engineered to provide a slow and controlled drug release profile by being incorporated with curcumin-loaded nanoparticles bearing high encapsulation efficiency. A core (alginate)–shell (chitosan) nanoparticle design was preferred to ensure the stability of the drug molecules encapsulated in the core and to provide slower drug release. Nanoparticle-embedded hydrogels were shown to release curcumin at least four times slower compared to the free nanoparticle itself and to possess high water uptake capacity and more mechanically stable viscoelastic behavior. Moreover, this therapy has the potential to specifically address tumor tissues over-expressing folate receptors like ovaries, as the nanoparticles target the receptors by folic acid conjugation to the periphery. Together with its temperature-driven injectability, it can be concluded that this hydrogel scaffold with drug-loaded and embedded folate-targeting nanoparticles would provide effective therapy for tumor tissues accessible via minimally invasive routes and be beneficial for post-operative drug administration after tumor resection.

Keywords: core–shell nanoparticles; drug-loaded scaffolds; injectable hydrogels; thermo-responsive polymers; controlled drug release

Citation: Ertugral-Samgar, E.G.; Ozmen, A.M.; Gok, O. Thermo-Responsive Hydrogels Encapsulating Targeted Core–Shell Nanoparticles as Injectable Drug Delivery Systems. *Pharmaceutics* **2023**, *15*, 2358. https://doi.org/10.3390/pharmaceutics15092358

Academic Editors: Ping Hu and Zheng Cai

Received: 10 August 2023
Revised: 1 September 2023
Accepted: 5 September 2023
Published: 21 September 2023

1. Introduction

Hydrogels are cross-linked, porous networks of hydrophilic polymer chains that serve as outstanding and effective 3D platforms with high water uptake capacity [1]. They allow the conjugation of various therapeutics, like drug molecules and peptide-based biomolecules, to either end groups or side chains due to the presence of functional moieties, such as amine, hydroxyl, carboxylic acid, maleimide, etc., in their structures [2–5]. Although their physicochemical properties are mainly affected by their swelling ratio for controlled delivery of encapsulated therapeutic agents inside, chemically or physically cross-linked smart polymers also contribute to the development of hydrogels with diverse stimuli responsiveness to temperature, pH, biomolecules, light, magnetic fields, etc. [6–9]. The drug release profile of these "intelligent hydrogels" is modulated by their polymer chain length, biodegradation rate, cross-linking degree, and pore size as well as where the drug molecules are encapsulated and stabilized against the host environment with regard to the presence of specific enzymes or pH value [10,11]. However, obtaining precise control over the pore size and biodegradation of hydrogel networks might emerge as a serious issue in obtaining controlled release profiles in the presence of a recurring and metastatic cancer type like ovarian cancer or glioma [12–16]. In particular, natural and hydrophilic pH-responsive polymers, such as alginate, chitosan, and gelatin, were shown to liberate internally loaded active agents more rapidly due to their high degradation rate in tumor environments [17–19] compared to polyanhydride- and polyester-based synthetic polymers (i.e., poly(glycolide-co-sebacate) (PGS), poly (caprolactone) (PCL), and poly (lactide-co-glycolide) (PLGA)) [20–24]. Thus, an urgent need has evolved for hydrogels with tunable properties for the slower and sustained release of therapeutic agents. Notably, recent literature revealed that the bioavailability and pharmacokinetic features of drug molecules can be improved by their incorporation into hydrogel systems via indirect methods, which mainly benefit from developments in nanotechnology [25].

Nanoparticle-embedded hydrogel scaffolds, which are also known as NP/gel systems, present innovative combinations that have emerged as powerful tools to provide more advantageous hybrid platforms for novel drug delivery systems [26]. The most recent literature covers many studies regarding the incorporation of nanoparticles into hydrogel systems to obtain more tunable drug release behavior [27–29]. Combinations of various types of nanoparticles, such as polymeric and metallic ones, as well as nanogels, liposomes, carbon nanotubes, and dendrimers into 3D hydrogel scaffolds have demonstrated the ability to provide not only enhanced drug loading efficiency but also different routes of administration via injectable hydrogels [30–35]. Natural polymers like polysaccharides (alginate, hyaluronic acid, chitosan, etc.) are mainly preferred for their excellent biocompatibility and hydrophilicity, whereas the incorporation of synthetic polymers, including PLGA and poly (lactide) (PLA), is more popular due to their controlled biodegradation ability and slow drug release tendency [36–39]. Their incorporation into polymeric scaffolds like hydrogels has been shown to improve not only the pharmacokinetic profiles of loaded drug molecules but also to enhance their stability and increase local drug concentration, allowing for a drug reservoir at the site of administration [40,41].

The diverse features provided by these multi-component NP/gel systems not only allow for increased local drug concentration at the site of injury after hydrogel implementation but also for the selective accumulation of drug molecules in nanoparticles due to the enhanced permeation and retention (EPR) effect. This effect is dependent upon nanosize or active targeting via the conjugation of a targeting unit like peptides (RGD (Arginylglycylaspartic acid), TAT (YGRKKRRQRRR), monoclonal antibodies, or ligands (folic acid, mannose) to the periphery of these nanoparticles [42–46]. These studies point out the superior effect of NP/gel systems in modulating drug release profiles over an extended period [28,47]. In particular, temperature-responsive hydrogels based on poly(N-isopropylacrylamide) (pNIPAM), poly(N,N-diethylacrylamide) (PDEAM), poly(2-(dimethylamino)ethyl methacrylate) (PDMAEMA), PEG methacrylate polymers (PEGMA), etc. are preferred as the main constructs for the preparation of injectable gels to slow the clearance rate of nanoparticles in the body, resulting in an improved bioavailability for therapeutic agents, such as chemotherapy drugs, antioxidants, anti-inflammatory drugs, and vaccines [48–51]. To the best of our knowledge, there is no example of a NP/gel system containing a targeted nanoparticle for delivering drug molecules to specific cells.

Therefore, we designed a novel drug-loaded nanoparticle system with a thermo-sensitive hydrogel scaffold to obtain an injectable biomaterial platform for a more controlled and slow drug release profile that could be administered in a minimally invasive manner to the injury site. For this purpose, pNIPAM-based thermo-responsive polymers were utilized to obtain an injectable hydrogel system, which was stabilized by an ethylene-glycol-based cross-linker. Employing polymeric core–shell type nanoparticles as carriers for the anti-inflammatory drug curcumin, this NP/gel system successfully increased the drug loading capacity and demonstrated improved viscoelastic properties. Visually observed in the pores of the hydrogel scaffold, nanoparticles were successfully embedded inside the

NP/gel system. Remarkably, this nanoparticle encapsulated hydrogel system resulted in a drug release profile that was four times slower compared to that of the free nanoparticle system. These nanoparticles comprised a core (alginate) and shell (chitosan) made from natural and pH-responsive polymers. The drug molecules were encapsulated at the core and were engineered to deliver the payload to the folate receptor over-expressing cells (such as ovarian and breast cancer) by being conjugated to folic acid molecules on the surface. Thus, we prepared an injectable nanoparticle-embedded hydrogel scaffold with a thermo-responsive feature that demonstrated rapid gelation, which can contribute to wound closure of damaged tissue, and embedded targeted polymeric nanoparticles to obtain the slow, controlled, and pH-responsive release of loaded drug molecules.

2. Materials and Methods

2.1. Materials

Alginic acid sodium salt from brown algae (low viscosity, Sigma-Aldrich A1112 (St. Louis, MO, USA), average molecular weight of 30,000–100,000), calcium chloride, sodium dodecyl sulfate (SDS), chitosan (low molecular weight [LMW], 50–190 kDa, 75–85% deacetylated); (high molecular weight [HMW], 310–375 kDa, >75% deacetylated), curcumin (from Curcuma longa (Turmeric) powder), and Tween 80 (for synthesis) were purchased from Sigma-Aldrich for the preparation of the nanoparticles. Poly(N-isopropyl acrylamide) (pNIPAM, Mwt: 40kDa), N,N,N′,N′-Tetramethylethylenediamine (TEMED, bioreagent, suitable for electrophoresis 99%), triethylene glycol dimethacrylate (containing 80–120 ppm inhibitor, 95%), folic acid (FA, 97%), diisopropylamine (DIPA, 99.5%), N,N Dimethylformamide (DMF, anhydrous, 99.8%), ammonium persulfate (APS, for molecular biology and for electrophoresis 99.8%), and poly-L-lysine (0.1% (*w*/*v*) in H_2O)) were purchased from Sigma-Aldrich for the preparation of the hydrogel scaffold. Aluminum oxide (90 active basic [0.063–0.200 mm] [activity stage I] for column chromatography) was purchased from Merck and used to filter the inhibitor in triethylene glycol dimethacrylate, as received. Acetate buffer (pH 5.5) was prepared with acetone and acetic acid (Merck, Rahway, NJ, USA) into distilled water, and phosphate saline buffer tablets (Biomatik Corporation, Kitchener, ON, Canada) were dissolved in distilled water; both solutions were used for the drug release profile experiments. Hexafluorophosphate azabenzotriazole tetramethyl uronium (HATU, 97%, Rahway, NJ, USA), diethyl ether, and sodium sulfate (anhydrous for analysis) were purchased from Merck. Spectrum™ Spectra/Por™ 6 (Pre-wetted Standard RC Dialysis Tubing, 1 kD MWCO) was purchased from Fisher Science (Waltham, MA USA) for dialysis.

2.2. Preparation of Alginate Nanoparticles (AA-NPs)

The empty (without drug) alginate nanoparticles were prepared according to procedures described in the literature with slight modifications [52]. Briefly, low viscosity sodium alginate (0.5% by weight) was physically cross-linked with calcium chloride at a ratio of 19:1 by volume for 2 h at room temperature to obtain nanoparticles. After 2 h, the mixture was centrifuged at 14,000 rpm for 30 min and rinsed with ultrapure water, followed by another centrifugation at 5000 rpm for 5 min. This washing step was repeated twice. The supernatant was decanted and filtered with a 0.22 µm cellulose acetate syringe filter for further measurements regarding the characterization of prepared nanoparticles. Both 50 and 75 mM $CaCl_2$ solutions were utilized for the cross-linking of alginate polymers; higher concentrations of Ca^{+2} ions seemed to fasten cross-linking to yield aggregates. Additionally, nanoparticles were stabilized by ionic balance obtained with the help of a commonly used surfactant, SDS, and a polycationic agent, poly-l-lysine, in differing amounts (Table 1).

Table 1. Preparation conditions for nanoparticles.

No *	$CaCl_2$ (50 mM) (mL)	NaAlg (0.5%) (mL)	L-Lysine (0.1%) (mL)	SDS (0.1%) (mL)	Temp (°C)
1	4.75	0.25	2	2	25
2	4.75	0.25	2	2	40
3	4.75	0.25	3	3	25
4	4.75	0.25	3	3	40

* All conditions were applied as using 0.5% (*w/v*) NaAlg and 50 mM $CaCl_2$.

2.3. Preparation of Curcumin-Loaded Alginate Nanoparticles (AA-Cur-NPs)

Curcumin-loaded alginate nanoparticles were prepared according to the procedure used to create the empty (without drug) nanoparticles but with the addition of 1 mg/mL curcumin (prepared in absolute ethanol) to the polymer solution [53]. After obtaining nanoparticles, the previously described centrifugation and washing steps were repeated, and the supernatant was collected and filtered with a 0.22 µm cellulose acetate syringe filter for further characterization measurements.

2.4. Preparation of Chitosan-Coated Curcumin-Loaded Alginate Nanoparticles (CS[AA-Cur-NPs])

The curcumin-loaded alginate nanoparticles were coated with the chitosan polymer according to the procedures described in previous literature with slight modifications [54]. Briefly, curcumin-loaded alginate nanoparticles were added dropwise into a 0.1% *w/v* (weight/volume) chitosan (LMW) solution by micropipette to achieve a chitosan to nanoparticle (CS:NP) ratio of 1:2 by *v*/*v* (volume/volume). The mixture was stirred magnetically for 2 h at room temperature. After 2h, the mixture was centrifuged at 14,000 rpm for 30 min and rinsed with ultrapure water (ddH_2O); then, it was centrifuged at 5000 rpm for 5 min. This step was repeated twice. Finally, the supernatant was collected and filtered with a 0.22 µm cellulose acetate syringe filter for further characterization measurements. The same procedure was utilized to coat the drug-loaded, alginate-based nanoparticles.

2.5. Conjugation of Folic Acid (FA) on the Surface of Nanoparticles (FA-CS[AA-Cur-NPs])

FA-conjugated NP synthesis was performed according to the procedure described in the literature [55]. First, HATU (3.9 mg, 10 µmol), FA (4.1 mg, 9.29 µmol), and DIPA (0.68 µL, 9.31 µmol) were dissolved in 1.5 mL of anhydrous DMF solution and stirred magnetically for 2 h at room temperature to activate the beta-carboxylic acid in FA. This solution was then transferred onto the nanoparticle powder, which was obtained by lyophilization of 1 mL of nanoparticle solution in a round-bottom flask. Suspended in DMF solution, the amine groups in the chitosan on the nanoparticle surface underwent the FA-conjugation reaction overnight and at room temperature. The next day, dialysis was performed against ddH_2O to remove free FA molecules and excess DMF in the nanoparticle solution.

2.6. Characterization Methods for Prepared Nanoparticles

Regarding the hydrodynamic volume measurement, the size determination of the nanoparticles was obtained using dynamic light scattering (DLS) measurements in water at 25 °C using the AntonPaar Litesizer500 and Wyatt Technologies Dynapro Nanostar. Hydrodynamic diameter and polydispersity index of nanoparticles (AA NP, Cur-AA NP, and CS(Cur-AA NP)) were measured in ddH_2O and at room temperature. A total of 1 mL of these solutions was transferred into a glass cuvette and run for 10 processes with 5 s equilibrium time for three repetitions.

The surface charge measurement was performed via the Anton Paar Litesizer500 at 25 °C with 100 runs for three repetitions. The morphology of obtained nanoparticles was evaluated with the aid of a transmission electron microscopic (TEM) (Thermo Fisher Scientific, Waltham, MA USA, Talos L120C) operated at 20 kV with 3.5 spot size; support–copper TEM grids were utilized to visualize nanoparticles. Freeze-dried nanoparticles were investigated for their primary functional groups via Fourier transform infrared (FT-IR) spectroscopy (Thermo Fisher Scientific Inc.; Nicolet 380, Madison, WI, USA). The stability of the nanoparticles was assessed according to the day-by-day change in hydrodynamic diameter obtained by the DLS instrument as described above. The hydrodynamic diameter of nanoparticles was run for 10 successive runs with a 5 s equilibrium time for three repetitions. Size measurements were taken at different time intervals for 10 days [56].

2.7. Determination of Drug Encapsulation Efficiency

Encapsulation efficiency values for drug-loaded nanoparticles were determined using liquid chromatography–mass spectrometry/mass spectrometry (LC-MS/MS) (Agilent Technologies (Santa Clara, CA, USA) 1260 Infinity II) [57]. Briefly, the multiple-reaction monitoring (MRM) method specific to the curcumin molecule was created in the LC-MS/MS instrument by taking its molecular ion peak with an *m/z* value of 365.2 $gmol^{-1}$. The standard curve of curcumin was plotted using this MRM method with serially diluted samples at concentrations of 25, 50, 100, 200, 500, 1000, 2500, 5000, 7500, and 10,000 ppb. The C18 column was used as the stationary phase, and 50%ACN:50%ddH_2O was passed through with a flow rate of 0.5 mL/min. To measure the amount of drug molecules loaded in the nanoparticles, dialysis-purified and drug-loaded nanoparticles were incubated in a DMF/water mixture at a ratio of 1:1:4 (NP:DMF:dH_2O) to dissociate and liberate the drug molecules in the solution. The amount of released curcumin was determined by the prepared calibration curve. For the drug-loaded nanoparticles, drug encapsulation efficiency (DEE) values were determined based on the following Equation (1):

$$\text{DEE: [mass of drug}_{\text{(loaded)}}/\text{mass of drug}_{\text{(feed)}}] \times 100 \quad (1)$$

2.8. Preparation of Nanoparticle-Embedded Hydrogel Scaffolds (HG/CS(AA-NPs))

Nanoparticle (with or without drug)-embedded hydrogels were prepared by the radical-based gelation of a dimethacrylate-containing monomer, into which the thermo-responsive polymer chains pNIPAM were entrapped and solidified due to the temperature increase (37 °C) above its T_g value (32 °C) to provide an interpenetrating hydrogel scaffold. In detail, the nanoparticle solution was added into a 0.14% pNIPAM (*w*/*v*) (Mwt: 40 kg mol^{-1}) solution at a 1:4 ratio (*v*/*v*). Al_2O_3-filtered tetraethylene glycol dimethacrylate (20.5 μL, 57.3 μmol) was mixed with the pNIPAM solution, and 20 μL of 5% (*w*/*v*) APS and 30 μL of TEMED (0.20 μmol) were added into the polymer mixture to start the cross-linking process. After vigorous vortexing, gelation was clearly observed. However, to characterize a completely gelated hydrogel structure, this mixture was incubated in a thermal shaker at 37 °C overnight. The blank hydrogel was prepared as a control using the same amount of dH_2O instead of the nanoparticle solution [58].

2.9. Characterization of Nanoparticle-Embedded Hydrogel Scaffolds (HG/CS(AA-NPs))

The degradation, swelling behavior, thermo-responsive (injectability) property, and morphology of nanoparticle-embedded hydrogel scaffolds were investigated using various techniques [59]. For the morphological analysis, scanning electron micrography (SEM) images were obtained using Thermo Fisher Scientific Quanta 650 FEG. SEM samples were coated with 20 nm of gold (Au/Pb) under vacuum and fixed on the stub with carbon tape. Regarding the mechanical analysis, the rheological properties of the hydrogels were assessed using the Malvern Kinexus rheometer. The gelation process and degradation properties of the hydrogel were evaluated using J2 SR 4703 SS geometry. The degradation property was studied by taking measurements at parameters between $\gamma = 0.001$ and $\gamma = 1$ at f = 1 Hz and 37 °C (30 data points). The gelation process was analyzed under CD-auto strain mode with $\gamma = 0.01$ at f = 1 Hz at 37 °C (30 data points.) The strain-dependent oscillatory rheology and frequency-dependent oscillatory rheology of hydrogel scaffolds were tested at 0.1 Hz, 50.5 Hz, and 100 Hz, with $\gamma = 0.01$, at 37 °C. The thermo-responsive property of the hydrogels was investigated with the use of a small piece of freshly obtained chicken breast tissue (4 cm × 4 cm). Briefly, a small scratch (1 cm) was made on the tissue surface to mimic a wound. The tissue sample was placed in a thermal shaker adjusted to 37 °C. Then, the mixture prepared for hydrogel formation was immediately injected into the scratch site with a syringe and allowed to spread. The tissue sample was then stored in the thermal shaker at 37 °C for further observation of the gelation process and wound closure [60,61]. The swelling behavior of the hydrogels (with and without nanoparticles) was investigated by calculating the water uptake percentage as a function of time until the equilibrium condition was observed. Briefly, a swollen piece of hydrogel was frozen at −20 °C, freeze-dried in a lyophilizer, then incubated in dH_2O. At different time points, the weight of the swollen hydrogel was measured. An increase in the weight of hydrogel was recorded as a function of time. Obtained data were used to plot the graphs showing swelling capacity. The swelling ratio, W, was calculated via Equation (2), where m_w and m_d are the weights of wet and dry samples, respectively.

$$W\ (\%) = ((m_w - m_d)/m_d) \times 100 \quad (2)$$

2.10. Drug Release Studies

Both targeted nanoparticles and nanoparticle-embedded hydrogels were analyzed for their drug release profiles at different pH values via the dialysis method with respect to time. The dialysis set-up utilized 10 mM of phosphate buffered saline (PBS, pH 7.4) and sodium acetate buffer (SAB, pH 5.5) as receptor solutions in the drug release experiments to mimic the human body conditions of healthy tissue and tumor microenvironment, respectively [62]. Dialysis membranes (Mwt cut-off: 1 kDa) containing either nanoparticles or NP-embedded hydrogels were placed in a thermal shaker and the temperature was adjusted to 37 °C. Dialysis set-ups were subjected to continuous shaking at 200 rpm. At different time intervals (0, 0.5, 1, 2, 4, 6, 8, 10, 24, 48 h, and so on), 50 µL from the receptor solutions was withdrawn and analyzed for its free drug content using the LC-MS/MS according to the MRM method, prepared specific to curcumin.

3. Results and Discussion

3.1. Preparation of Drug-Loaded Nanoparticles

Alginate nanoparticles were prepared via the ionic gelation method with slight modifications [52]. It was observed that as the amount of surfactant increased in the nanoparticle solution, the nanoparticles obtained were of smaller size with a lower polydispersity index. Regarding the effect of gelation temperature on the size of nanoparticles, a higher temperature, close to body conditions, seemed to provide better DLS results for the obtained nanoparticles compared with the ones prepared at room temperature.

The alginate nanoparticles were coated with a positively charged chitosan polymer to introduce functional groups on the surface for further conjugation studies and to positively charge the surface for better cellular uptake. Different molecular weights of the chitosan polymers, HMW (310–375 kDa, >75% deacetylated) and LMW (50–190 kDa, 75–85% deacetylated); different concentrations (1, 0.5, and 0.1% *w*/*v*); and different mixing ratios (1:1, 1:2, and 2:1 (CS:NP)) were investigated in this study to assess a suitable size and surface charge. Since an HMW chitosan has longer polymer chains, its viscous solution resulted in the agglomeration of nanoparticles, despite its positive surface charge (detected by zeta potential measurements). DLS results revealed that the LMW chitosan can cover the surface of particles without a significant size increase and with a more positive surface charge (Table 2). Curcumin molecules were loaded into the core alginate of the prepared nanoparticle to prevent a burst release and provide a more controlled drug release based on the swelling of the polymeric carrier. For both drug-loaded and empty nanoparticles, the chitosan coating resulted in an increase in surface charge and the obtained nanoparticles remained in the range of 230–260 nm, which is suitable to benefit from the EPR effect after their release into the circulation system all the way to their targeted tissue.

Table 2. Characterization details of prepared nanoparticles.

Nanoparticle	Hydrodynamic Volume (nm) [1]	PDI [1]	Zeta Potential (mV) [2]	EE% [3]
AA NP	249.2	0.79	-0.4 ± 0.4	-
CS (AA NP)	261.4	0.64	1.7 ± 0.6	-
AA-Cur NP	233.1	0.67	-2.1 ± 0.4	94
CS (AA-Cur NP)	245.2	0.75	1.9 ± 0.5	88
FA-CS(AA-Cur NP)	264.2	0.19	0.8 ± 0.3	75

[1] Size and PDI values were measured in ddH_2O by DLS instrument. [2] Surface charge values were measured using 1:10 dilution factor (*v/v*) in 1 mM NaCl. [3] Encapsulation efficiency values were measured by LC-MS/MS instrument.

For this study, the nanoparticles were designed to be efficient carriers for antioxidants to ovarian tissue in particular, which is why the surface of the obtained nanoparticles was decorated with a folic acid molecule that can bind to folate receptors, which are over-expressed in ovarian cancer tissues in general. Free primary amine groups from the chitosan layer on the nanoparticles were successfully utilized for FA conjugation from its beta-carboxylic acid group through an amidation reaction. According to the DLS results, the FA conjugation did not substantially affect the size of nanoparticles; however, the decrease in the surface charge value indicates the conjugation of FA molecules onto the nanoparticles.

For the drug-loaded nanoparticles, the assembly was disturbed by dissociating the polymer–drug complex in the excess PBS/DMF mixture, and the amount of revealed drug molecules was measured by LC-MS/MS using the MRM method specifically prepared for curcumin molecular ion. As shown in Table 2, each step performed on the surface of nanoparticles resulted in a slight decrease in the amount of encapsulated drug at the alginate core (from 94% to 75%). However, the electrostatic interaction between the alginate surface and the chitosan layer may have ameliorated the stability of the nanoparticles and prevented burst drug release. By this strategy, the obtained core–shell nanoparticles bear a high potential to provide not only a sustained release of encapsulated drug molecules but also efficient delivery to the target.

Chemical characterization of prepared curcumin-loaded and chitosan-coated nanoparticles was performed using FT-IR spectroscopy analysis. After purification of nanoparticles via the dialysis method, the solution was lyophilized to perform the analysis in powder form. It is clearly seen in Figure 1 that the intensity of the carbonyl peak (1633 cm^{-1}) belonging to the primary amide increased for the FA-conjugated nanoparticle compared with the non-conjugated one. In addition, the newly formed peak at 1686 cm^{-1} for the FA-conjugated nanoparticles indicates the presence of a carboxylic acid group of FA incorporated onto the nanoparticle surface. Multiple peaks around 700–800 cm^{-1} (representing aromatic group bending in the spectrum of FA) are also detectable in the FA-conjugated nanoparticle spectrum. Moreover, characteristic peaks of alginate like –C–O–C– bonds (around 1050 cm^{-1}) and -N-H peaks of chitosan polymer (around 3300 cm^{-1}) can be observed in the spectrum of FA-conjugated nanoparticles.

Morphological evaluation of the prepared nanoparticles was performed via TEM analysis. Figure 2A clearly illustrates the spherical shape of the nanoparticles. The empty nanoparticles appear to be a lighter color, whereas the drug-loaded particles can be distinguished with a dark color at the bottom. The stability behavior of the nanoparticles was evaluated by measuring their size change for 5 days. The comparative stability profiles of chitosan-coated empty and drug-loaded nanoparticles revealed a 15–20% change in size compared with that of their initial state (day 0) (Figure 2B), which might be attributed to their swelling and the dissociation of polymer chains from the nanoparticle structure.

Targeted nanoparticles with folic acid molecules conjugated to their surface were 264.2 nm in diameter with a symmetrical size distribution (Figure 3A). While the stability study revealed a slight increase in diameter due to their swelling in the aqueous media over 15 days of incubation (Figure 3B), the nanoparticles were observed to be spherical in shape in the TEM image (Figure 3C).

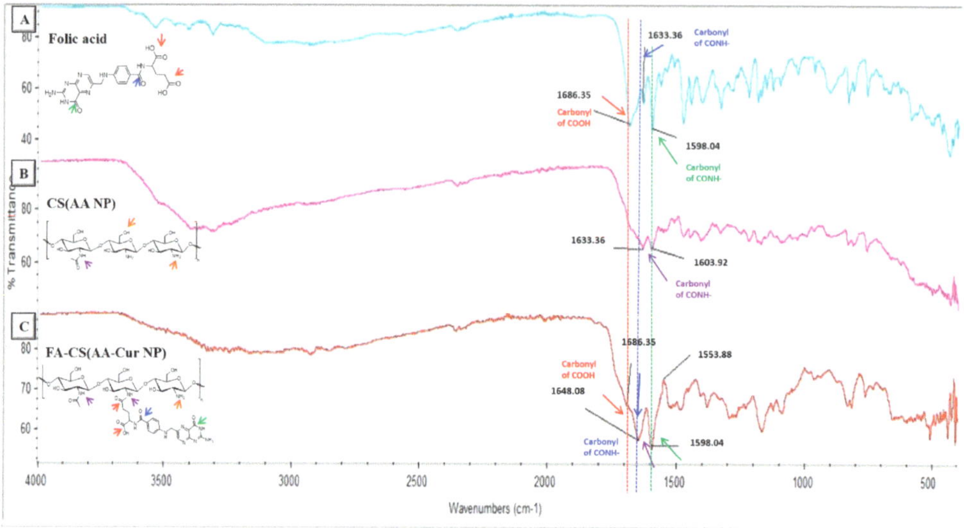

Figure 1. FT-IR spectra of FA molecule (**A**), CS(AA NP) (**B**), and FA-CS(AA-Cur NP)(**C**).

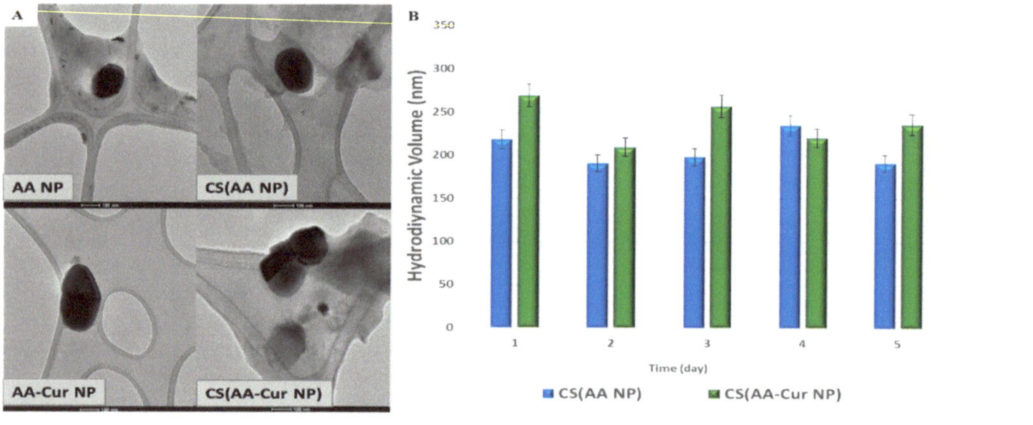

Figure 2. TEM images of prepared nanoparticles (**A**) and their stability behavior (**B**) (scale bar: 100 nm).

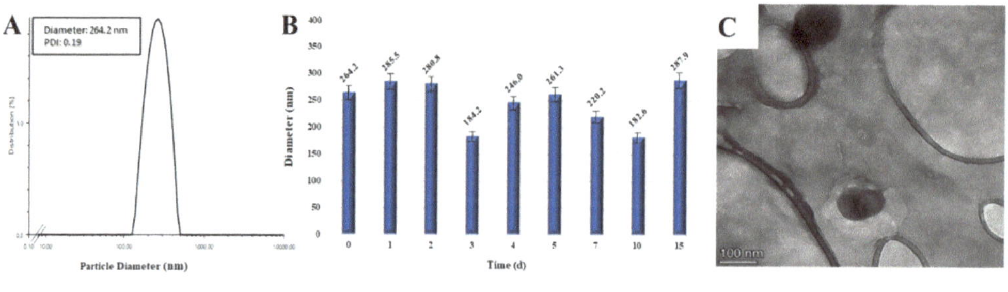

Figure 3. Size distribution (**A**), stability (**B**), and morphological evaluation (**C**) of FA-CS(AA-Cur NP).

3.2. Characterization of Nanoparticle-Embedded Hydrogel Scaffolds (HG/CS(AA-Cur NPs))

3.2.1. Morphological Characterization

The pNIPAM-based hydrogel scaffolds were prepared according to the literature procedures with slight modifications [34]. Gelation of thermo-responsive pNIPAM polymer chains was stabilized by cross-linking with a methacrylated ethylene-glycol-based monomer (TEG-MA), which was initiated based on the radical generation by APS and TEMED couple and fastened by increasing the temperature to human body temperature. Hydrogels without nanoparticles (control) were also prepared for comparison with the drug-loaded, nanoparticle-embedded hydrogel scaffolds. Morphological evaluation of the hydrogel scaffolds was performed by SEM analysis to confirm the porous structure. In Figure 4A, a lyophilized control hydrogel was observed to have a uniform porous structure, whereas the SEM image of a nanoparticle-embedded hydrogel scaffold confirms the presence of nanoparticles encapsulated during the gelation process (Figure 4C). A closer look at the SEM image shows the diameter of round-shaped nanoparticles inside the hydrogel to be in the range of 120–150 nm, which might be due to the shrinkage of nanoparticles due to the lyophilization process under high *vacuo*.

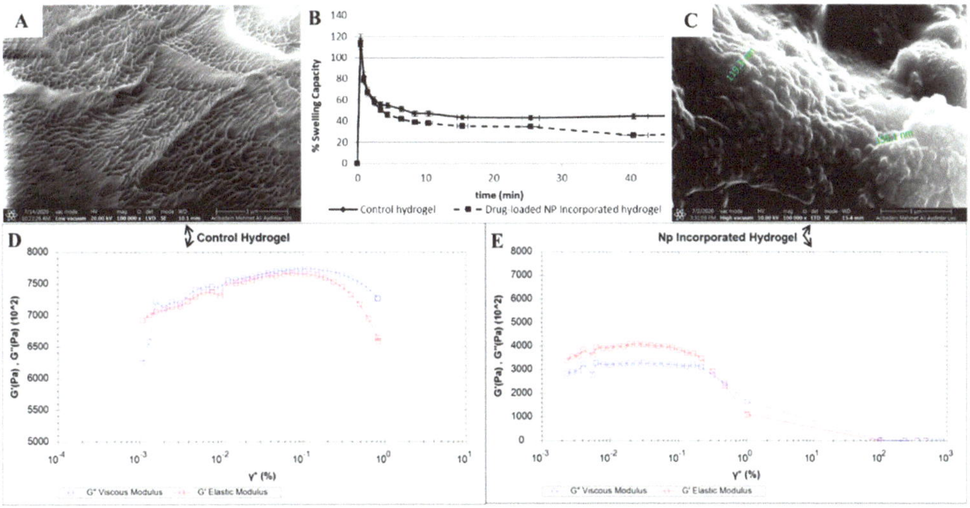

Figure 4. Morphological and mechanical evaluations for blank pNIPAM-based hydrogel (**A**,**D**), FA-CS(AA-Cur NP)-incorporated hydrogel (**C**,**E**), and their comparative swelling profiles (**B**).

3.2.2. Water Uptake Capacity

The swelling profiles of the hydrogels were investigated to determine their water uptake capacity over time and provide insight into their degradation behavior. Figure 4B demonstrates the percent swelling ratios of both the control and nanoparticle-embedded hydrogels scaffolds. A sudden and sharp increase in hydrogel weight was initially observed for both, followed by a sustained and slow decrease. This trend might be an indication of the slow degradation of obtained scaffolds, in spite of their less hydrophilic nature due to their pNIPAM chains and ethylene glycol units.

3.2.3. Mechanical Characterization

The degradation behavior of control and nanoparticle-embedded hydrogel scaffolds were studied via an amplitude sweep test (Figures 4D and 4E, respectively) using a rheometer. When a 0.001 to 100% strain was applied on the hydrogels, the nanoparticle-embedded hydrogel clearly demonstrated a linear viscoelastic behavior with a stiffness of 0.36 MPa up to 0.9% strain under 1 Hz frequency as a general method. Although the control hydrogel showed better stiffness at the beginning of the analysis, with a value of 0.70 MPa for elastic modulus, it switched to its yield point as the cross point at which G″ and G′ overlap at 0.005% strain, indicating a lack of structural integrity very quickly. The gelation profiles of these hydrogel scaffolds were also analyzed at three different frequencies (0.1, 50, and 100 Hz) that cover the stiffness range of human tissues [63]. These tests were applied to the hydrogel mixture solution, in which the strain was gradually increased. For the control hydrogel, as the frequency increased, stiffer gels were obtained, with increasing G′ storage modules value (Figure S1). Furthermore, for the nanoparticle-incorporated hydrogels, as the frequency of the analysis increased, loss and storage modules grew closer to each other compared with those of the control group, suggesting faster, better organization and assembly of the polymer chains to provide stiffer scaffolds, which is more obvious for the case at 100 Hz (Figure S2).

3.3. *Drug Release Studies of Nanoparticles and Nanoparticle-Embedded Hydrogel Scaffolds*

The release profiles of loaded curcumin either from only nanoparticles or nanoparticle-embedded hydrogels were investigated at body temperature and under two different conditions with pH values of 7.4 and 5.5 to represent normal physiological conditions and inflammation at the tumor microenvironment, respectively. Based on the measured drug amounts that were released at different time points through the dialysis membrane, the percentages with respect to the initial loaded drug amounts were calculated. Figure 5 clearly reveals not only the effect of lower pH value but also the effect of hydrogel encapsulation on the drug release profile. It is well-known that an acidic environment leads to accelerated degradation of natural polymers, resulting in faster drug release. This is the case for both the nanoparticles themselves and their hydrogel-encapsulated versions. At a pH of 7.4, there was a negligible amount of drug released over 4 days, whereas at a pH of 5.5, the nanoparticles and nanoparticle-incorporated hydrogel appeared to liberate the drug molecules in a sustained manner, with almost four times more drug released from the free nanoparticles. This difference obviously originates from the fact that the encapsulation of the nanoparticles in the hydrogel scaffolds has a direct impact on the drug release profile such that the encapsulated drug molecules in the nanoparticles embedded in hydrogels were liberated through the hydrogel pores in a slower fashion, which may provide better control and a continuous supply of the drug payload.

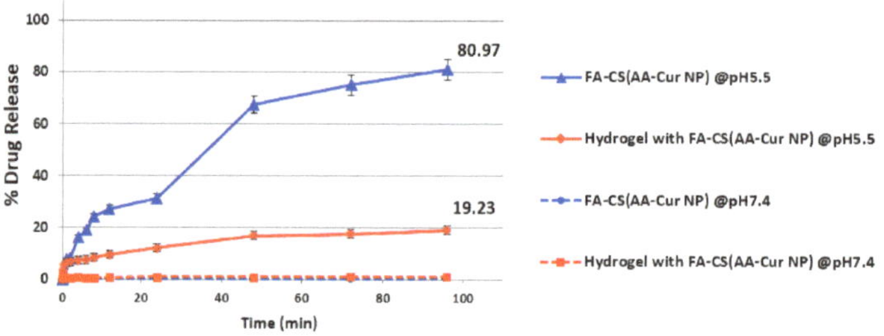

Figure 5. Release profiles of curcumin from NP alone and NP-incorporated hydrogels at different pH conditions.

3.4. *Thermo-Responsiveness and Injectability of Nanoparticle-Embedded Hydrogel Scaffolds*

Designed as an injectable hydrogel system, this scaffold was prepared via temperature-initiated gelation of pNIPAM chains and stabilized by simultaneous cross-linking with a methacrylate-based ethylene glycol monomer. Homogeneous mixing of this solution with drug-loaded nanoparticles provided encapsulation into the pores generated by polymer chains connected to each other by a cross-linked network of ethylene-glycol-based monomers to form the resultant hydrogel scaffold. Together with the abovementioned characterization of hydrogels prepared with or without nanoparticles, their thermo-responsive feature was evaluated via an ex vivo-like condition generated by freshly obtained chicken breast tissue (4 cm × 4 cm). At body temperature, a deep scratch was made on the tissue sample, followed by the application of nanoparticle-containing hydrogel solution with a syringe. As expected, gelation at 37 °C occurred within 30 s (Figure 6), and the generated hydrogel covered the scar completely. Moreover, incubation of this assembly was continued for 2 days at body temperature to assess the stability of the obtained scaffold at the scratch site, positively contributing to its ameliorating effect on wound closure.

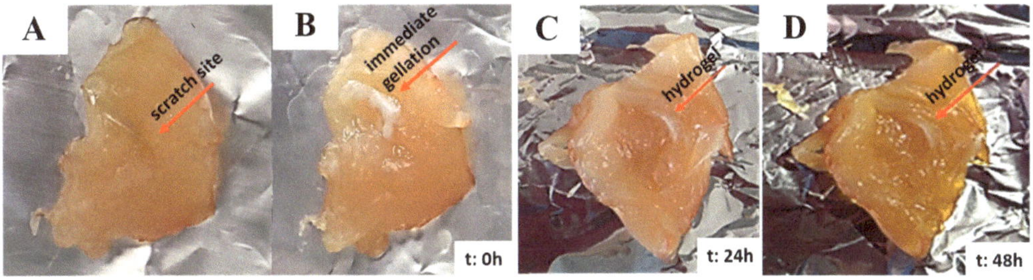

Figure 6. Scratch before the injection (**A**) and after the injection (**B**) of NP-incorporated, thermo-responsive pNIPAM hydrogel and its degradation behavior (**C**,**D**) on chicken breast tissue incubated at 37 °C.

4. Conclusions

The nanoparticle-incorporated hydrogels prepared in this study were designed as effective drug delivery systems with multifunctional features, including rapid injectability at body temperature, slower drug release profile, and direct targeting to cancerous cells with over-expressed folate receptors. For this purpose, curcumin was selected not only for its anti–carcinogenic but also for its anti-inflammatory activity. Alginate nanoparticles with an encapsulation efficiency of ~94% were loaded with curcumin to create a drug reservoir core, which was coated with another natural polymer, chitosan, to increase its stability. By benefiting from the functional groups of chitosan, folic acid was conjugated to the surface of these core–shell nanoparticles, providing targeted and drug-loaded carriers with a diameter (264.2 nm) suitable for the EPR effect. Incorporation of these nanostructures into the pNIPAM-based hydrogels with a swelling ratio of approximately 70% provided fast injectability (within 30 s) against a freshly obtained chicken breast tissue and demonstrated an almost four times slower drug release profile compared with that of free nanoparticles in slightly acidic media, which mimics the tumor microenvironment. The incorporation of nanoparticles clearly contributed to prolonged viscoelastic behavior. In conclusion, these nanoparticle-integrated hydrogel scaffolds have the potential to serve as efficacious therapeutic tools for delivering drug molecules to tumor sites with a simple injection, post-operational procedures, and wound closure.

Supplementary Materials: The following supporting information can be downloaded at https://www.mdpi.com/article/10.3390/pharmaceutics15092358/s1, Figure S1: Mechanical evaluations for FA-CS(AA-Cur NP)-incorporated hydrogel under different oscillation pressures, 0.1 Hz (A), 50.5 Hz (B), and 100 Hz (C); Figure S2: Degradation of drug-loaded NP-embedded hydrogel and its comparison with empty NP-embedded hydrogel, 24 h after their injection into tissue sample.

Author Contributions: Conceptualization and methodology, E.G.E.-S., A.M.O. and O.G.; validation and formal analysis, E.G.E.-S. and O.G.; writing—original draft preparation and writing—review and editing, E.G.E.-S. and O.G.; supervision, project administration, investigation, and resources, O.G.; funding acquisition, E.G.E.-S. and O.G. All authors have read and agreed to the published version of the manuscript.

Funding: This study was supported by ABAPKO (Acibadem University Scientific Research Projects Commission) with project number 2019/04-04.

Institutional Review Board Statement: Not applicable.

Informed Consent Statement: Not applicable.

Data Availability Statement: Not applicable.

Acknowledgments: The authors would like to thank Selçuk Birdoğan for his endless help and valuable expertise in taking SEM and TEM images of prepared nanoparticles and hydrogel scaffolds at Acibadem Mehmet Ali Aydinlar University Electron Microscopy Facility.

Conflicts of Interest: The authors declare no conflict of interest.

References

1. Mahinroosta, M.; Jomeh Farsangi, Z.; Allahverdi, A.; Shakoori, Z. Hydrogels as Intelligent Materials: A Brief Review of Synthesis, Properties and Applications. *Mater. Today Chem.* **2018**, *8*, 42–55. [CrossRef]
2. He, Y.; Tsao, H.K.; Jiang, S. Improved Mechanical Properties of Zwitterionic Hydrogels with Hydroxyl Groups. *J. Phys. Chem. B* **2012**, *116*, 5766–5770. [CrossRef]
3. Summonte, S.; Racaniello, G.F.; Lopedota, A.; Denora, N.; Bernkop-Schnürch, A. Thiolated Polymeric Hydrogels for Biomedical Application: Cross-Linking Mechanisms. *J. Control. Release* **2021**, *330*, 470–482. [CrossRef] [PubMed]
4. Tang, C.; Holt, B.D.; Wright, Z.M.; Arnold, A.M.; Moy, A.C.; Sydlik, S.A. Injectable Amine Functionalized Graphene and Chondroitin Sulfate Hydrogel with Potential for Cartilage Regeneration. *J. Mater. Chem. B* **2019**, *7*, 2442–2453. [CrossRef]
5. Jain, E.; Neal, S.; Graf, H.; Tan, X.; Balasubramaniam, R.; Huebsch, N. Copper-Free Azide–Alkyne Cycloaddition for Peptide Modification of Alginate Hydrogels. *ACS Appl. Bio. Mater.* **2021**, *4*, 1229–1237. [CrossRef] [PubMed]
6. Yan, S.; Chai, L.; Li, W.; Xiao, L.P.; Chen, X.; Sun, R.C. Tunning the Properties of PH-Responsive Lignin-Based Hydrogels by Regulating Hydroxyl Content. *Colloids Surf. A Physicochem. Eng. Asp.* **2022**, *643*, 128815. [CrossRef]
7. Thornton, P.D.; Mart, R.J.; Webb, S.J.; Ulijn, R.V. Enzyme-Responsive Hydrogel Particles for the Controlled Release of Proteins: Designing Peptide Actuators to Match Payload. *Soft Matter* **2008**, *4*, 821–827. [CrossRef]
8. Emam, H.E.; Shaheen, T.I. Design of a Dual PH and Temperature Responsive Hydrogel Based on Esterified Cellulose Nanocrystals for Potential Drug Release. *Carbohydr. Polym.* **2022**, *278*, 118925. [CrossRef]
9. Li, Z.; Li, Y.; Chen, C.; Cheng, Y. Magnetic-Responsive Hydrogels: From Strategic Design to Biomedical Applications. *J. Control. Release* **2021**, *335*, 541–556. [CrossRef]
10. Bustamante-Torres, M.; Romero-Fierro, D.; Arcentales-Vera, B.; Palomino, K.; Magaña, H.; Bucio, E. Hydrogels Classification According to the Physical or Chemical Interactions and as Stimuli-Sensitive Materials. *Gels* **2021**, *7*, 182. [CrossRef]
11. Koetting, M.C.; Peters, J.T.; Steichen, S.D.; Peppas, N.A. Stimulus-Responsive Hydrogels: Theory, Modern Advances, and Applications. *Mater. Sci. Eng. R Rep.* **2015**, *93*, 1–49. [CrossRef]
12. Varghese, J.S.; Chellappa, N.; Fathima, N.N. Colloids and Surfaces B: Biointerfaces Gelatin—Carrageenan Hydrogels: Role of Pore Size Distribution on Drug Delivery Process. *Colloids Surf. B Biointerfaces* **2014**, *113*, 346–351. [CrossRef] [PubMed]
13. Liaw, C.; Ji, S.; Guvendiren, M. Engineering 3D Hydrogels for Personalized In Vitro Human Tissue Models. *Adv. Healthc. Mater.* **2018**, *7*, 1701165. [CrossRef]
14. Markwell, S.M.; Mukherjee, S.; Brat, D.J.; Olson, C.L. Methods for in Vitro Modeling of Glioma Invasion: Choosing Tools to Meet the Need. *Glia* **2020**, *68*, 2173–2191.
15. Hauck, M.; Hellmold, D.; Kubelt, C.; Synowitz, M.; Adelung, R.; Schütt, F.; Held-Feindt, J. Localized Drug Delivery Systems in High-Grade Glioma Therapy—From Construction to Application. *Adv. Healthcare Mater.* **2022**, *5*, 2200013. [CrossRef]
16. Braccini, S.; Tacchini, C.; Chiellini, F.; Puppi, D. Polymeric Hydrogels for In Vitro 3D Ovarian Cancer Modeling. *Int. J. Mol. Sci.* **2022**, *23*, 3265. [CrossRef]
17. Daud, H.; Ghani, A.; Najaf, D.; Ahmad, N.; Nazir, S. Preparation and Characterization of Guar Gum Based Biopolymeric Hydrogels for Controlled Release of Antihypertensive Drug. *Arab. J. Chem.* **2021**, *14*, 103111. [CrossRef]
18. Aslzad, S.; Savadi, P.; Dalir, E.; Omidi, Y.; Fathi, M.; Barar, J. Chitosan/Dialdehyde Starch Hybrid in Situ Forming Hydrogel for Ocular Delivery of Betamethasone. *Mater. Today Commun.* **2022**, *33*, 104873. [CrossRef]
19. Cheon, S.; Keun, I.; Park, K. Hydrogels for Delivery of Bioactive Agents: A Historical Perspective. *Adv. Drug Deliv. Rev.* **2013**, *65*, 17–20.
20. Afzal, A.; Jalalah, M.; Noor, A.; Khaliq, Z.; Qadir, M.B.; Masood, R.; Nazir, A.; Ahmad, S.; Ahmad, F.; Irfan, M.; et al. Development and Characterization of Drug Loaded PVA/PCL Fibres for Wound Dressing Applications. *Polymers* **2023**, *15*, 1355. [CrossRef]
21. Ghasemiyeh, P.; Mohammadi-Samani, S. Polymers Blending as Release Modulating Tool in Drug Delivery. *Front. Mater.* **2021**, *8*, 752813. [CrossRef]
22. Raza, M.A. Irradiated Ch/GG/PVP-Based Stimuli-Responsive Hydrogels for Controlled Drug Release. *J. Appl. Polym. Sci.* **2020**, *137*, 49041. [CrossRef]
23. Spizzirri, U.G. Functional Polymers for Controlled Drug Release. *Pharmaceutics* **2020**, *12*, 135. [CrossRef]
24. Alexis, V.; Jorge, S.; Johanna, A.R.; Julio, C.; Investigación, G. De Use of Hydrogels as Controlled Drug Release Systems in Breast Cancer. *Eur. Chem. Bull.* **2023**, *94*, e2023100.
25. Huang, G.; Gao, J.; Hu, Z.; John, J.V.S.; Ponder, B.C.; Moro, D. Controlled Drug Release from Hydrogel Nanoparticle Networks. *J. Control. Release* **2004**, *94*, 303–311. [CrossRef]

26. Thoniyot, P.; Tan, M.J.; Karim, A.A.; Young, D.J. Nanoparticle—Hydrogel Composites: Concept, Design, and Applications of These Promising, Multi-Functional Materials. *Adv. Sci.* **2015**, *2*, 1400010. [CrossRef] [PubMed]
27. Hu, Z.; Xia, X.; Marquez, M.; Weng, H.; Tang, L. Controlled Release from and Tissue Response to Physically Bonded Hydrogel Nanoparticle Assembly. *Macromol. Symp.* **2005**, *227*, 275–284. [CrossRef]
28. Mook, S.; Se, L.; Oh, H.; Hoon, H. Dual Growth Factor-Releasing Nanoparticle/Hydrogel System for Cartilage Tissue Engineering. *J. Mater. Sci. Mater. Med.* **2010**, *21*, 2593–2600.
29. Jiang, Y.; Krishnan, N.; Heo, J.; Fang, R.H.; Zhang, L. Nanoparticle—Hydrogel Superstructures for Biomedical Applications. *J. Control. Release* **2020**, *324*, 505–521. [CrossRef]
30. Yang, H.; Tyagi, P.; Kadam, R.S.; Holden, C.A.; Kompella, U.B. Hybrid Dendrimer Hydrogel/PLGA Nanoparticle Platform Sustains Drug Delivery for One Week and Anti-Glaucoma Effects for Four Days Following One-Time Topical Administration. *ACS Nano* **2012**, *6*, 7595–7606. [CrossRef]
31. Machado, N.D.; Fernandez, M.A.; Haring, M.; Saldias, C.; Diaz, D.D. Niosomes encapsulated in biohydrogels for tunable delivery of phytoalexin resveratrol. *RSC Adv.* **2019**, *9*, 7601–7609. [CrossRef]
32. Zhang, Y.; Zhang, J.; Chen, M.; Gong, H.; Thamphiwatana, S.; Eckmann, L.; Gao, W.; Zhang, L. A Bioadhesive Nanoparticle—Hydrogel Hybrid System for Localized Antimicrobial Drug Delivery. *ACS Appl. Mater. Interfaces.* **2016**, *8*, 18367–18374. [CrossRef] [PubMed]
33. Khoee, S.; Kardani, M. Preparation of PCL/PEG Superporous Hydrogel Containing Drug-Loaded Nanoparticles: The Effect of Hydrophobic-Hydrophilic Interface on the Physical Properties. *Eur. Polym. J.* **2014**, *58*, 180–190. [CrossRef]
34. Chen, Y.; Tan, Z.; Wang, W.; Peng, Y.Y.; Narain, R. Injectable, Self-Healing, and Multi-Responsive Hydrogels via Dynamic Covalent Bond Formation between Benzoxaborole and Hydroxyl Groups. *Biomacromolecules* **2019**, *20*, 1028–1035. [CrossRef] [PubMed]
35. Mellati, A.; Akhtari, J. Injectable Hydrogels: A Review of Injectability Mechanisms and Biomedical Applications. *Res. Mol. Med.* **2019**, *6*, 1–14. [CrossRef]
36. Zhang, Y.; Chen, Y.; Shen, X.; Hu, J.; Jan, J. Reduction- and PH-Sensitive Lipoic Acid-Modi Fi Ed Poly (L-Lysine) and Polypeptide/Silica Hybrid Hydrogels/Nanogels. *Polymers* **2016**, *86*, 32–41. [CrossRef]
37. Zhu, J.; Li, F.; Wang, X.; Yu, J.; Wu, D. Hyaluronic Acid and Polyethylene Glycol Hybrid Hydrogel Encapsulating Nanogel with Hemostasis and Sustainable Antibacterial Property for Wound Healing. *ACS Appl. Mater. Interfaces* **2018**, *10*, 13304–13316. [CrossRef] [PubMed]
38. Dadashzadeh, A.; Imani, R.; Moghassemi, S.; Omidfar, K.; Abolfathi, N. Study of Hybrid Alginate/Gelatin Hydrogel-Incorporated Niosomal Aloe Vera Capable of Sustained Release of Aloe Vera as Potential Skin Wound Dressing. *Polym. Bull.* **2020**, *77*, 387–403. [CrossRef]
39. Diego, S.; Jolla, L. Nanoparticle-Hydrogel: A Hybrid Biomaterial System for Localized Drug Delivery. *Ann. Biomed. Eng.* **2016**, *44*, 2049–2061.
40. Kostarelos, K.; Prato, M.; Va, E. Nanocomposite Hydrogels: 3D Polymer À Nanoparticle Synergies for On-Demand Drug Delivery. *ACS Nano* **2015**, *9*, 4686–4697.
41. Hsu, X.L.; Wu, L.C.; Hsieh, J.Y.; Huang, Y.Y. Nanoparticle-Hydrogel Composite Drug Delivery System for Potential Ocular Applications. *Polymers* **2021**, *13*, 642. [CrossRef] [PubMed]
42. Sultana, A.; Zare, M.; Thomas, V.; Kumar, T.S.S.; Ramakrishna, S. Nano-Based Drug Delivery Systems: Conventional Drug Delivery Routes, Recent Developments and Future Prospects. *Med. Drug Discov.* **2022**, *15*, 100134. [CrossRef]
43. Elliott, I.; Shoichet, M.S. Acta Biomaterialia Controlled Release of Bioactive PDGF-AA from a Hydrogel/Nanoparticle Composite. *Acta Biomater.* **2015**, *25*, 35–42. [CrossRef]
44. Du, W.; Zong, Q.; Guo, R.; Ling, G.; Zhang, P. Injectable Nanocomposite Hydrogels for Cancer Therapy. *Macromol. Biosci.* **2021**, *21*, 202100186. [CrossRef] [PubMed]
45. Vyas, D.; Patel, M.; Wairkar, S. Strategies for Active Tumor Targeting-an Update. *Eur. J. Pharmacol.* **2022**, *915*, 174512. [CrossRef]
46. Iyer, K.S. Distinction Between Active and Passive Targeting of Nanoparticles Dictate Their Overall Therapeutic Efficacy. *Langmuir* **2018**, *34*, 15343–15349.
47. Wang, X.; Ye, L.; He, W.; Teng, C.; Sun, S.; Lu, H.; Li, S.; Lv, L.; Cao, X.; Yin, H.; et al. In Situ Targeting Nanoparticles-Hydrogel Hybrid System for Combined Chemo-Immunotherapy of Glioma. *J. Control. Release* **2022**, *345*, 786–797. [CrossRef]
48. Chatterjee, S.; Hui, P.C.L. Review of Applications and Future Prospects of Stimuli-Responsive Hydrogel Based on Thermo-Responsive Biopolymers in Drug Delivery Systems. *Polymers* **2021**, *13*, 2086. [CrossRef]
49. Alexander, A.; Ajazuddin; Khan, J.; Saraf, S.; Saraf, S. Polyethylene Glycol (PEG)-Poly(N-Isopropylacrylamide) (PNIPAAm) Based Thermosensitive Injectable Hydrogels for Biomedical Applications. *Eur. J. Pharm. Biopharm.* **2014**, *88*, 575–585. [CrossRef]
50. Navath, R.S.; Menjoge, A.R.; Dai, H.; Romero, R.; Kannan, S.; Kannan, R.M. Injectable PAMAM Dendrimer-PEG Hydrogels for the Treatment of Genital Infections: Formulation and in Vitro and in Vivo Evaluation. *Mol. Pharm.* **2011**, *8*, 1209–1223. [CrossRef]
51. Ward, M.A.; Georgiou, T.K. Thermoresponsive Polymers for Biomedical Applications. *Polymers* **2011**, *3*, 1215–1242. [CrossRef]
52. Bavel, N.V.; Lewrenz, A.; Issler, T.; Pang, L.; Anikovskiy, M.; Prenner, E.J. Synthesis of Alginate Nanoparticles Using Hydrolyzed and Enzyme-Digested Alginate Using the Ionic Gelation and Water-in-Oil Emulsion Method. *Polymers* **2023**, *15*, 1319. [CrossRef] [PubMed]
53. Venkata, V.; Reddy, S.; Kuppusamy, G. International Journal of Biological Macromolecules Curcumin Loaded Chitosan Nanoparticles Impregnated into Collagen-Alginate Scaffolds for Diabetic Wound Healing. *Int. J. Biol. Macromol.* **2016**, *93*, 1519–1529.

54. Access, O. Preparation and Characterization of Magnetic Nanoparticles with Chitosan Coating Preparation and Characterization of Magnetic Nanoparticles with Chitosan Coating. *J. Phys. Conf. Ser.* **2009**, *187*, 012036.
55. Song, H.; Su, C.; Cui, W.; Zhu, B.; Liu, L.; Chen, Z.; Zhao, L. Folic Acid-Chitosan Conjugated Nanoparticles for Improving Tumor-Targeted Drug Delivery. *BioMed Res. Int.* **2013**, *2013*, 723158. [CrossRef] [PubMed]
56. Mourdikoudis, S.; Pallares, R.M. Characterization Techniques for Nanoparticles: Comparison and Complementarity upon Studying. *Nanoscale* **2018**, *10*, 12871–12934. [CrossRef]
57. Li, X.; Su, J.; Kamal, Z.; Guo, P.; Wu, X.; Lu, L.; Wu, H.; Qiu, M. Odorranalectin Modified PEGPLGA/PEG—PBLG Curcumin-Loaded Nanoparticle for Intranasal Administration. *Drug Dev. Ind. Pharm.* **2020**, *46*, 899–909. [CrossRef]
58. Zhao, J.; Zhao, X.; Guo, B. Multifunctional Interpenetrating Polymer Network Hydrogels Based on Methacrylated Alginate for the Delivery of Small Molecule Drugs and Sustained Release of Protein. *Biomacromolecules* **2014**, *15*, 3246–3252. [CrossRef]
59. Sokker, H.H.; Ghaffar, A.M.A.; Gad, Y.H.; Aly, A.S. Synthesis and Characterization of Hydrogels Based on Grafted Chitosan for the Controlled Drug Release. *Carbohydr. Polym.* **2009**, *75*, 222–229. [CrossRef]
60. Drapala, P.W.; Brey, E.M.; Mieler, W.F.; Venerus, D.C.; Derwent, J.J.K.; Pérez-luna, V.H.; Drapala, P.W.; Brey, E.M.; Mieler, W.F.; Venerus, D.C.; et al. Role of Thermo-Responsiveness and Poly (Ethylene Glycol) Diacrylate Cross-Link Density on Protein Release from Poly (N-Isopropylacrylamide) Hydrogels Diacrylate Cross-Link Density on Protein Release From. *J. Biomater. Sci. Polym. Ed.* **2021**, *22*, 59–75. [CrossRef]
61. Safakas, K.; Saravanou, S.-F.; Iatridi, Z.; Tsitsilianis, C. Thermo-Responsive Injectable Hydrogels Formed by Self-Assembly of Alginate-Based Heterograft Copolymers. *Gels* **2023**, *9*, 236. [CrossRef] [PubMed]
62. Qindeel, M.; Ahmed, N.; Sabir, F.; Khan, S.; Ur-Rehman, A. Development of novel pH-sensitive nanoparticles loaded hydrogel for transdermal drug delivery. *Drug Dev. Ind. Pharm.* **2019**, *45*, 629–641. [CrossRef] [PubMed]
63. Matsuzaki, S. Mechanobiology of the Female Reproductive System. *Reprod. Med. Biol.* **2021**, *20*, 371–401. [CrossRef] [PubMed]

pharmaceutics

Review

Engineered Extracellular Vesicles for Drug Delivery in Therapy of Stroke

Waqas Ahmed [1,2], Muhammed Shibil Kuniyan [2], Aqil Mohammad Jawed [2] and Lukui Chen [1,*]

[1] Department of Neurosurgery, Neuroscience Center, Integrated Hospital of Traditional Chinese Medicine, Southern Medical University, Guangzhou 510310, China; ahmed.waqas3@gmail.com
[2] School of Medicine, Southeast University, Nanjing 210009, China; shibil1996@gmail.com (M.S.K.); doctorjawedaqil@gmail.com (A.M.J.)
* Correspondence: neuro_clk@hotmail.com

Abstract: Extracellular vesicles (EVs) are promising therapeutic modalities for treating neurological conditions. EVs facilitate intercellular communication among brain cells under normal and abnormal physiological conditions. The potential capability of EVs to pass through the blood–brain barrier (BBB) makes them highly promising as nanocarrier contenders for managing stroke. EVs possess several potential advantages compared to existing drug-delivery vehicles. These advantages include their capacity to surpass natural barriers, target specific cells, and stability within the circulatory system. This review explores the trafficking and cellular uptake of EVs and evaluates recent findings in the field of EVs research. Additionally, an overview is provided of the techniques researchers utilize to bioengineer EVs for stroke therapy, new results on EV–BBB interactions, and the limitations and prospects of clinically using EVs for brain therapies. The primary objective of this study is to provide a comprehensive analysis of the advantages and challenges related to engineered EVs drug delivery, specifically focusing on their application in the treatment of stroke.

Keywords: extracellular vesicles; engineering; stroke; blood-brain-barrier; drug delivery

Citation: Ahmed, W.; Kuniyan, M.S.; Jawed, A.M.; Chen, L. Engineered Extracellular Vesicles for Drug Delivery in Therapy of Stroke. *Pharmaceutics* **2023**, *15*, 2173. https://doi.org/10.3390/pharmaceutics15092173

Academic Editor: Ruggero Bettini

Received: 18 July 2023
Revised: 10 August 2023
Accepted: 17 August 2023
Published: 22 August 2023

1. Introduction

EVs are nanoscale heterogeneous structures released constitutively into the extracellular space by nearly all prokaryotic and eukaryotic cell types [1–4]. EVs are lipidic vesicles that develop in cells naturally. They facilitate cell-to-cell interaction by transferring various bioactive molecules from the mother cell, such as microRNAs, messenger RNAs, long noncoding RNAs (LncRNAs), circular RNAs (circRNAs) proteins, and lipids [5] (Figure 1). They are divided into three distinct categories: (i) Exosomes, (ii) Microvesicles, and (iii) Apoptotic bodies (Figure 2). Exosomes are a minor type of EVs, and prior electron microscopy studies have shown that they have a cup-like structure with a diameter ranging from 40 to 100 nm. During the development of multivesicular endosomes, an inward budding of the endosomal membrane produces exosomes [6]. Microvesicles, the second most significant type of vesicle, are formed when the plasma membrane buds and splits apart, with diameters between 100 and 1000 nm [7]. Apoptotic bodies represent the most abundant type of vesicles, exhibiting a size range of 1–5 μm and a diverse range of morphological characteristics. They are generated during the process of apoptosis. As a result, they possess a wide variety of constituents inherited from their progenitor cells, such as organelles and fragments of DNA [8].

Stroke is a prevalent neurological condition that can lead to permanent disability [9,10]. Annually, approximately 6.7 million individuals globally experience a stroke, with ischemic stroke comprising 87% of all mortalities [11]. The pathophysiological responses that occur after a stroke are complicated, and at present, tissue plasminogen activator remains the most efficacious treatment option for stroke [12,13], effective only when taken within 4–6 h of the onset of symptoms [14,15]. Despite this, due to its limited treatment window, it benefits less than 5% of patients [16]. Recent studies suggest that utilizing anti-inflammatory methods has considerable potential for expanding the time frame for treatment and decreasing severe brain damage following reperfusion [17,18]. Still, there is a constant demand for effective and cutting-edge medications that may prevent ischemia cascades and the diseases they cause.

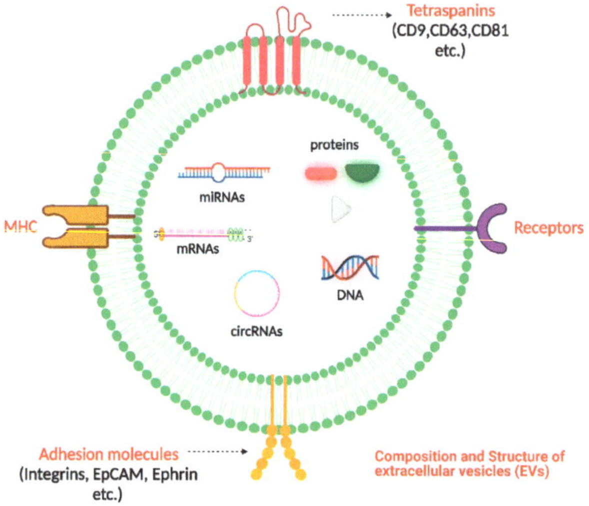

Figure 1. Composition and Structure of EVs. The structure of EVs consists of a phospholipid bilayer that encloses proteins (membrane protein and cargo protein) and nucleic acids. Membrane proteins encompass a variety of molecules, such as tetraspanins (including CD9, CD63, and CD81, among others), adhesion molecules (such as integrins, EpCAM, and Ephrin), the major histocompatibility complex (MHC), and receptors. Nucleic acids encompass DNA and RNA, which consist of various types of RNA molecules, such as messenger RNA (mRNA), microRNA (miRNA), long non-coding RNA (lncRNA), and circular RNA (circRNA). The phospholipid bilayer confers protection to the contents enclosed within. Created with BioRender.com (https://app.biorender.com/illustrations/649b3cd0422a45d3d7cc3c29, accessed date: 7 July 2023).

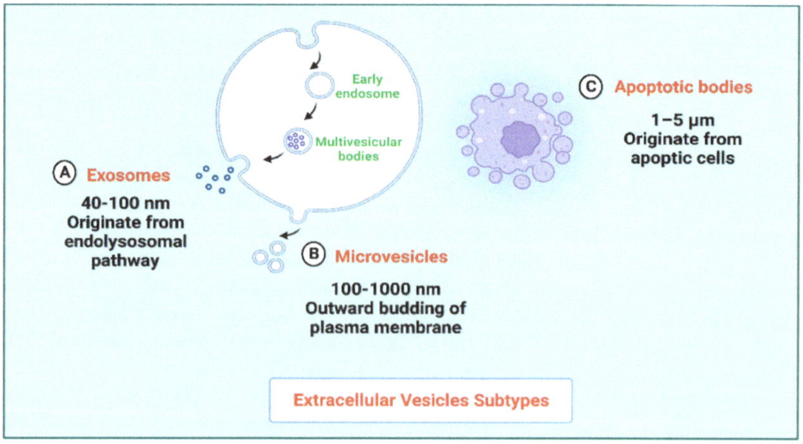

Figure 2. Schematic of EV Subtypes. (**A**) Exosomes and their formation. (**B**) Microvesicles and their formation. (**C**) Apoptotic bodies and their formation. Created with BioRender.com (https://app.biorender.com/illustrations/64d0be423f71706d207a7881, accessed date: 7 August 2023).

EVs significantly function in the complex intercellular communication among neurons, glia, and vascular cells. They are essential in regulating homeostasis and influencing the development and prognosis of pathological conditions. EVs are involved in various physiological processes, including the maintenance and restoration of neurons [19], synaptic function [20], neurovascular stability [21], and the preservation of myelination [22]. In recent years, several studies have demonstrated the potential of EVs as nanotherapeutics for treating brain pathologies [23–25]. The scientific world has taken a keen interest in this topic, with numerous studies demonstrating the neuroprotective and regenerative effects of natural EVs from various resources [23,26,27].

The present review suggests that engineered EVs can enhance the curative effectiveness of EV-based treatments for stroke. We will explore the curative abilities of natural EVs for neurological applications, including crucial factors for their therapeutic success. We also discuss recent advances in regulating the BBB by EVs and their movement throughout the BBB. In our final part, we summarized the many scientific approaches discovered for modulating the content and surface of EVs, with a particular emphasis on the tactics employed for various therapeutic and targeting drugs.

2. Analysis Criteria

A digital database and search tool were utilized to thoroughly review scientific literature, including original articles regarding experimental and observational studies, case series, and reports, among other relevant sources. PubMed, Google Scholar, Scopus, Web of Science, bioRxiv, medRxiv, CNKI, and WanFang Data are central databanks utilized for medical studies. (The latter two databases are particularly significant within the Chinese mainland.) The study analyzed a total of 42 articles that were published or in preprint form between December 2017 and June 2023. A brief overview of the connection between EVs and stroke was found.

3. Isolation and Characterization of EVs

The primary challenge in isolating and characterizing EVs lies in their small size and heterogeneous nature. In 2018, the International Society for Extracellular Vesicles updated its "Minimum information for studies of extracellular vesicles" (MISEV) standards, which can be summed up as follows: (I) give a quantitative description of the EV source; (II) show the existence of the functioning bilayers of lipids and describe their purity; (III) use a mixture of EV analysis methods, ideally one optical and one biophysical/biochemical; and (IV) use a solid and accurate experimental design when figuring out how EVs work in the body [28,28].

The methodologies used for EV separation exhibit a wide range of diversity. Moreover, every single technique may possess unique parameters and configurations designed to enrich specific subtypes of EVs. The workflow of EV analysis is shown in (Figure 3), along with typical methods for EV size, concentration, and cargo measurement. The selection of the EV separation method, or a combination of methods, is significantly impacted by the research purpose, as well as considerations of time, costs, and applicability. This is particularly important when considering potential clinical applications [29].

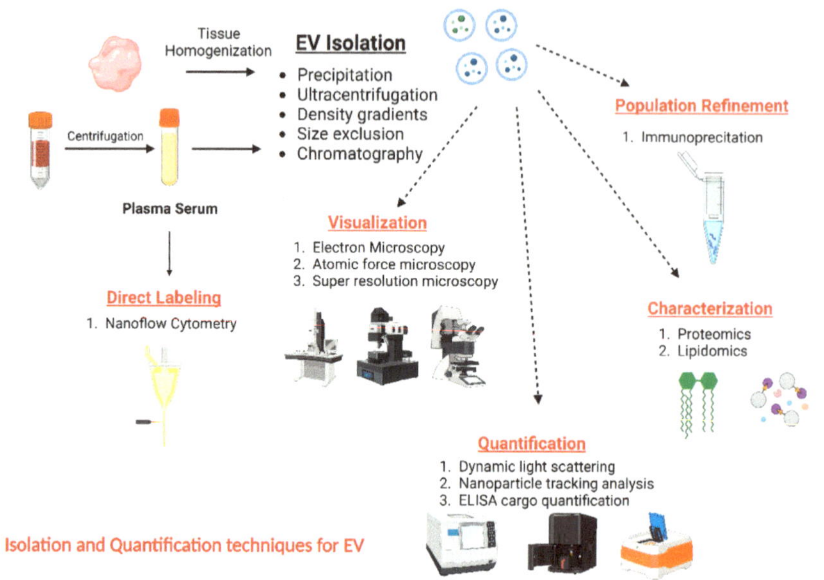

Figure 3. Isolation and quantification techniques for EVs. The diagram illustrates frequently employed methods for analyzing EVs. EVs can be quantified in tissue homogenates and natural fluids, such as urine, saliva, and blood. The isolation of plasma or serum from blood is utilized in this context as an illustrative case. Nanoflow cytometry enables direct labeling and quantifying EVs in various fluid samples. In contrast, EVs have the potential to be separated and subsequently utilized for further analysis. Immunoprecipitation is a technique that can be employed to enhance the specificity of EV populations. EVs can be observed using electron microscopy (EM) or alternative high-resolution microscopy methodologies. Lipidomics and proteomics methodologies can also be utilized to analyze and describe the composition of EVs populations. Ultimately, EV concentration and size measurement can now be achieved through dynamic light scattering and nanoparticle tracking analysis. Additionally, EV products can be measured by employing susceptible protein or RNA assays. Created with BioRender.com (https://app.biorender.com/illustrations/649b163862468f1db106b519, Accessed date: 7 August 2023).

4. EV Extraction from Biological Specimens

EVs have been extracted from a wide range of biological fluids, such as blood, urine, saliva, breast milk, cerebrospinal fluid, ascitic fluid, gastric juice, bile, sputum, bronchoalveolar lavage, semen, and tears [30,30–34]. They are actively released by cells throughout various tissues and organs, exhibiting their presence in physiological and pathological conditions [35,36]. The primary contributors to the population of blood microvesicles are platelets, which constitute a significant proportion of blood, with EVs ranging from 70% to 90% [35]. In addition to the mentioned hematopoietic cells, many other cell types, including reticulocytes, B lymphocytes, T cells, neutrophils, mast cells, dendritic cells, and macrophages, also play a significant role. Moreover, cells originating from different bodily tissues, such as epithelial cells, also contribute to this process [37]. The use of standardized pre-analytical procedures (Figure 3) is of the greatest significance to minimize the presence of mistakes in the analysis of EVs, mainly when these EVs are obtained from complex body fluids, such as blood. The composition, concentration, and characteristics of EVs produced from biofluids can be influenced by various factors, such as age, gender, ethnicity, body mass index, disease status, medication usage, overall lifestyle, and dietary lifestyles [38]. These variables must be considered and modified across all study participants (patients and any relevant controls).

5. Natural EVs for Treating Stroke

The significance of EV signaling within the brain's framework was initially recorded in the early 1950s through electron microscopy studies [39–42]. Since then, researchers have discovered that EVs produced by nerve cells, like astrocytes and microglia, play an important role in immune signaling during synaptic plasticity [43–45]; in the specialized nature of neural cell interaction [46,47]; and in the diffusion of various neurological diseases, like neurodegenerative diseases and cerebral tumors [48]. Stroke [24], traumatic brain injury (TBI) [49], Alzheimer's disease (AD) [50], autism [51], and schizophrenia [52] are just a few of the brain disorders where the therapeutic effects of EVs have been described since 2011. Over the past decade, a notable transition has been from cell-based treatments to EVs treatments. Several clinical investigations have exhibited the potential of EVs to protect and regenerate in various therapeutic applications in stroke (Table 1).

Table 1. Natural EVs for the treatment of stroke.

Disease	Model	EV Source	Route	Dose	Outcome	Reference
Stroke	MCAO in mouse	Human MSCs	IV	Multiple administrations	↑ Neurogenesis ↑ Angiogenesis	[53]
		M2 Microglia	IV	100 µg	↑ Neuron protection ↓ Volume of infarction	[54]
		Mouse NSCs	IV	100 µg	↑ Availability of astrocytes ↓ Volume of infarction	[27]
		Mouse NSCs and MSCs	RO	1–100 µg (multiple administrations)	↓ Impaired motor coordination ↑ Neuro-regeneration	[55,56]
	TE-MCAO in mouse	Human NSCs	IV	2.7×10^{11} EVs/kg (multiple administrations)	↓ Cerebral atrophy ↑ Motor recovery	[57,58]
	MCAO in rat	Porcine MSCs	IV	100 µg	↑ Functional recovery ↓ Volume of infarct ↑ Angiogenesis	[59]
		Human MSCs	IA	200 µg/kg	↑ Functional recovery ↓ Volume of infarct ↑ Angiogenesis	[60]
		Rat NSCs	ICV	30 µg	↑ Neural protection ↓ Microgliosis ↓ Size of infarct ↓ Behavioral deficits	[61,62]
		Rat MSCs	ICV	100 µg	↓ Size of infarct ↑ Functional recovery	[63]
		Rat MSCs	IV	100 µg	↑ Neuron transformation	[24]

MSCs—Mesenchymal stem cells; **IV**—intravenous injection; **MCAO**—middle cerebral artery occlusion; **NSCs**—neural stem cells; **TE-MCAO**—thromboembolic middle cerebral artery occlusion; **RO**—retro-orbital; **ICV**—intracerebroventricularly. ↑ Increase, ↓ Decrease.

5.1. EV Origin

According to current research, the origin of EVs after systemic treatment affects their biodistribution [64]. This aspect has yet to be thoroughly investigated when designing EVs as therapies for stroke. A natural brain stereotype could be employed to enhance the therapeutic benefit of an EV. As far as current knowledge goes, research has yet to be conducted to directly contrast the brain tropism of extracellular vesicles derived from various origins. Research on native EVs for stroke has focused on their therapeutic potential rather than their specific ability to target the brain. According to experimental evidence, the mechanism by which EVs are derived from mesenchymal stem cells (MSCs) targeting damaged areas in the brain may be influenced by inflammatory processes [65]. Previous research has utilized EVs released by neural stem cells (NSCs) sourced from the subventricular area of mice [6,46,66] or from human NSCs [57] that were derived following the division of induced embryonic stem cells (Figure 4). Initial research utilizing mouse NSC-EVs indicated that these EVs are more likely to build in the liver and lung than the brain following intravenous or retro-orbital administration [55].

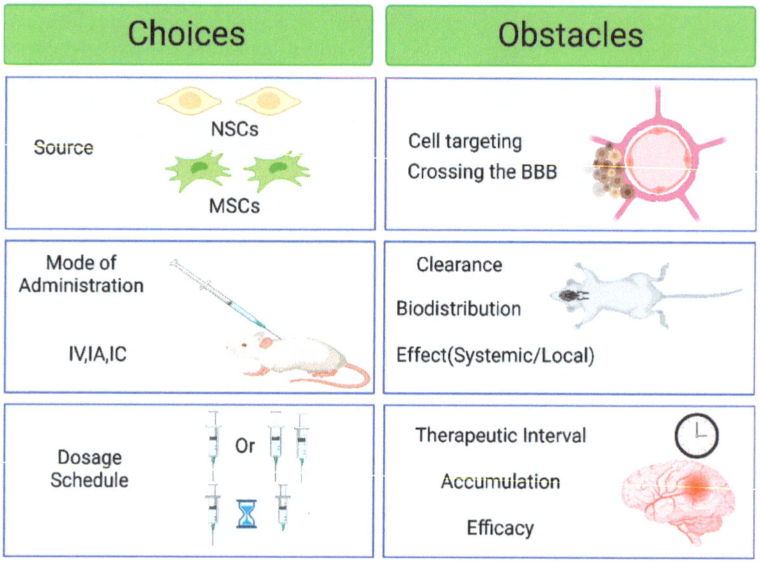

Figure 4. Choices and obstacles while using EVs. The application of EVs originating from diverse cellular origins is commonly observed in managing stroke. The properties of EVs associated with each cell type may have varying levels of tropism for brain vasculature or neuronal cells, which could impact their ability to target the brain effectively. However, a complete evaluation of these properties has yet to be conducted. Crossing the blood–brain barrier (BBB) poses a significant challenge. The method of administration affects the biodistribution and clearance of EVs and can also impact the effect's nature, i.e., whether it is localized or systematic. Lastly, the dosing schedule can be single or repeated, affecting accumulation and efficacy. Created with BioRender.com (https://app.biorender.com/illustrations/647df1821b2f09af295c29aa, accessed Date: 5 June 2023).

Substances on their surface mediate the natural targeting capability of EVs [67,68]. Findings from the report of metastatic progression have revealed that the brain tropism of EVs originating from breast tissue cells [68] is determined by expressing Integrin Beta3. Additional research on surface molecules that facilitate brain targeting may offer insights into selecting cell sources or developing engineering techniques to improve cerebral tropism.

5.2. Route of Administration

The route of administration is an essential factor to consider when investigating the biodistribution of a drug. This is also applicable to the investigation of EVs. (Figure 4). In a variety of animal experiments, EVs have been given to the animals intracerebrally [69–73], intravenously [74], intranasally [75], intra-arterially, intraperitoneally [76], and via retro-orbital [77] routes. Limited research has been conducted to compare the number of EVs produced in the nervous system through various delivery methods.

Administering EVs through the intra-arterial route is more productive for targeting the brain than the other routes. This is because the EVs are delivered near the brain, which reduces their elimination by other organs in the body [64]. EVs generated from human mesenchymal stem cells isolated from human bone marrow were administered intravenously to mice with acute brain lesions resembling ischemic stroke conditions [78]. Following treatment with EVs, a reduction in the presence of macrophages was observed in the affected area compared to the control group. In addition, there was a decline in the expression of pro-inflammatory cytokines and astrocyte activation.

5.3. EV Dose Comparisons

In addition to the delivery pathway and cellular origin, the number of EVs and the schedule of administration are critical factors that significantly impact the therapeutic effectiveness of the treatment (Figure 4). Various doses and administration regimens have been utilized to treat stroke using native EVs (Table 1). In stroke therapy, Aβ oligomers have been reduced in rats and a transgenic mouse model by administering native EVs at concentrations ranging from 10 to 100 μg and 30 to 30 μg, respectively [60,61,63,72,79]. Some studies administer EVs only once, while others administer them multiple times due to the quick elimination of EVs from the infarcted region within twenty-four hours of the initial intravenous injection [80] to achieve sustained brain accumulation. The administration time varied between 2 and 48 h post-ischemic stroke for single-dose therapies and 2 h weekly for multiple-dose regimens [23,60,81]. It has been suggested that reducing systemic inflammation in the blood after a stroke can be achieved by increasing the number of M2-type macrophages and Treg populations and decreasing the number of Th17 cells within 2 h of treatment. This creates a favorable environment for successful brain remodeling [57]. Importantly, from a therapeutic standpoint, higher concentrations of EVs are not always preferable. NPC-EVs or MSC-EVs at an average dose boosted neuronal densities in stroke mice but not at either low or high doses.

5.4. Mechanism of Action

The purpose of current study aims to examine the functional benefits of vesicles that are secreted from mesenchymal stem cells (MSCs) [82] and neural stem cells [57], which have been identified in rodents, rats, and pigs [60] models of cerebral ischemia that were caused by the blockage of the middle cerebral artery. It has been demonstrated that MSC-derived EVs have similar outcomes to those described with MSC transplantation in terms of decreasing infarct volume, enhancing functional recovery, increasing angiogenesis and neovascularization [83,84], decreasing astrocyte stimulation [60], and modulating peripheral immune system responses (Figure 5).

Most reported therapeutic effects of EVs in treating stroke are believed to be passive, mediated explicitly through extracranial organs. EVs facilitate a reduction in the overall inflammatory response following stroke, which might decrease leukocyte infiltration in the brain, ultimately reducing blood–brain permeation and neuronal inflammation [57,85]. The study reveals that NSC-EVs can induce the polarization of macrophages toward an M2 genotype with anti-inflammatory properties. Additionally, NSC-EVs were found to increase the population of regulatory T cells while reducing the number of proinflammatory T helper 17 cells [57].

The fact that EVs can cross the BBB and retain their functional cargo has significantly contributed to the development of biomarker research using EVs and their potential application as a vehicle for drug delivery. Alvarez-Erviti et al. showed that mice injected with EVs delivered siRNA to the brain. Dendritic cells were modified to express EVs membrane protein Lamp2b26. Genetically pairing Lamp2b with a CNS-specific rabies virus glycoprotein (RVG) peptide targeted EVs exclusively to the brain [50]. In another study, researchers utilized rats as subjects to investigate the presence of a fluorescently labeled protein specifically expressed in brain tissue. The study found this protein could be detected in microscopic EVs in the rats' blood. This research study presents empirical support for intercellular communication facilitated by EVs originating from the CNS and disseminating throughout the peripheral tissues [86]. The studies provide evidence that supports the concept of EV crossing the BBB in a bidirectional manner. However, the precise mechanism by which this crossing occurs remains uncertain.

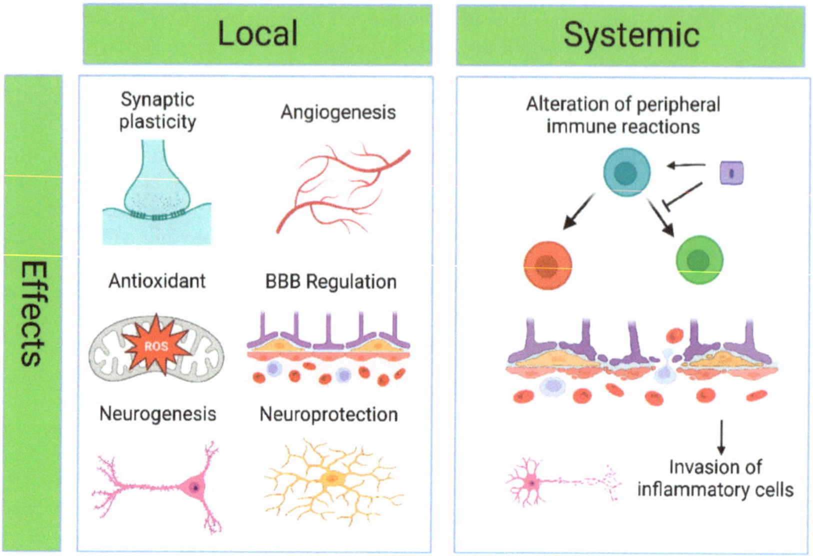

Figure 5. The role of natural EVs in the pathophysiology of stroke. The management of stroke has shown benefits through direct local effects in the brain, such as neuroprotection, neurogenesis, angiogenesis, antioxidant and anti-inflammatory properties, and systemic effects by modulating peripheral immune system responses. These effects may create a favorable environment for cerebral regeneration. Created with BioRender.com (https://app.biorender.com/illustrations/647df0bfe74d4f82a5bc4ade, accessed: 11 June 2023).

The therapeutic efficacy of EVs in stroke is primarily attributed to the molecular mechanisms involving microRNAs (miRNAs) present within these vesicles. Typically, in vitro experiments evaluate the direct impact of EVs on neuronal cells. They promote neurite outgrowth in nerve cells, and the inhibition of the growth factor for connective tissue in astrocytes was observed upon exposure to miR-133b-containing EVs released by mesenchymal stem cells (MSCs). This effect was attributed to the suppression of RhoA by the EVs [87,88]. Furthermore, it has been discovered that EVs containing miR-124, released by M2 microglia cells, can increase neuronal survival in vivo. The downregulation of ubiquitin-specific protease 14 is regulated to achieve the desired result. However, whether the effect is direct or systemic is still being determined since there is no apparent connection between transfected cells and the downregulation of ubiquitin-specific protease 14 (Figure 6).

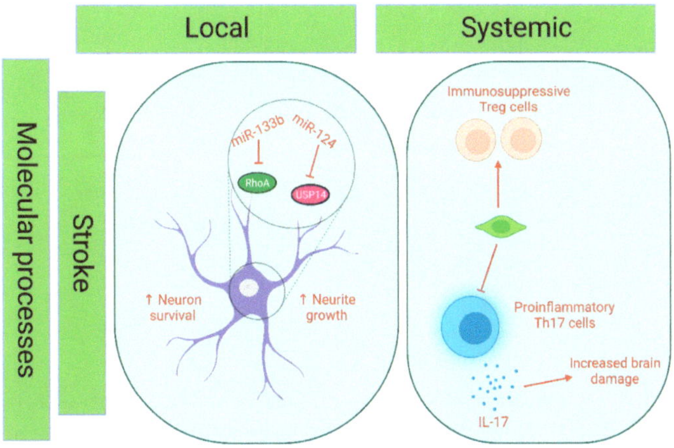

Figure 6. Natural EV modes of action in stroke. The transfer of MiR-133b through EVs originating from mesenchymal stem cells (MSCs) has been found to facilitate the growth of neurites. This effect is achieved through the targeting of the converting protein RhoA. Additionally, miR-124 is linked to increased neuronal viability by targeting USP-14, a ubiquitin-specific protease. Systemically, it has been demonstrated that EVs from NSC reduce pro-inflammatory Th17 cells while improving immunosuppressive Treg cells. Created with BioRender.com (https://app.biorender.com/illustrations/647ca600a95ee7a5e7fd6757, accessed: 11 June 2023).

6. Neuronal Regeneration via Sustained EV/NP Delivery

Over several decades, extensive research has been conducted on utilizing the body's inherent regenerative capacity. Numerous studies have investigated the utilization of various therapeutic approaches to induce endogenous regeneration. These approaches include instructive biomaterial scaffolds, EVs, nanoparticles (NPs), small molecules, and other similar interventions [89]. Therapeutic EVs have been utilized for potential regenerative uses primarily due to their adaptability in modifying size and capacity to serve as carriers for transporting drugs, growth factors, tiny molecules, or genetic information [90,91].

Nerve injuries pose significant clinical challenges as a result of their inherent limitations in terms of regenerative capacity. Conventional treatments for nerve injuries have traditionally relied on autologous nerve grafts. However, these grafts are gradually being supplanted by artificial nerve guidance conduits (NGCs) due to limitations, such as the limited availability of nerve grafts, the need for multiple surgeries to isolate donor grafts, and the potential risk of developing neuromas. The primary objective of a recent research study on managing peripheral nerve injury was to explore the potential of targeted therapeutics. This was achieved by utilizing alginate hydrogels composed of laminin-coated poly(l-lactide-co-glycolide) (PLGA) conduits. These conduits were designed to contain a mixture of gold nanoparticles (NPs), brain-derived neurotropic growth factor (BDNF), and adipose-derived stem cells [92].

A separate investigation examined the administration of conductive poly(3,4-ethylenedioxythiophene) nanoparticles/EVs modified with cell adhesive tetrapeptide. These nanoparticles were delivered using a biocompatible chitin scaffold. The study's results indicate that the conductive scaffold exhibited high porosity and compatibility with biological systems. Upon introduction into an in vivo model, a notable enhancement in nerve regeneration was observed, as evidenced by an increase in the regenerated myelin's thickness and the muscle fibers' area. An augmentation in the adhesive capacity of Schwann cells, along with enhanced angiogenesis, was also noted at the site of the injury (Figure 7). Hence, the utilization of this chitin scaffold with electrical activity has been proposed as a promising alternative for a nerve guidance conduit, as well as a suitable material for the administration of therapeutics to facilitate nerve regeneration [93].

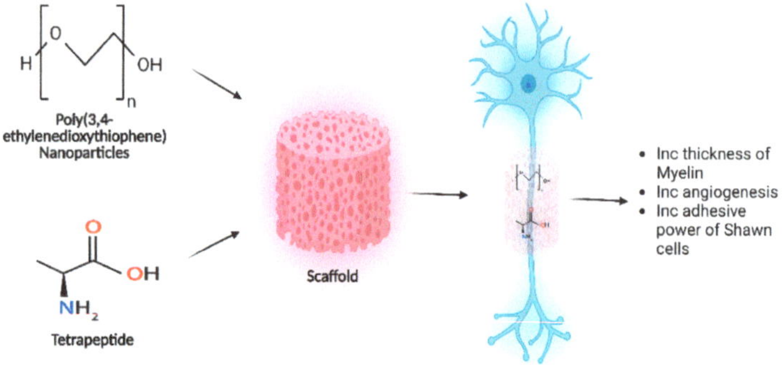

Figure 7. EV/NP. Transport Neural Remodeling. Poly(3,4-ethylenedioxythiophene) modified with tetrapeptide was administered utilizing a biocompatible chitin scaffold. In an in vivo model, myelin thickness increased, indicating nerve regeneration. At the injury's site, Schwann cell adhesiveness and angiogenesis increased. Created with BioRender.com (https://app.biorender.com/illustrations/64a80816d2fc5a3659e189a9, accessed: 7 July 2023).

7. Drug Loading Techniques

The effectiveness of EVs as a new class of nanocarriers arises from their unique qualities as information carriers, including their inherent homing ability, widespread distribution in biological fluids, biological compatibility, cell-specific targeting, non-immunogenicity, and easy penetration through physiological barriers. Pre-loading and post-loading are the two primary strategies for transferring cargo into EVs. Pre-loading refers to loading cargo into parent cells before the isolation of EVs, which releases o EVs that are loaded with cargo. Post-loading refers to loading cargo directly into EVs using either passive or active means after EVs have been isolated (Figure 8). Table 2 provides a comprehensive overview of various cargo loading tactics and procedures employed for extracellular vesicles, along with their advantages and disadvantages.

Table 2. Methods for loading EVs with drugs.

Loading Strategies	Loading Methods	Advantages	Disadvantages	Reference
Pre-loading	Co-incubation	1. Simple 2. Cost-effective 3. EV-friendly	1. Low encapsulation efficiency 2. Strict cargo selection	[94–96]
	Transfection	Target molecule overexpression	1. Time-consuming 2. Highly dependent on cell viability 3. Potential toxicity and genetic changes	[97,98]
Post-loading	Co-incubation	1. Easy operation 2. No extra equipment is required 3. Minimal destruction to EVs	1. Low loading efficiency 2. Limited variety	[99–101]
	Electroporation	1. Effective loading efficiency 2. Loading of large biomolecules	1. Affect EVs integrity 2. Risk of EVs aggregation 3. Heat can cause damage	[102,103]
	Sonication	High loading efficiency	1. EVs membrane degradation 2. EV aggregation risk	[104,105]
	Freeze–thawing cycle	1. Cost-effective 2. Applicable for most cargoes	1. Low loading efficiency 2. EVs membrane damage 3. EVs aggregation risk	[106,107]
	Surfactant administration	1. Affordable 2. Applicable for most cargoes	EVs surface potential and functionality may be altered	[76,108]

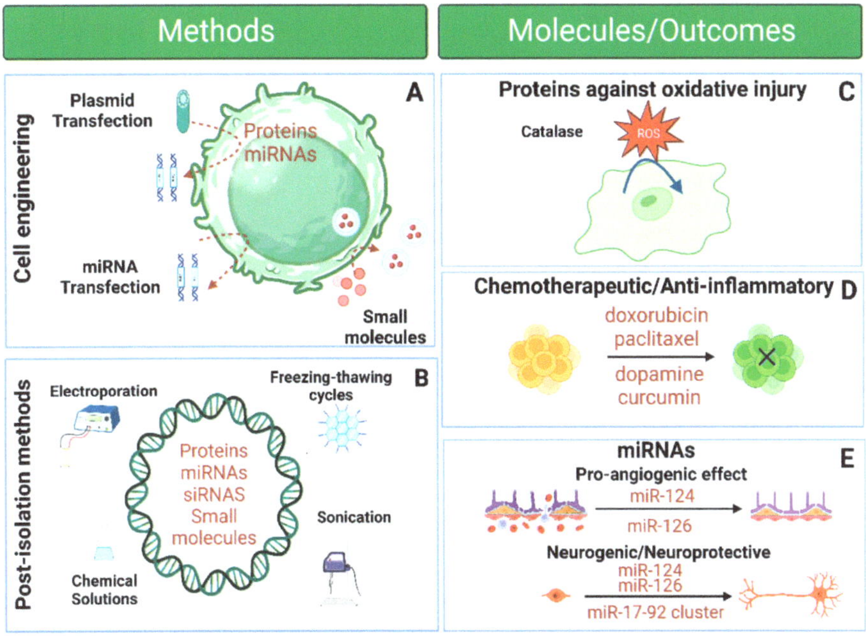

Figure 8. Engineering strategies for modifying EV content. Cellular engineering techniques can regulate EVs, including altering primitive cells or directly loading them via various post-isolation methods. (**A**) Cell engineering uses genetic manipulation techniques, such as plasmid transfection or enriching cells with miRNAs or small compounds, to load a parent cell indirectly. (**B**) Electroporation, sonication, freeze–thaw cycles, and chemical agents modulate isolated EVs post-isolation. Therapeutic substances and loading efficiency determine the optimum EV modulation strategy. EVs cargo manipulation can treat stroke by acting on cargo type. (**C**) Proteins. (**D**) Small molecules. (**E**) miRNAs. Created with BioRender.com (https://app.biorender.com/illustrations/647dfe244f0c62bb59ac8cb8, accessed: 6 June 2023).

8. Engineered EVs for Stroke Treatment

Despite advancements in the preclinical application of endogenous EVs as therapeutic agents for stroke over the past decade, additional enhancements are required to optimize their therapeutic efficacy and expedite their clinical implementation. The first involves the biological effects of EVs. The EVs of native origin exhibit heterogeneity, even if obtained from an identical cell resource. Therefore, concentrating the EV material into a singular therapeutic entity with the most potent neuronal activity can enhance the efficacy of their treatment. The second is related to the focus on EV targeting. After being administered systemically, very few EVs (usually less than 5%) end up in the brain [109–111]. To have the most significant local or direct effect on the brain, we need to make strides in the surface engineering of EVs to improve their range and target particular cell membrane receptors. On the other hand, assessing the in vivo targeting and therapeutic mechanisms of EVs demands the creation of analytical and imaging platforms that are highly sensitive and have high resolution, respectively.

Consequently, engineering techniques to modify EV bioactivity [27,112–121], targeting [122–130], and tracking [123] have been created to tackle past difficulties. The earlier approaches can be implemented in EVs after isolation or within the cells responsible for EV production. This can be achieved through the use of gene editing [112], metabolic and residue-specific protein packaging [131], or the process of incubating cells with external compounds [132] or nanoparticles [133] (Figures 8 and 9; Tables 2 and 3). Numerous techniques are available for rapidly and efficiently engineering EVs with functional groups, genetic material, biologically active proteins, and peptides. However, the development of methods that do not adversely affect the function of EVs remains a challenging task. The present section investigates various methodologies, including genetics, exogenous delivery, and chemically inspired techniques, that can alter EVs' outside appearance and composition to facilitate drug delivery to the brain.

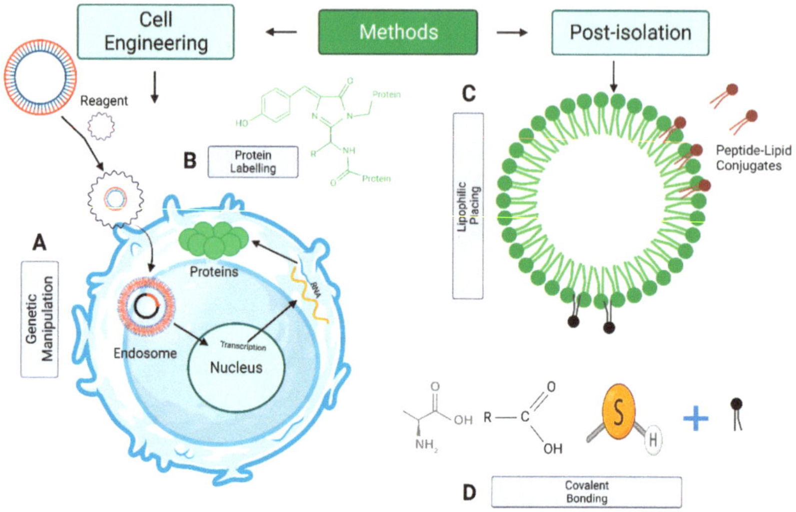

Figure 9. Surface modulation of EVs. The modulation of EV surfaces can be accomplished by genetically modifying the cells that produce them. (**A**) Protein plasmids or (**B**) Protein-residues (**C**) directly conjugated to lipids that are then integrated into EV membranes. (**D**) Bio-orthogonal chemistry identifies extracellular vesicle functional groups. Created with BioRender.com (https://app.biorender.com/illustrations/6480cf6ae6947f82704ea72e, accessed: 11 June 2023).

Table 3. Techniques for modifying EVs cargo in stroke.

Origin of EVs	Method	Model	Result	Reference
Rat MSCs	miR-17-92 cluster overexpression	MCAO rat model	↑ Neurogenesis ↑ Neurological function	[119]
Rat MSCs	miR-133b overexpression	MCAO rat model	↑ Neuroprotection	[116]
Human ADSCs	miR-126 overexpression	Rat MCAO	↑ Neurogenesis ↑ Angiogenesis ↓ Inflammation	[113,134]
Mouse EPCs	miR-126 overexpression	Mouse MCAO	↓ Infarct size ↑ Neurogenesis ↑ Angiogenesis	[135]
Mouse MSCs	Diffusion of curcumin-loaded EVs	Mouse MCAO model	↓ Inflammation ↓ Neuronal apoptosis	[122]
Human MSCs	Diffusion of leucocyte-loaded EVs	Mouse MCAO model	↓ Brain leukocyte infiltration ↑ Neuroprotection	[136]

Table 3. *Cont.*

Origin of EVs	Method	Model	Result	Reference
Rat-blood-derived EVs	PCSK9 overexpression	Mouse ICH model	↑ Neuroprotection ↑ Myelination ↑ Angiogenesis	[137]
Human umbilical cord blood (UCB)–MSC-derived EVs	Diffusion of BDNF-Loaded EVs	Rat IVH model	↑ Neuroprotection ↓ Inflammatory response/ Apoptosis/ ↑ Myelination and neurogenesis	[138]
Bone-marrow–MSCs derived EVs	miR-21-5p overexpression	Rat SAH model	↓ Neuronal apoptosis ↑ Neuroprotection	[139]
BMSC-derived EVs	miR-183-5p overexpression	Rat model of db-ICH	↓ Neuroinflammation ↓ Neurological deficit	[140]
EVs from angiotensin-converting enzyme 2 (ACE 2)	Endothelial progenitor cells overexpression	Mouse ICH model	↓ Decreased hemorrhage volume ↓ Brain edema Improved Neurological Deficit Score (NDS)	[141]

MSCs—Mesenchymal stem cells; **ADSCs**—adipose-derived stem cells; **EPCs**—endothelial progenitor cells; **EVs**—extracellular vesicles; **MCAO**—middle cerebral artery occlusion; **ICH**—intracerebral hemorrhage; **IVH**—intraventricular hemorrhage; **SAH**—subarachnoid hemorrhage; **BMSCs**—bone marrow mesenchymal stem cells; **db-ICH**—diabetic intracerebral hemorrhage. ↑ Increase, ↓ Decrease.

8.1. Modulation of Content

Over the past five years, a remarkable increase in the number of described techniques for loading functional molecules into EVs has been seen [27,116,118,142,143]. The predominant approach employed in such methods involves genetic modification via plasmid transfection of the cells that secrete extracellular vesicles, thereby effectively regulating the composition of the EVs [27,114,116,119,144]. Plasmid transfection can be accomplished through electroporation or incubation with transfection reagents [117]. Therefore, EVs have modulated the expression of genes in human disease models, both in vitro and in vivo, by incorporating functional proteins, mRNAs, microRNAs (miRNAs), and other short noncoding RNAs [119,145]. The direct modulation technique has been implemented in manipulating isolated EVs to incorporate small drug molecules and for encapsulating proteins and small amounts of non-coding RNA within EVs (Figure 8) [106,146–148]. When implementing these strategies, it is essential to consider certain factors. The molecules' size determines the material type that EVs can transport. Numerous molecules, such as miRNAs or small drugs, can be encapsulated within EVs. However, the capacity of EVs is restricted when it comes to larger molecules such as mRNA or proteins. Furthermore, a more significant amount of cargo sometimes equates with increased biological value. Additionally, genetically modified EVs' effectiveness on the target cell is influenced by internalization efficiency, intracellular trafficking, and channels altered by the EV-based molecules.

The fact that these studies were performed on animal models is the only thing that could be considered a limitation. On the other hand, there is no evidence of this therapeutic possibility in the human field due to the challenges involved in the preparation of engineered EVs and the challenges related to the methods of administration needed to achieve a significant enough result to be considered a valid therapeutic strategy. Although there are plenty of issues to be resolved, the development of standardized techniques and guidelines for EV engineering, isolation, and storage has brought EV-based therapies closer to being utilized for stroke and other neurological illnesses (Table 4).

Table 4. EV cargo modification in other neurological conditions.

Origin of EVs	Method	Model	Result	Reference
Mouse embryonic fibroblasts	Cre recombinase enzyme overexpression	Transgenic mouse model	Intranasal transport of brain-active proteins	[117]
Human HEK-293 T	Overexpression of the catalase enzyme	PD mouse model	↓ Neuronal inflammation	[112]
Mouse astrocytes	Transfection with lincRNA-Cox2-siRNA	In vitro/in vivo lincRNA-Cox2 knockout model Intranasal	↓ Expression of lincRNA-Cox2; LPS-induced microglial proliferation	[114]
Human astrocytes	Transfection with lincRNA-Cox2-siRNA	In vitro/in vivo lincRNA-Cox2 knockout model Intranasal	Microglial phagocytic activity restored	[149]
Mouse macrophages	Transfection with curcumin	Rat AD model	↑ Neuron survival; ↓ Tau phosphorylation	[118]
Mouse macrophages	EV loading with catalase: sonication, extrusion, or saponin	Mouse PD model	↓ Oxidative stress ↑ Neuron survival	[106]
Human ESCs	EV loading with paclitaxel: diffusion	Orthotopic mouse xenografts	↑ Accumulation at the glioma spot ↑ Mouse survival	[147]
Mouse BECs	EV loading with paclitaxel or doxorubicin: diffusion	Xenotransplanted brain cancer zebrafish model	↑ Brain cancer cell elimination	[148]
Mouse blood serum	EV loading with dopamine: diffusion	Mouse PD model	↑ Dopaminergic neurogenesis ↑ Symptomatic performance	[150,151]

PD—Parkinson's disease; **AD**—Alzheimer's disease; **ESCs**—embryonic stem cells; **BECs**—brain endothelial cells. ↑ Increase, ↓ Decrease.

8.1.1. Nanoparticle

EVs are being utilized to enclose tiny therapeutic particles, typically comprising a medicinal substance, with sizes ranging from 10 nm [123] to 150 nm [152]. This approach aims to enhance the transportation of such nanoparticles across the blood–brain barrier (BBB). The loading of EVs can be achieved through two distinct processes: The first involves isolating the EVs and subsequently subjecting them to an electroporation procedure with nanoparticles [123]. The second process entails transfecting EV-secreting cells with nanoparticles and loading the EVs [68]. Recent research has indicated that EVs exhibit comparable therapeutic efficacy to stem cells derived from ischemic stroke treatment [56,81,153,154]. One central area for improvement in utilizing exosomes is the inability to target the ischemic lesion within the brain specifically. It has been found that using magnetic nanovesicles (MNVs) made from mesenchymal stem cells (MSCs) and filled with iron oxide nanoparticles makes it easier to target the area of the brain that is ischemic. This is achieved by applying an external magnetic field, which facilitates magnetic navigation. Using magnetic navigation resulted in a 5.1-fold increase in the EVs' capacity to target the ischemic lesion specifically. The MNVs were found to have a significant impact on reducing the infarct volume and enhancing motor function. Additionally, they were observed to stimulate a defensive response, promote vascular development, and prevent cell death in cerebral ischemia [88,155–157].

An animal stroke model utilized gold nanoparticles coated with glucose to facilitate non-invasive neurological imaging and EV tracking. This approach aided in identifying the most effective administration route and size parameter [158,159]. The diagnosis and treatment of numerous neurological disorders are impeded due to the limited ability of diagnostic agents to penetrate the blood–brain barrier (BBB) [160]. Following the idea of the Nature Biotechnology Group, which involved the production of EVs as vehicles for genetic treatment with selective targets in the brain [50], gold-coated vesicles targeted brain cells by enhancing nanoparticle permeability to cross the BBB [161].

8.1.2. Proteins

Determining the appropriate approach for encapsulating therapeutic proteins within EVs is based on their intended utilization. The method of transfecting cells that secrete extracellular vesicles (EVs) with plasmids is utilized to produce enzyme-loaded EVs, including catalase [106], Cre-recombinase [117], and the lysosomal enzyme tripeptidylpeptidase-1 (TPP-1) [76]. Following a stroke, there is a change in the proportions of pro-inflammatory and anti-inflammatory proteins, impacting the size of the infarct and the individual's functional outcome [162,163]. EVs containing IFN-ɣ have been utilized in treating neurodegenerative conditions such as multiple sclerosis. The study demonstrated that IFN-ɣ-stimulated extracellular vesicles (EVs) decreased demyelination and neurological inflammation in a murine model [158,164]. They investigated the impact of TNFα and interleukin-1β cytokines on the molecular composition and release of astrocyte-derived extracellular vesicles. The findings indicate that vesicles derived from astrocytes treated with TNFα and IL-1β contained a high concentration of miR-125a-5p and miR-16-5p, which are known to target proteins that regulate neurotrophin signaling.

Furthermore, it was noted that EVs injected with cytokines reduced the neuronal expression of NTKR3 and Bcl2 [165]. The inflammatory cytokine IL-1β, which affects the brain's inflammatory response to injury, was administered into the brain. An IL-1β injection into the striatum led to more Ly6b+ leukocytes going to the lesion site and more circulating vesicles in the plasma of mice compared to controls. IL-1β also caused astrocytes to release EVs, which quickly passed the BBB [166].

An additional study examined the pro-angiogenic effects of microglial BV2 cells that were polarized by IL-4 and lipopolysaccharide. The cells polarized by IL-4 demonstrated an increase in endothelial cell tube formation through the secretion of EVs. Furthermore, the miRNA-26a profile was observed to be higher in comparison to the LPS-polarized group [167]. Researchers found that preconditioning neural stem cells with IL-6, a proinflammatory cytokine that promotes prosurvival signaling, reduced ischemic injury in a mouse stroke model [167,168].

8.1.3. Small Non-Coding RNAs

The study of EVs in the context of nervous system disorders is a relatively developing area of research. The blood–brain barrier (BBB) is formed by the tightly joined endothelial cells of brain capillaries, which effectively limit the passage of small molecules that are lipid-insoluble (90–98%) into the brain [132,169,170]. Two distinct approaches can be employed for the loading of non-coding RNAs in EVs: (I) chemical (e.g., chemically induced transfection) [106,171] or physical (e.g., electroporation) [50,132] strategies following EV separation; and (II) the introduction of plasmid-encoded non-coding RNAs or non-coding RNAs directly into EV-secreting cells through transfection [113,119,149].

The researcher Yang et al. employed EVs to transport circular RNA to the ischemic area of stroke. The study's authors used a targeted approach to deliver Circ-SCMHI RNA to neuronal cells. This was achieved by expressing RVG peptides on exosome membranes, which served as a cargo-delivering vehicle system for the Circ-SCMHI RNA of interest. The RVG-circSCMH1-EVs have been found to enhance neuronal plasticity through their binding to MeCP2 and subsequent upregulation of downstream gene expression (Mobp, Igfbp3, Fxyd1, and Prodh). This mechanism is believed to contribute to the maintenance of proper brain function. The administration of RVG-CircSCMH1-EVs via intravenous injection enhanced motor recovery, digit movement, and functional recovery in rodent and non-human primate experimental models. The authors proposed that RVG-CircSCMH1-EVs may possess a broader therapeutic window compared to existing treatments, as it could be administered up to 24 h following the onset of stroke [172].

MiR-124 is recognized for its propensity to promote neuronal development in the developing and mature brain. EVs containing miR-124 facilitate the acquisition of neuronal identity by cortical neural progenitors and confer post-ischemic recovery by promoting reliable cortical neurogenesis [132]. The BACE1 gene was effectively knocked down through siRNA delivery via EVs. This resulted in a significant decrease in β-amyloid levels in the brains of mice with wild-type mutations [50]. MiRNA-210 exhibits promising prospects for enhancing angiogenesis in the context of brain area restoration after ischemic events. The enhancement of miRNA-210 expression resulted in a more excellent restoration of function after stroke. The delivery of miRNA-210 to the ischemic area was achieved by linking EVs with the c(RGDyK) peptide and adding miRNA-210.

This resulted in an upregulation of miR-210 at the ischemic site and increased the expression of integrinβ3, vascular endothelial growth factor, and CD34, significantly improving animal survival rates [130].

8.1.4. Neurotrophic Factors (NTFs)

The neurotrophic factor is being researched as a protective factor in neurological diseases [173,174]. They control the development of neural stem cells, which are accountable for restoring neurological function and repairing vascular damage caused by stroke [175,176]. Neurotrophic factors (NTFs) are a promising therapeutic option for stroke repair. Their diverse neuroprotective functions following ischemic events have been acknowledged [177,178]. The clinical application of NTF is currently not feasible due to the absence of an effective method for delivering it systemically to the ischemic area. Brain-derived neurotrophic factor (BDNF) is extensively studied for its neuroprotective and anti-inflammatory effects. BDNF was packed within naive exosomes and administered intravenously to rats to combat brain inflammation [179]. MiR-206 knockdown EVs reduced early damage to the brain by increasing BDNF levels following the treatment [180]. This suggests that bioengineering vesicles with BDNF could help with brain diseases like stroke. More research is needed to understand how EVs and NTFs work in stroke treatment. It would be highly beneficial to prioritize exploring this area in the future.

9. Conclusions and Future Prospective

The domain of EVs is presently considered a rapidly advancing field in fundamental science and applied research [181]. EVs derived from various cellular origins have demonstrated therapeutic efficacy in stroke. Over the past decade, significant progress has been achieved in the field (i) by demonstrating the curative value of specific groups of EVs in preclinical studies for cognitive and behavioral brain diseases; (ii) by discovering the systemic [57] and local [61] actions that characterize EV brain regeneration processes; (iii) by showing the effects of EVs in neurogenesis [132], neural protection, angiogenesis, and cerebral remodeling; and (iv) by describing how EVs are transported through the BBB [132,182]. Based on empirical evidence, EVs are swiftly eliminated from the brain, leading to a significant absence of EVs within a short time. So, experts are working on bioengineering EVs to improve their half-life in circulation, make them more available at the disease site, make it easier to deliver them to specific cells, and use them to provide therapeutic molecules or regenerative medicine.

According to a study [57], treating ischemic stroke with innate EVs resulted in particular outcomes, primarily attributed to the alteration of the immune response rather than a localized effect in the brain. However, high growth in the lesion area could produce a greater neuroprotective and pro-angiogenic impact. Numerous investigations have been conducted, primarily in vitro, wherein the culture environment may influence the EV's biochemical and biophysical characteristics. Consequently, further research is needed to comprehend the engineered EVs physiological impacts on human well-being comprehensively.

In short, EVs possess significant potential for therapeutic applications. Clinical trials have exclusively involved endogenous EVs, while engineered EVs designed to target the brain have yet to undergo clinical testing. This is primarily due to challenges associated with the large-scale production of EVs and the production of EVs with similar characteristics. Collectively, EV-derived therapeutics and diagnostics have exhibited encouraging outcomes in diverse phases of clinical trials. Nevertheless, most clinical trials on EVs are underway, and the available published data regarding their current progress or results could be much better.

Translating modified EVs into clinical settings presents significant obstacles, including restricted techniques for versatile isolation and purification, EV variability, poor storage conditions, potential immunogenic adverse effects, and batch-to-batch variations. Therefore, much work must be done to utilize EVs' therapeutic effects properly.

Author Contributions: W.A. conceived, designed, and wrote the manuscript. M.S.K. and A.M.J. provided critical revision and helped in the analysis of the manuscript. L.C. supervised and contributed to the concepts, the perspectives, and the discussion of ideas, helped in the correction, and proofread the manuscript. All authors have read and agreed to the published version of the manuscript.

Funding: This work was sponsored by the National Key R&D Program of China (2022YFA1104900 and 2022YFA1104904), the Natural Science Foundation of Guangdong Province (2021A1515010013), the Department of Education of Guangdong Province (2021ZDZX2011), the Traditional Chinese Medicine Bureau of Guangdong Province (20221275), the Guangzhou Municipal Science and Technology Project (202201011760), and the President Foundation of the Integrated Hospital of Traditional Chinese Medicine of Southern Medical University (1202101003).

Conflicts of Interest: The authors declare no conflict of interest.

References

1. Brown, L.; Wolf, J.M.; Prados-Rosales, R.; Casadevall, A. Through the wall: Extracellular vesicles in Gram-positive bacteria, mycobacteria and fungi. *Nat. Rev. Microbiol.* **2015**, *13*, 620–630. [CrossRef]
2. Raposo, G.; Stoorvogel, W. Extracellular vesicles: Exosomes, microvesicles, and friends. *J. Cell Biol.* **2013**, *200*, 373–383. [CrossRef] [PubMed]
3. Colombo, M.; Raposo, G.; Théry, C. Biogenesis, secretion, and intercellular interactions of exosomes and other extracellular vesicles. *Annu. Rev. Cell Dev. Biol.* **2014**, *30*, 255–289. [CrossRef]
4. Schwechheimer, C.; Kuehn, M.J. Outer-membrane vesicles from Gram-negative bacteria: Biogenesis and functions. *Nat. Rev. Microbiol.* **2015**, *13*, 605–619. [CrossRef]
5. Kalluri, R.; LeBleu, V.S. The biology, function, and biomedical applications of exosomes. *Science* **2020**, *367*, eaau6977. [CrossRef] [PubMed]
6. Van Niel, G.; d'Angelo, G.; Raposo, G. Shedding light on the cell biology of extracellular vesicles. *Nat. Rev. Mol. Cell Biol.* **2018**, *19*, 213–228. [CrossRef]
7. Gharbi, T.; Zhang, Z.; Yang, G.-Y. The function of astrocyte mediated extracellular vesicles in central nervous system diseases. *Front. Cell Dev. Biol.* **2020**, *8*, 568889. [CrossRef]
8. Lu, M.; DiBernardo, E.; Parks, E.; Fox, H.; Zheng, S.-Y.; Wayne, E. The role of extracellular vesicles in the pathogenesis and treatment of autoimmune disorders. *Front. Immunol.* **2021**, *12*, 566299. [CrossRef]
9. Murphy, T.H.; Corbett, D. Plasticity during stroke recovery: From synapse to behaviour. *Nat. Rev. Neurosci.* **2009**, *10*, 861–872. [CrossRef]
10. Dimyan, M.A.; Cohen, L.G. Neuroplasticity in the context of motor rehabilitation after stroke. *Nat. Rev. Neurol.* **2011**, *7*, 76–85. [CrossRef]
11. Cunningham, C.J.; Wong, R.; Barrington, J.; Tamburrano, S.; Pinteaux, E.; Allan, S.M. Systemic conditioned medium treatment from interleukin-1 primed mesenchymal stem cells promotes recovery after stroke. *Stem Cell Res. Ther.* **2020**, *11*, 1–12. [CrossRef] [PubMed]
12. Otero-Ortega, L.; Laso-García, F.; Gómez-de Frutos, M.; Fuentes, B.; Diekhorst, L.; Díez-Tejedor, E.; Gutiérrez-Fernández, M. Role of exosomes as a treatment and potential biomarker for stroke. *Transl. Stroke Res.* **2019**, *10*, 241–249. [CrossRef] [PubMed]
13. Pan, J.; Qu, M.; Li, Y.; Wang, L.; Zhang, L.; Wang, Y.; Tang, Y.; Tian, H.-L.; Zhang, Z.; Yang, G.-Y. MicroRNA-126-3p/-5p overexpression attenuates blood-brain barrier disruption in a mouse model of middle cerebral artery occlusion. *Stroke* **2020**, *51*, 619–627. [CrossRef] [PubMed]
14. Malone, K.; Amu, S.; Moore, A.C.; Waeber, C. The immune system and stroke: From current targets to future therapy. *Immunol. Cell Biol.* **2019**, *97*, 5–16. [CrossRef]
15. Wang, J.; Liu, H.; Chen, S.; Zhang, W.; Chen, Y.; Yang, Y. Moderate exercise has beneficial effects on mouse ischemic stroke by enhancing the functions of circulating endothelial progenitor cell-derived exosomes. *Exp. Neurol.* **2020**, *330*, 113325. [CrossRef]
16. Wang, F.; Tang, H.; Zhu, J.; Zhang, J.H. Transplanting mesenchymal stem cells for treatment of ischemic stroke. *Cell Transplant.* **2018**, *27*, 1825–1834. [CrossRef]

17. Iadecola, C.; Anrather, J. The immunology of stroke: From mechanisms to translation. *Nat. Med.* **2011**, *17*, 796–808. [CrossRef]
18. Kelly, P.J.; Murphy, S.; Coveney, S.; Purroy, F.; Lemmens, R.; Tsivgoulis, G.; Price, C. Anti-inflammatory approaches to ischaemic stroke prevention. *J. Neurol. Neurosurg. Psychiatry* **2018**, *89*, 211–218. [CrossRef]
19. Pascua-Maestro, R.; González, E.; Lillo, C.; Ganfornina, M.D.; Falcón-Pérez, J.M.; Sanchez, D. Extracellular vesicles secreted by astroglial cells transport apolipoprotein D to neurons and mediate neuronal survival upon oxidative stress. *Front. Cell. Neurosci.* **2019**, *12*, 526. [CrossRef]
20. Antonucci, F.; Turola, E.; Riganti, L.; Caleo, M.; Gabrielli, M.; Perrotta, C.; Novellino, L.; Clementi, E.; Giussani, P.; Viani, P. Microvesicles released from microglia stimulate synaptic activity via enhanced sphingolipid metabolism. *EMBO J.* **2012**, *31*, 1231–1240. [CrossRef]
21. Xu, B.; Zhang, Y.; Du, X.-F.; Li, J.; Zi, H.-X.; Bu, J.-W.; Yan, Y.; Han, H.; Du, J.-L. Neurons secrete miR-132-containing exosomes to regulate brain vascular integrity. *Cell Res.* **2017**, *27*, 882–897. [CrossRef] [PubMed]
22. Prada, I.; Gabrielli, M.; Turola, E.; Iorio, A.; D'Arrigo, G.; Parolisi, R.; De Luca, M.; Pacifici, M.; Bastoni, M.; Lombardi, M. Glia-to-neuron transfer of miRNAs via extracellular vesicles: A new mechanism underlying inflammation-induced synaptic alterations. *Acta Neuropathol.* **2018**, *135*, 529–550. [CrossRef] [PubMed]
23. Webb, R.L.; Kaiser, E.E.; Jurgielewicz, B.J.; Spellicy, S.; Scoville, S.L.; Thompson, T.A.; Swetenburg, R.L.; Hess, D.C.; West, F.D.; Stice, S.L. Human neural stem cell extracellular vesicles improve recovery in a porcine model of ischemic stroke. *Stroke* **2018**, *49*, 1248–1256. [CrossRef] [PubMed]
24. Xin, H.; Li, Y.; Cui, Y.; Yang, J.J.; Zhang, Z.G.; Chopp, M. Systemic administration of exosomes released from mesenchymal stromal cells promote functional recovery and neurovascular plasticity after stroke in rats. *J. Cereb. Blood Flow Metab.* **2013**, *33*, 1711–1715. [CrossRef]
25. Feng, J.; Waqas, A.; Zhu, Z.; Chen, L. Exosomes: Applications in respiratory infectious diseases and prospects for coronavirus disease 2019 (COVID-19). *J. Biomed. Nanotechnol.* **2020**, *16*, 399–418. [CrossRef]
26. Upadhya, D.; Shetty, A.K. Extracellular vesicles as therapeutics for brain injury and disease. *Curr. Pharm. Des.* **2019**, *25*, 3500–3505. [CrossRef] [PubMed]
27. Sun, X.; Jung, J.-H.; Arvola, O.; Santoso, M.R.; Giffard, R.G.; Yang, P.C.; Stary, C.M. Stem cell-derived exosomes protect astrocyte cultures from in vitro ischemia and decrease injury as post-stroke intravenous therapy. *Front. Cell. Neurosci.* **2019**, *13*, 394. [CrossRef] [PubMed]
28. Théry, C.; Witwer, K.W.; Aikawa, E.; Alcaraz, M.J.; Anderson, J.D.; Andriantsitohaina, R.; Antoniou, A.; Arab, T.; Archer, F.; Atkin-Smith, G.K.; et al. Minimal information for studies of extracellular vesicles 2018 (MISEV2018): A position statement of the International Society for Extracellular Vesicles and update of the MISEV2014 guidelines. *J. Extracell. Vesicles* **2018**, *7*, 1535750. [CrossRef]
29. Sáenz-Cuesta, M.; Arbelaiz, A.; Oregi, A.; Irizar, H.; Osorio-Querejeta, I.; Muñoz-Culla, M.; Banales, J.M.; Falcón-Pérez, J.M.; Olascoaga, J.; Otaegui, D. Methods for extracellular vesicles isolation in a hospital setting. *Front. Immunol.* **2015**, *6*, 50. [CrossRef]
30. Caby, M.P.; Lankar, D.; Vincendeau-Scherrer, C.; Raposo, G.; Bonnerot, C. Exosomal-like vesicles are present in human blood plasma. *Int. Immunol.* **2005**, *17*, 879–887. [CrossRef]
31. Lässer, C.; Alikhani, V.S.; Ekström, K.; Eldh, M.; Paredes, P.T.; Bossios, A.; Sjöstrand, M.; Gabrielsson, S.; Lötvall, J.; Valadi, H. Human saliva, plasma and breast milk exosomes contain RNA: Uptake by macrophages. *J. Transl. Med.* **2011**, *9*, 9. [CrossRef] [PubMed]
32. Akers, J.C.; Ramakrishnan, V.; Kim, R.; Phillips, S.; Kaimal, V.; Mao, Y.; Hua, W.; Yang, I.; Fu, C.C.; Nolan, J.; et al. miRNA contents of cerebrospinal fluid extracellular vesicles in glioblastoma patients. *J. Neuro-Oncol.* **2015**, *123*, 205–216. [CrossRef] [PubMed]
33. Choi, H.I.; Choi, J.P.; Seo, J.; Kim, B.J.; Rho, M.; Han, J.K.; Kim, J.G. Helicobacter pylori-derived extracellular vesicles increased in the gastric juices of gastric adenocarcinoma patients and induced inflammation mainly via specific targeting of gastric epithelial cells. *Exp. Mol. Med.* **2017**, *49*, e330. [CrossRef]
34. Wahlund, C.J.E.; Eklund, A.; Grunewald, J.; Gabrielsson, S. Pulmonary Extracellular Vesicles as Mediators of Local and Systemic Inflammation. *Front. Cell Dev. Biol.* **2017**, *5*, 39. [CrossRef] [PubMed]
35. Żmigrodzka, M.; Guzera, M.; Miśkiewicz, A.; Jagielski, D.; Winnicka, A. The biology of extracellular vesicles with focus on platelet microparticles and their role in cancer development and progression. *Tumor Biol.* **2016**, *37*, 14391–14401. [CrossRef]
36. Ciardiello, C.; Cavallini, L.; Spinelli, C.; Yang, J.; Reis-Sobreiro, M.; De Candia, P.; Minciacchi, V.R.; Di Vizio, D. Focus on extracellular vesicles: New frontiers of cell-to-cell communication in cancer. *Int. J. Mol. Sci.* **2016**, *17*, 175. [CrossRef]
37. Frydrychowicz, M.; Kolecka-Bednarczyk, A.; Madejczyk, M.; Yasar, S.; Dworacki, G. Exosomes–structure, biogenesis and biological role in non-small-cell lung cancer. *Scand. J. Immunol.* **2015**, *81*, 2–10. [CrossRef]
38. Barteneva, N.S.; Fasler-Kan, E.; Bernimoulin, M.; Stern, J.N.; Ponomarev, E.D.; Duckett, L.; Vorobjev, I.A. Circulating microparticles: Square the circle. *BMC Cell Biol.* **2013**, *14*, 15. [CrossRef]
39. Maxwell, D.S.; Pease, D.C. The electron microscopy of the choroid plexus. *J. Biophys. Biochem. Cytol.* **1956**, *2*, 467. [CrossRef]
40. Jorge, L.R. Morphological evidence for possible functional role of supra-ependymal nerves on ependyma. *Brain Res.* **1977**, *125*, 362–368. [CrossRef]
41. Cupédo, R. The surface ultrastructure of the habenular complex of the rat. *Anat. Embryol.* **1977**, *152*, 43–64. [CrossRef] [PubMed]

42. Chen, L.; Zhang, G.; Feng, S.; Xue, M.; Cai, J.; Chen, L.; Deng, Y.; Wang, Y.; Chinese Association of Neurorestoratology (Preparatory); China Committee of International Association of Neurorestoratology. Preparation and quality control standard of clinical-grade neural progenitor/precursor cells-derived exosomes (2022 China version). *J. Neurorestoratology* **2022**, *10*, 100001. [CrossRef]
43. Bianco, F.; Perrotta, C.; Novellino, L.; Francolini, M.; Riganti, L.; Menna, E.; Saglietti, L.; Schuchman, E.H.; Furlan, R.; Clementi, E. Acid sphingomyelinase activity triggers microparticle release from glial cells. *EMBO J.* **2009**, *28*, 1043–1054. [CrossRef] [PubMed]
44. Potolicchio, I.; Carven, G.J.; Xu, X.; Stipp, C.; Riese, R.J.; Stern, L.J.; Santambrogio, L. Proteomic analysis of microglia-derived exosomes: Metabolic role of the aminopeptidase CD13 in neuropeptide catabolism. *J. Immunol.* **2005**, *175*, 2237–2243. [CrossRef]
45. Belykh, E.; Shaffer, K.V.; Lin, C.; Byvaltsev, V.A.; Preul, M.C.; Chen, L. Blood-brain barrier, blood-brain tumor barrier, and fluorescence-guided neurosurgical oncology: Delivering optical labels to brain tumors. *Front. Oncol.* **2020**, *10*, 739. [CrossRef]
46. Chivet, M.; Javalet, C.; Laulagnier, K.; Blot, B.; Hemming, F.J.; Sadoul, R. Exosomes secreted by cortical neurons upon glutamatergic synapse activation specifically interact with neurons. *J. Extracell. Vesicles* **2014**, *3*, 24722. [CrossRef]
47. Chen, W.; Li, Q.; Zhang, G.; Wang, H.; Zhu, Z.; Chen, L. LncRNA HOXA-AS3 promotes the malignancy of glioblastoma through regulating miR-455-5p/USP3 axis. *J. Cell. Mol. Med.* **2020**, *24*, 11755–11767. [CrossRef]
48. Budnik, V.; Ruiz-Cañada, C.; Wendler, F. Extracellular vesicles round off communication in the nervous system. *Nat. Rev. Neurosci.* **2016**, *17*, 160–172. [CrossRef]
49. Zhang, Y.; Chopp, M.; Meng, Y.; Katakowski, M.; Xin, H.; Mahmood, A.; Xiong, Y. Effect of exosomes derived from multipluripotent mesenchymal stromal cells on functional recovery and neurovascular plasticity in rats after traumatic brain injury. *J. Neurosurg.* **2015**, *122*, 856–867. [CrossRef]
50. Alvarez-Erviti, L.; Seow, Y.; Yin, H.; Betts, C.; Lakhal, S.; Wood, M.J. Delivery of siRNA to the mouse brain by systemic injection of targeted exosomes. *Nat. Biotechnol.* **2011**, *29*, 341–345. [CrossRef]
51. Geffen, Y.; Perets, N.; Horev, R.; Yudin, D.; Oron, O.; Elliott, E.; Marom, E.; Danon, U.; Offen, D. Exosomes derived from adipose mesenchymal stem cells: A potential non-invasive intranasal treatment for autism. *Cytotherapy* **2020**, *22*, S49. [CrossRef]
52. Tsivion-Visbord, H.; Perets, N.; Sofer, T.; Bikovski, L.; Goldshmit, Y.; Ruban, A.; Offen, D. Mesenchymal stem cells derived extracellular vesicles improve behavioral and biochemical deficits in a phencyclidine model of schizophrenia. *Transl. Psychiatry* **2020**, *10*, 305. [CrossRef] [PubMed]
53. Doeppner, T.R.; Herz, J.; Görgens, A.; Schlechter, J.; Ludwig, A.-K.; Radtke, S.; de Miroschedji, K.; Horn, P.A.; Giebel, B.; Hermann, D.M. Extracellular Vesicles Improve Post-Stroke Neuroregeneration and Prevent Postischemic Immunosuppression. *Stem Cells Transl. Med.* **2015**, *4*, 1131–1143. [CrossRef] [PubMed]
54. Song, Y.; Li, Z.; He, T.; Qu, M.; Jiang, L.; Li, W.; Shi, X.; Pan, J.; Zhang, L.; Wang, Y.; et al. M2 microglia-derived exosomes protect the mouse brain from ischemia-reperfusion injury via exosomal miR-124. *Theranostics* **2019**, *9*, 2910–2923. [CrossRef]
55. Zheng, X.; Zhang, L.; Kuang, Y.; Venkataramani, V.; Jin, F.; Hein, K.; Zafeiriou, M.P.; Lenz, C.; Moebius, W.; Kilic, E. Extracellular Vesicles Derived from Neural Progenitor Cells—A Preclinical Evaluation for Stroke Treatment in Mice. *Transl. Stroke Res.* **2021**, *12*, 185–203. [CrossRef] [PubMed]
56. Long, J.; Gu, C.; Zhang, Q.; Liu, J.; Huang, J.; Li, Y.; Zhang, Y.; Li, R.; Ahmed, W.; Zhang, J. Extracellular vesicles from medicated plasma of Buyang Huanwu decoction-preconditioned neural stem cells accelerate neurological recovery following ischemic stroke. *Front. Cell Dev. Biol.* **2023**, *11*, 1096329. [CrossRef] [PubMed]
57. Webb, R.L.; Kaiser, E.E.; Scoville, S.L.; Thompson, T.A.; Fatima, S.; Pandya, C.; Sriram, K.; Swetenburg, R.L.; Vaibhav, K.; Arbab, A.S. Human neural stem cell extracellular vesicles improve tissue and functional recovery in the murine thromboembolic stroke model. *Transl. Stroke Res.* **2018**, *9*, 530–539. [CrossRef]
58. Chen, L. Exosomes Derived from Human Neural Stem Cell Improve Recovery in a Cynomolgus Monkey Model of Ischemic Stroke. *J. Neurosurg.* **2020**, *132*, 12.
59. Chen, K.-H.; Chen, C.-H.; Wallace, C.G.; Yuen, C.-M.; Kao, G.-S.; Chen, Y.-L.; Shao, P.-L.; Chen, Y.-L.; Chai, H.-T.; Lin, K.-C. Intravenous administration of xenogenic adipose-derived mesenchymal stem cells (ADMSC) and ADMSC-derived exosomes markedly reduced brain infarct volume and preserved neurological function in rat after acute ischemic stroke. *Oncotarget* **2016**, *7*, 74537. [CrossRef]
60. Lee, J.Y.; Kim, E.; Choi, S.-M.; Kim, D.-W.; Kim, K.P.; Lee, I.; Kim, H.-S. Microvesicles from brain-extract—Treated mesenchymal stem cells improve neurological functions in a rat model of ischemic stroke. *Sci. Rep.* **2016**, *6*, 1–14. [CrossRef]
61. Mahdavipour, M.; Hassanzadeh, G.; Seifali, E.; Mortezaee, K.; Aligholi, H.; Shekari, F.; Sarkoohi, P.; Zeraatpisheh, Z.; Nazari, A.; Movassaghi, S. Effects of neural stem cell-derived extracellular vesicles on neuronal protection and functional recovery in the rat model of middle cerebral artery occlusion. *Cell Biochem. Funct.* **2020**, *38*, 373–383. [CrossRef] [PubMed]
62. Lin, C.; Huang, S.; Zhang, J.; Yuan, H.; Yao, T.; Chen, L. Dl-3-N-butylphthalide attenuates hypoxic injury of neural stem cells by increasing hypoxia-inducible factor-1alpha. *J. Stroke Cerebrovasc. Dis.* **2022**, *31*, 106221. [CrossRef] [PubMed]
63. Safakheil, M.; Safakheil, H. The effect of exosomes derived from bone marrow stem cells in combination with rosuvastatin on functional recovery and neuroprotection in rats after ischemic stroke. *J. Mol. Neurosci.* **2020**, *70*, 724–737. [CrossRef] [PubMed]
64. Wiklander, O.P.; Nordin, J.Z.; O'Loughlin, A.; Gustafsson, Y.; Corso, G.; Mäger, I.; Vader, P.; Lee, Y.; Sork, H.; Seow, Y. Extracellular vesicle in vivo biodistribution is determined by cell source, route of administration and targeting. *J. Extracell. Vesicles* **2015**, *4*, 26316. [CrossRef]

65. Perets, N.; Betzer, O.; Shapira, R.; Brenstein, S.; Angel, A.; Sadan, T.; Ashery, U.; Popovtzer, R.; Offen, D. Golden exosomes selectively target brain pathologies in neurodegenerative and neurodevelopmental disorders. *Nano Lett.* **2019**, *19*, 3422–3431. [CrossRef]
66. Chen, W.; Wang, H.; Feng, J.; Chen, L. Overexpression of circRNA circUCK2 attenuates cell apoptosis in cerebral ischemia-reperfusion injury via miR-125b-5p/GDF11 signaling. *Mol. Ther.-Nucleic Acids* **2020**, *22*, 673–683. [CrossRef]
67. Cossetti, C.; Iraci, N.; Mercer, T.R.; Leonardi, T.; Alpi, E.; Drago, D.; Alfaro-Cervello, C.; Saini, H.K.; Davis, M.P.; Schaeffer, J. Extracellular vesicles from neural stem cells transfer IFN-γ via Ifngr1 to activate Stat1 signaling in target cells. *Mol. Cell* **2014**, *56*, 193–204. [CrossRef]
68. Hoshino, A.; Costa-Silva, B.; Shen, T.-L.; Rodrigues, G.; Hashimoto, A.; Tesic Mark, M.; Molina, H.; Kohsaka, S.; Di Giannatale, A.; Ceder, S.; et al. Tumour exosome integrins determine organotropic metastasis. *Nature* **2015**, *527*, 329–335. [CrossRef]
69. Zheng, T.; Pu, J.; Chen, Y.; Mao, Y.; Guo, Z.; Pan, H.; Zhang, L.; Zhang, H.; Sun, B.; Zhang, B. Plasma exosomes spread and cluster around β-amyloid plaques in an animal model of Alzheimer's disease. *Front. Aging Neurosci.* **2017**, *9*, 12. [CrossRef]
70. Orefice, N.S.; Souchet, B.; Braudeau, J.; Alves, S.; Piguet, F.; Collaud, F.; Ronzitti, G.; Tada, S.; Hantraye, P.; Mingozzi, F. Real-time monitoring of exosome enveloped-AAV spreading by endomicroscopy approach: A new tool for gene delivery in the brain. *Mol. Ther.-Methods Clin. Dev.* **2019**, *14*, 237–251. [CrossRef]
71. Elia, C.A.; Tamborini, M.; Rasile, M.; Desiato, G.; Marchetti, S.; Swuec, P.; Mazzitelli, S.; Clemente, F.; Anselmo, A.; Matteoli, M. Intracerebral injection of extracellular vesicles from mesenchymal stem cells exerts reduced Aβ plaque burden in early stages of a preclinical model of Alzheimer's disease. *Cells* **2019**, *8*, 1059. [CrossRef] [PubMed]
72. An, K.; Klyubin, I.; Kim, Y.; Jung, J.H.; Mably, A.J.; O'Dowd, S.T.; Lynch, T.; Kanmert, D.; Lemere, C.A.; Finan, G.M. Exosomes neutralize synaptic-plasticity-disrupting activity of Aβ assemblies in vivo. *Mol. Brain* **2013**, *6*, 47 . [CrossRef] [PubMed]
73. Gu, C.; Feng, J.; Waqas, A.; Deng, Y.; Zhang, Y.; Chen, W.; Long, J.; Huang, S.; Chen, L. Technological advances of 3D scaffold-based stem cell/exosome therapy in tissues and organs. *Front. Cell Dev. Biol.* **2021**, *9*, 709204. [CrossRef] [PubMed]
74. Zhang, Y.; Chopp, M.; Zhang, Z.G.; Katakowski, M.; Xin, H.; Qu, C.; Ali, M.; Mahmood, A.; Xiong, Y. Systemic administration of cell-free exosomes generated by human bone marrow derived mesenchymal stem cells cultured under 2D and 3D conditions improves functional recovery in rats after traumatic brain injury. *Neurochem. Int.* **2017**, *111*, 69–81. [CrossRef] [PubMed]
75. Betzer, O.; Perets, N.; Angel, A.; Motiei, M.; Sadan, T.; Yadid, G.; Offen, D.; Popovtzer, R. In vivo neuroimaging of exosomes using gold nanoparticles. *ACS Nano* **2017**, *11*, 10883–10893. [CrossRef] [PubMed]
76. Haney, M.J.; Klyachko, N.L.; Harrison, E.B.; Zhao, Y.; Kabanov, A.V.; Batrakova, E.V. TPP1 delivery to lysosomes with extracellular vesicles and their enhanced brain distribution in the animal model of batten disease. *Adv. Healthc. Mater.* **2019**, *8*, 1801271. [CrossRef]
77. Ni, H.; Yang, S.; Siaw-Debrah, F.; Hu, J.; Wu, K.; He, Z.; Yang, J.; Pan, S.; Lin, X.; Ye, H. Exosomes derived from bone mesenchymal stem cells ameliorate early inflammatory responses following traumatic brain injury. *Front. Neurosci.* **2019**, *13*, 14. [CrossRef]
78. Dabrowska, S.; Andrzejewska, A.; Strzemecki, D.; Muraca, M.; Janowski, M.; Lukomska, B. Human bone marrow mesenchymal stem cell-derived extracellular vesicles attenuate neuroinflammation evoked by focal brain injury in rats. *J. Neuroinflammation* **2019**, *16*, 1–15. [CrossRef]
79. Huang, H.; Bach, J.R.; Sharma, H.S.; Saberi, H.; Jeon, S.R.; Guo, X.; Shetty, A.; Hawamdeh, Z.; Sharma, A.; von Wild, K. The 2022 yearbook of Neurorestoratology. *J. Neurorestoratology* **2023**, *11*, 100054. [CrossRef]
80. Aboody, K.S.; Brown, A.; Rainov, N.G.; Bower, K.A.; Liu, S.; Yang, W.; Small, J.E.; Herrlinger, U.; Ourednik, V.; Black, P.M. Neural stem cells display extensive tropism for pathology in adult brain: Evidence from intracranial gliomas. *Proc. Natl. Acad. Sci. USA* **2000**, *97*, 12846–12851. [CrossRef]
81. Chen, W.; Wang, H.; Zhu, Z.; Feng, J.; Chen, L. Exosome-shuttled circSHOC2 from IPASs regulates neuronal autophagy and ameliorates ischemic brain injury via the miR-7670-3p/SIRT1 axis. *Mol. Ther.-Nucleic Acids* **2020**, *22*, 657–672. [CrossRef]
82. Otero-Ortega, L.; Laso-García, F.; Gómez-de Frutos, M.d.C.; Rodríguez-Frutos, B.; Pascual-Guerra, J.; Fuentes, B.; Díez-Tejedor, E.; Gutiérrez-Fernández, M. White matter repair after extracellular vesicles administration in an experimental animal model of subcortical stroke. *Sci. Rep.* **2017**, *7*, 44433. [CrossRef] [PubMed]
83. Zhao, T.; Sun, F.; Liu, J.; Ding, T.; She, J.; Mao, F.; Xu, W.; Qian, H.; Yan, Y. Emerging role of mesenchymal stem cell-derived exosomes in regenerative medicine. *Curr. Stem Cell Res. Ther.* **2019**, *14*, 482–494. [CrossRef] [PubMed]
84. Lin, C.-Q.; Chen, L.-K. Effect of differential hypoxia-related gene expression on glioblastoma. *J. Int. Med. Res.* **2021**, *49*, 03000605211013774. [CrossRef]
85. Gu, C.; Liu, J.; Li, Y.; Zhang, Q.; Lin, C.; Huang, J.; Duan, W.; Deng, Y.; Ahmed, W.; Li, R. Comparison of ketamine/xylazine and isoflurane anesthesia on the establishment of mouse middle cerebral artery occlusion model. *Exp. Anim.* **2023**, *72*, 209–217. [CrossRef] [PubMed]
86. Gómez-Molina, C.; Sandoval, M.; Henzi, R.; Ramírez, J.P.; Varas-Godoy, M.; Luarte, A.; Lafourcade, C.A.; Lopez-Verrilli, A.; Smalla, K.-H.; Kaehne, T. Small extracellular vesicles in rat serum contain astrocyte-derived protein biomarkers of repetitive stress. *Int. J. Neuropsychopharmacol.* **2019**, *22*, 232–246. [CrossRef]
87. Xin, H.; Li, Y.; Buller, B.; Katakowski, M.; Zhang, Y.; Wang, X.; Shang, X.; Zhang, Z.G.; Chopp, M. Exosome-mediated transfer of miR-133b from multipotent mesenchymal stromal cells to neural cells contributes to neurite outgrowth. *Stem Cells* **2012**, *30*, 1556–1564. [CrossRef]

88. Yu, Y.; Zheng, Y.; Dong, X.; Qiao, X.; Tao, Y. Efficacy and safety of tirofiban in patients with acute ischemic stroke without large-vessel occlusion and not receiving intravenous thrombolysis: A randomized controlled open-label trial. *J. Neurorestoratology* **2022**, *10*, 100026. [CrossRef]
89. van Rijt, S.; Habibovic, P. Enhancing regenerative approaches with nanoparticles. *J. R. Soc. Interface* **2017**, *14*, 20170093. [CrossRef]
90. Saleh, B.; Dhaliwal, H.K.; Portillo-Lara, R.; Shirzaei Sani, E.; Abdi, R.; Amiji, M.M.; Annabi, N. Local immunomodulation using an adhesive hydrogel loaded with miRNA-laden nanoparticles promotes wound healing. *Small* **2019**, *15*, 1902232. [CrossRef]
91. Tan, H.-L.; Teow, S.-Y.; Pushpamalar, J. Application of metal nanoparticle–hydrogel composites in tissue regeneration. *Bioengineering* **2019**, *6*, 17. [CrossRef] [PubMed]
92. Jahromi, M.; Razavi, S.; Seyedebrahimi, R.; Reisi, P.; Kazemi, M. Regeneration of Rat Sciatic Nerve Using PLGA Conduit Containing Rat ADSCs with Controlled Release of BDNF and Gold Nanoparticles. *J. Mol. Neurosci.* **2021**, *71*, 746–760. [CrossRef] [PubMed]
93. Huang, L.; Yang, X.; Deng, L.; Ying, D.; Lu, A.; Zhang, L.; Yu, A.; Duan, B. Biocompatible chitin hydrogel incorporated with PEDOT nanoparticles for peripheral nerve repair. *ACS Appl. Mater. Interfaces* **2021**, *13*, 16106–16117. [CrossRef]
94. Sun, D.; Zhuang, X.; Xiang, X.; Liu, Y.; Zhang, S.; Liu, C.; Barnes, S.; Grizzle, W.; Miller, D.; Zhang, H.-G. A Novel Nanoparticle Drug Delivery System: The Anti-inflammatory Activity of Curcumin Is Enhanced When Encapsulated in Exosomes. *Mol. Ther.* **2010**, *18*, 1606–1614. [CrossRef] [PubMed]
95. Zhuang, X.; Xiang, X.; Grizzle, W.; Sun, D.; Zhang, S.; Axtell, R.C.; Ju, S.; Mu, J.; Zhang, L.; Steinman, L.; et al. Treatment of Brain Inflammatory Diseases by Delivering Exosome Encapsulated Anti-inflammatory Drugs From the Nasal Region to the Brain. *Mol. Ther.* **2011**, *19*, 1769–1779. [CrossRef] [PubMed]
96. Tang, T.-T.; Lv, L.-L.; Wang, B.; Cao, J.-Y.; Feng, Y.; Li, Z.-L.; Wu, M.; Wang, F.-M.; Wen, Y.; Zhou, L.-T.; et al. Employing Macrophage-Derived Microvesicle for Kidney-Targeted Delivery of Dexamethasone: An Efficient Therapeutic Strategy against Renal Inflammation and Fibrosis. *Theranostics* **2019**, *9*, 4740–4755. [CrossRef]
97. Lang, F.M.; Hossain, A.; Gumin, J.; Momin, E.N.; Shimizu, Y.; Ledbetter, D.; Shahar, T.; Yamashita, S.; Parker Kerrigan, B.; Fueyo, J. Mesenchymal stem cells as natural biofactories for exosomes carrying miR-124a in the treatment of gliomas. *Neuro-Oncology* **2018**, *20*, 380–390. [CrossRef]
98. Monfared, H.; Jahangard, Y.; Nikkhah, M.; Mirnajafi-Zadeh, J.; Mowla, S.J. Potential therapeutic effects of exosomes packed with a miR-21-sponge construct in a rat model of glioblastoma. *Front. Oncol.* **2019**, *9*, 782. [CrossRef]
99. Piffoux, M.; Silva, A.K.A.; Wilhelm, C.; Gazeau, F.; Tareste, D. Modification of Extracellular Vesicles by Fusion with Liposomes for the Design of Personalized Biogenic Drug Delivery Systems. *ACS Nano* **2018**, *12*, 6830–6842. [CrossRef]
100. Kooijmans, S.A.A.; Fliervoet, L.A.L.; van der Meel, R.; Fens, M.H.A.M.; Heijnen, H.F.G.; van Bergen en Henegouwen, P.M.P.; Vader, P.; Schiffelers, R.M. PEGylated and targeted extracellular vesicles display enhanced cell specificity and circulation time. *J. Control. Release* **2016**, *224*, 77–85. [CrossRef]
101. O'Loughlin, A.J.; Mäger, I.; de Jong, O.G.; Varela, M.A.; Schiffelers, R.M.; El Andaloussi, S.; Wood, M.J.A.; Vader, P. Functional Delivery of Lipid-Conjugated siRNA by Extracellular Vesicles. *Mol. Ther.* **2017**, *25*, 1580–1587. [CrossRef]
102. de Abreu, R.C.; Ramos, C.V.; Becher, C.; Lino, M.; Jesus, C.; da Costa Martins, P.A.; Martins, P.A.; Moreno, M.J.; Fernandes, H.; Ferreira, L. Exogenous loading of miRNAs into small extracellular vesicles. *J. Extracell. Vesicles* **2021**, *10*, e12111. [CrossRef] [PubMed]
103. Liu, J.; Yi, K.; Zhang, Q.; Xu, H.; Zhang, X.; He, D.; Wang, F.; Xiao, X. Strong Penetration-Induced Effective Photothermal Therapy by Exosome-Mediated Black Phosphorus Quantum Dots. *Small* **2021**, *17*, 2104585. [CrossRef] [PubMed]
104. Kim, M.S.; Haney, M.J.; Zhao, Y.; Yuan, D.; Deygen, I.; Klyachko, N.L.; Kabanov, A.V.; Batrakova, E.V. Engineering macrophage-derived exosomes for targeted paclitaxel delivery to pulmonary metastases: In vitro and in vivo evaluations. *Nanomed. Nanotechnol. Biol. Med.* **2018**, *14*, 195–204. [CrossRef] [PubMed]
105. Haney, M.J.; Zhao, Y.; Jin, Y.S.; Li, S.M.; Bago, J.R.; Klyachko, N.L.; Kabanov, A.V.; Batrakova, E.V. Macrophage-derived extracellular vesicles as drug delivery systems for triple negative breast cancer (TNBC) therapy. *J. Neuroimmune Pharmacol.* **2020**, *15*, 487–500. [CrossRef] [PubMed]
106. Haney, M.J.; Klyachko, N.L.; Zhao, Y.; Gupta, R.; Plotnikova, E.G.; He, Z.; Patel, T.; Piroyan, A.; Sokolsky, M.; Kabanov, A.V.; et al. Exosomes as drug delivery vehicles for Parkinson's disease therapy. *J. Control. Release* **2015**, *207*, 18–30. [CrossRef]
107. Chen, C.; Sun, M.; Wang, J.; Su, L.; Lin, J.; Yan, X. Active cargo loading into extracellular vesicles: Highlights the heterogeneous encapsulation behaviour. *J. Extracell. Vesicles* **2021**, *10*, e12163. [CrossRef]
108. Ahmed, F.; Tamma, M.; Pathigadapa, U.; Reddanna, P.; Yenuganti, V.R. Drug loading and functional efficacy of cow, buffalo, and goat milk-derived exosomes: A comparative study. *Mol. Pharm.* **2022**, *19*, 763–774. [CrossRef]
109. Banerjee, A.; Alves, V.; Rondão, T.; Sereno, J.; Neves, Â.; Lino, M.; Ribeiro, A.; Abrunhosa, A.J.; Ferreira, L.S. A positron-emission tomography (PET)/magnetic resonance imaging (MRI) platform to track in vivo small extracellular vesicles. *Nanoscale* **2019**, *11*, 13243–13248. [CrossRef]
110. Lai, C.P.; Mardini, O.; Ericsson, M.; Prabhakar, S.; Maguire, C.A.; Chen, J.W.; Tannous, B.A.; Breakefield, X.O. Dynamic biodistribution of extracellular vesicles in vivo using a multimodal imaging reporter. *ACS Nano* **2014**, *8*, 483–494. [CrossRef]
111. Hwang, D.W.; Choi, H.; Jang, S.C.; Yoo, M.Y.; Park, J.Y.; Choi, N.E.; Oh, H.J.; Ha, S.; Lee, Y.-S.; Jeong, J.M. Noninvasive imaging of radiolabeled exosome-mimetic nanovesicle using 99mTc-HMPAO. *Sci. Rep.* **2015**, *5*, 15636. [CrossRef]

112. Kojima, R.; Bojar, D.; Rizzi, G.; Hamri, G.C.-E.; El-Baba, M.D.; Saxena, P.; Ausländer, S.; Tan, K.R.; Fussenegger, M. Designer exosomes produced by implanted cells intracerebrally deliver therapeutic cargo for Parkinson's disease treatment. *Nat. Commun.* **2018**, *9*, 1305. [CrossRef] [PubMed]
113. Geng, W.; Tang, H.; Luo, S.; Lv, Y.; Liang, D.; Kang, X.; Hong, W. Exosomes from miRNA-126-modified ADSCs promotes functional recovery after stroke in rats by improving neurogenesis and suppressing microglia activation. *Am. J. Transl. Res.* **2019**, *11*, 780.
114. Liao, X.; Gao, Z.; Xia, Y.; Zhai, W.; Pan, C.; Zhang, Y.; Yan, S.; Han, J. Micellization behavior of anionic gemini surfactants-templated manufacture of cerium oxide nanoparticles. *J. Dispers. Sci. Technol.* **2019**, *40*, 390–402. [CrossRef]
115. Schindler, C.; Collinson, A.; Matthews, C.; Pointon, A.; Jenkinson, L.; Minter, R.R.; Vaughan, T.J.; Tigue, N.J. Exosomal delivery of doxorubicin enables rapid cell entry and enhanced in vitro potency. *PLoS ONE* **2019**, *14*, e0214545. [CrossRef] [PubMed]
116. Shen, H.; Yao, X.; Li, H.; Li, X.; Zhang, T.; Sun, Q.; Ji, C.; Chen, G. Role of Exosomes Derived from miR-133b Modified MSCs in an Experimental Rat Model of Intracerebral Hemorrhage. *J. Mol. Neurosci.* **2018**, *64*, 421–430. [CrossRef]
117. Sterzenbach, U.; Putz, U.; Low, L.-H.; Silke, J.; Tan, S.-S.; Howitt, J. Engineered exosomes as vehicles for biologically active proteins. *Mol. Ther.* **2017**, *25*, 1269–1278. [CrossRef]
118. Wang, H.; Sui, H.; Zheng, Y.; Jiang, Y.; Shi, Y.; Liang, J.; Zhao, L. Curcumin-primed exosomes potently ameliorate cognitive function in AD mice by inhibiting hyperphosphorylation of the Tau protein through the AKT/GSK-3β pathway. *Nanoscale* **2019**, *11*, 7481–7496. [CrossRef]
119. Xin, H.; Katakowski, M.; Wang, F.; Qian, J.-Y.; Liu, X.S.; Ali, M.M.; Buller, B.; Zhang, Z.G.; Chopp, M. MicroRNA-17–92 cluster in exosomes enhance neuroplasticity and functional recovery after stroke in rats. *Stroke* **2017**, *48*, 747–753. [CrossRef]
120. Yim, N.; Ryu, S.-W.; Choi, K.; Lee, K.R.; Lee, S.; Choi, H.; Kim, J.; Shaker, M.R.; Sun, W.; Park, J.-H. Exosome engineering for efficient intracellular delivery of soluble proteins using optically reversible protein–protein interaction module. *Nat. Commun.* **2016**, *7*, 12277. [CrossRef]
121. Zheng, Y.; He, R.; Wang, P.; Shi, Y.; Zhao, L.; Liang, J. Exosomes from LPS-stimulated macrophages induce neuroprotection and functional improvement after ischemic stroke by modulating microglial polarization. *Biomater. Sci.* **2019**, *7*, 2037–2049. [CrossRef] [PubMed]
122. Tian, T.; Zhang, H.-X.; He, C.-P.; Fan, S.; Zhu, Y.-L.; Qi, C.; Huang, N.-P.; Xiao, Z.-D.; Lu, Z.-H.; Tannous, B.A.; et al. Surface functionalized exosomes as targeted drug delivery vehicles for cerebral ischemia therapy. *Biomaterials* **2018**, *150*, 137–149. [CrossRef] [PubMed]
123. Jia, G.; Han, Y.; An, Y.; Ding, Y.; He, C.; Wang, X.; Tang, Q. NRP-1 targeted and cargo-loaded exosomes facilitate simultaneous imaging and therapy of glioma in vitro and in vivo. *Biomaterials* **2018**, *178*, 302–316. [CrossRef] [PubMed]
124. Khongkow, M.; Yata, T.; Boonrungsiman, S.; Ruktanonchai, U.R.; Graham, D.; Namdee, K. Surface modification of gold nanoparticles with neuron-targeted exosome for enhanced blood–brain barrier penetration. *Sci. Rep.* **2019**, *9*, 8278. [CrossRef]
125. Kooijmans, S.A.; Aleza, C.G.; Roffler, S.R.; van Solinge, W.W.; Vader, P.; Schiffelers, R.M. Display of GPI-anchored anti-EGFR nanobodies on extracellular vesicles promotes tumour cell targeting. *J. Extracell. Vesicles* **2016**, *5*, 31053. [CrossRef] [PubMed]
126. Lee, J.; Lee, H.; Goh, U.; Kim, J.; Jeong, M.; Lee, J.; Park, J.-H. Cellular engineering with membrane fusogenic liposomes to produce functionalized extracellular vesicles. *ACS Appl. Mater. Interfaces* **2016**, *8*, 6790–6795. [CrossRef]
127. Nakase, I.; Futaki, S. Combined treatment with a pH-sensitive fusogenic peptide and cationic lipids achieves enhanced cytosolic delivery of exosomes. *Sci. Rep.* **2015**, *5*, 10112. [CrossRef]
128. Qi, H.; Liu, C.; Long, L.; Ren, Y.; Zhang, S.; Chang, X.; Qian, X.; Jia, H.; Zhao, J.; Sun, J. Blood exosomes endowed with magnetic and targeting properties for cancer therapy. *ACS Nano* **2016**, *10*, 3323–3333. [CrossRef]
129. Smyth, T.; Petrova, K.; Payton, N.M.; Persaud, I.; Redzic, J.S.; Graner, M.W.; Smith-Jones, P.; Anchordoquy, T.J. Surface functionalization of exosomes using click chemistry. *Bioconjugate Chem.* **2014**, *25*, 1777–1784. [CrossRef]
130. Zhang, H.; Wu, J.; Wu, J.; Fan, Q.; Zhou, J.; Wu, J.; Liu, S.; Zang, J.; Ye, J.; Xiao, M. Exosome-mediated targeted delivery of miR-210 for angiogenic therapy after cerebral ischemia in mice. *J. Nanobiotechnol.* **2019**, *17*, 29. [CrossRef]
131. Wang, M.; Altinoglu, S.; Takeda, Y.S.; Xu, Q. Integrating Protein Engineering and Bioorthogonal Click Conjugation for Extracellular Vesicle Modulation and Intracellular Delivery. *PLoS ONE* **2015**, *10*, e0141860. [CrossRef]
132. Yang, J.; Zhang, X.; Chen, X.; Wang, L.; Yang, G. Exosome mediated delivery of miR-124 promotes neurogenesis after ischemia. *Mol. Ther.-Nucleic Acids* **2017**, *7*, 278–287. [CrossRef] [PubMed]
133. Silva, A.K.A.; Luciani, N.; Gazeau, F.; Aubertin, K.; Bonneau, S.; Chauvierre, C.; Letourneur, D.; Wilhelm, C. Combining magnetic nanoparticles with cell derived microvesicles for drug loading and targeting. *Nanomed. Nanotechnol. Biol. Med.* **2015**, *11*, 645–655. [CrossRef]
134. Zhang, G.; Chen, L.; Guo, X.; Wang, H.; Chen, W.; Wu, G.; Gu, B.; Miao, W.; Kong, J.; Jin, X. Comparative analysis of microRNA expression profiles of exosomes derived from normal and hypoxic preconditioning human neural stem cells by next generation sequencing. *J. Biomed. Nanotechnol.* **2018**, *14*, 1075–1089. [CrossRef] [PubMed]
135. Wang, J.; Chen, S.; Zhang, W.; Chen, Y.; Bihl, J.C. Exosomes from miRNA-126-modified endothelial progenitor cells alleviate brain injury and promote functional recovery after stroke. *CNS Neurosci. Ther.* **2020**, *26*, 1255–1265. [CrossRef] [PubMed]
136. Wang, C.; Börger, V.; Sardari, M.; Murke, F.; Skuljec, J.; Pul, R.; Hagemann, N.; Dzyubenko, E.; Dittrich, R.; Gregorius, J. Mesenchymal Stromal Cell–Derived Small Extracellular Vesicles Induce Ischemic Neuroprotection by Modulating Leukocytes and Specifically Neutrophils. *Stroke* **2020**, *51*, 1825–1834. [CrossRef] [PubMed]

137. Laso-García, F.; Casado-Fernández, L.; Piniella, D.; Gómez-de Frutos, M.C.; Arizaga-Echebarria, J.K.; Pérez-Mato, M.; Alonso-López, E.; Otero-Ortega, L.; Bravo, S.B.; del Pilar Chantada-Vázquez, M. Circulating extracellular vesicles promote recovery in a preclinical model of intracerebral hemorrhage. *Mol. Ther.-Nucleic Acids* **2023**, *32*, 247–262. [CrossRef] [PubMed]
138. Ahn, S.Y.; Sung, D.K.; Kim, Y.E.; Sung, S.; Chang, Y.S.; Park, W.S. Brain-derived neurotropic factor mediates neuroprotection of mesenchymal stem cell-derived extracellular vesicles against severe intraventricular hemorrhage in newborn rats. *Stem Cells Transl. Med.* **2021**, *10*, 374–384. [CrossRef]
139. Gao, X.; Xiong, Y.; Li, Q.; Han, M.; Shan, D.; Yang, G.; Zhang, S.; Xin, D.; Zhao, R.; Wang, Z.; et al. Extracellular vesicle-mediated transfer of miR-21-5p from mesenchymal stromal cells to neurons alleviates early brain injury to improve cognitive function via the PTEN/Akt pathway after subarachnoid hemorrhage. *Cell Death Dis.* **2020**, *11*, 363. [CrossRef]
140. Ding, H.; Jia, Y.; Lv, H.; Chang, W.; Liu, F.; Wang, D. Extracellular vesicles derived from bone marrow mesenchymal stem cells alleviate neuroinflammation after diabetic intracerebral hemorrhage via the miR-183-5p/PDCD4/NLRP3 pathway. *J. Endocrinol. Investig.* **2021**, *44*, 2685–2698. [CrossRef]
141. Wang, J.; Chen, S.; Meghana Yerrapragada, S.; Zhang, W.; Bihl, J.C. Therapeutic effects of exosomes from angiotensin-converting enzyme 2 -overexpressed endothelial progenitor cells on intracerebral hemorrhagic stroke. *Brain Hemorrhages* **2021**, *2*, 57–62. [CrossRef]
142. Liao, K.; Niu, F.; Dagur, R.S.; He, M.; Tian, C.; Hu, G. Intranasal delivery of lincRNA-Cox2 siRNA loaded extracellular vesicles decreases lipopolysaccharide-induced microglial proliferation in mice. *J. Neuroimmune Pharmacol.* **2020**, *15*, 390–399. [CrossRef] [PubMed]
143. Xin, H.; Li, Y.; Chopp, M. Exosomes/miRNAs as mediating cell-based therapy of stroke. *Front. Cell. Neurosci.* **2014**, *8*, 377. [CrossRef]
144. Liu, Y.; Li, D.; Liu, Z.; Zhou, Y.; Chu, D.; Li, X.; Jiang, X.; Hou, D.; Chen, X.; Chen, Y. Targeted exosome-mediated delivery of opioid receptor Mu siRNA for the treatment of morphine relapse. *Sci. Rep.* **2015**, *5*, 17543. [CrossRef]
145. Ahmed, W.; Khan, A.; Sundar, W.H.; Naseem, H.; Chen, W.; Feng, J.; Durrani, S.; Chen, L. Neurological diseases caused by coronavirus infection of the respiratory airways. *Brain Sci. Adv.* **2020**, *6*, 324–343. [CrossRef]
146. Qi, Y.; Guo, L.; Jiang, Y.; Shi, Y.; Sui, H.; Zhao, L. Brain delivery of quercetin-loaded exosomes improved cognitive function in AD mice by inhibiting phosphorylated tau-mediated neurofibrillary tangles. *Drug Deliv.* **2020**, *27*, 745–755. [CrossRef] [PubMed]
147. Zhu, Q.; Ling, X.; Yang, Y.; Zhang, J.; Li, Q.; Niu, X.; Hu, G.; Chen, B.; Li, H.; Wang, Y.; et al. Embryonic stem cells-derived exosomes endowed with targeting properties as chemotherapeutics delivery vehicles for glioblastoma therapy. *Adv. Sci.* **2019**, *6*, 1801899. [CrossRef]
148. Yang, T.; Martin, P.; Fogarty, B.; Brown, A.; Schurman, K.; Phipps, R.; Yin, V.P.; Lockman, P.; Bai, S. Exosome delivered anticancer drugs across the blood-brain barrier for brain cancer therapy in Danio rerio. *Pharm. Res.* **2015**, *32*, 2003–2014. [CrossRef]
149. Hu, G.; Liao, K.; Niu, F.; Yang, L.; Dallon, B.W.; Callen, S.; Tian, C.; Shu, J.; Cui, J.; Sun, Z.; et al. Astrocyte EV-Induced lincRNA-Cox2 Regulates Microglial Phagocytosis: Implications for Morphine-Mediated Neurodegeneration. *Mol. Ther.-Nucleic Acids* **2018**, *13*, 450–463. [CrossRef]
150. Qu, M.; Lin, Q.; Huang, L.; Fu, Y.; Wang, L.; He, S.; Fu, Y.; Yang, S.; Zhang, Z.; Zhang, L.; et al. Dopamine-loaded blood exosomes targeted to brain for better treatment of Parkinson's disease. *J. Control. Release* **2018**, *287*, 156–166. [CrossRef]
151. Liu, J.; Duan, W.; Deng, Y.; Zhang, Q.; Li, R.; Long, J.; Ahmed, W.; Gu, C.; Qiu, Y.; Cai, H. New Insights into Molecular Mechanisms Underlying Neurodegenerative Disorders. *J. Integr. Neurosci.* **2023**, *22*, 58. [CrossRef] [PubMed]
152. Yong, T.; Zhang, X.; Bie, N.; Zhang, H.; Zhang, X.; Li, F.; Hakeem, A.; Hu, J.; Gan, L.; Santos, H.A. Tumor exosome-based nanoparticles are efficient drug carriers for chemotherapy. *Nat. Commun.* **2019**, *10*, 3838. [CrossRef] [PubMed]
153. Zhang, Z.G.; Buller, B.; Chopp, M. Exosomes—Beyond stem cells for restorative therapy in stroke and neurological injury. *Nat. Rev. Neurol.* **2019**, *15*, 193–203. [CrossRef] [PubMed]
154. Xu, L.; Yang, X.; Gao, H.; Wang, X.; Zhou, B.; Li, Y.; Li, L.; Guo, X.; Ren, L. Clinical efficacy and safety analysis of argatroban and alteplase treatment regimens for acute cerebral infarction. *J. Neurorestoratology* **2022**, *10*, 100017. [CrossRef]
155. Kim, H.Y.; Kim, T.J.; Kang, L.; Kim, Y.-J.; Kang, M.K.; Kim, J.; Ryu, J.H.; Hyeon, T.; Yoon, B.-W.; Ko, S.-B. Mesenchymal stem cell-derived magnetic extracellular nanovesicles for targeting and treatment of ischemic stroke. *Biomaterials* **2020**, *243*, 119942. [CrossRef] [PubMed]
156. Zhu, Z.; Kalyan, B.S.; Chen, L. Therapeutic potential role of exosomes for ischemic stroke. *Brain Sci. Adv.* **2019**, *5*, 128–143. [CrossRef]
157. Feng, J.; Zhang, Y.; Zhu, Z.; Gu, C.; Waqas, A.; Chen, L. Emerging exosomes and exosomal MiRNAs in spinal cord injury. *Front. Cell Dev. Biol.* **2021**, *9*, 703989. [CrossRef]
158. Xu, T.; Ma, Y.; Yuan, Q.; Hu, H.; Hu, X.; Qian, Z.; Rolle, J.K.; Gu, Y.; Li, S. Enhanced ferroptosis by oxygen-boosted phototherapy based on a 2-in-1 nanoplatform of ferrous hemoglobin for tumor synergistic therapy. *ACS Nano* **2020**, *14*, 3414–3425. [CrossRef]
159. Gu, C.; Zhang, Q.; Li, Y.; Li, R.; Feng, J.; Chen, W.; Ahmed, W.; Soufiany, I.; Huang, S.; Long, J. The PI3K/AKT Pathway—The Potential Key Mechanisms of Traditional Chinese Medicine for Stroke. *Front. Med.* **2022**, *9*, 900809. [CrossRef]
160. Moura, R.P.; Sousa, F.; Almeida, A.; Pinto, S.; Sarmento, B. Theranostic biomaterials for regulation of the blood–brain barrier. In *Theranostic Bionanomaterials*; Elsevier: Amsterdam, The Netherlands, 2019; pp. 303–319.
161. Yang, D.; Shao, J.; Hu, R.; Chen, H.; Xie, P.; Liu, C. Angiotensin II promotes the anticoagulant effects of rivaroxaban via angiotensin type 2 receptor signaling in mice. *Sci. Rep.* **2017**, *7*, 369. [CrossRef]

162. Doll, D.N.; Barr, T.L.; Simpkins, J.W. Cytokines: Their role in stroke and potential use as biomarkers and therapeutic targets. *Aging Dis.* **2014**, *5*, 294. [CrossRef]
163. Klimiec-Moskal, E.; Piechota, M.; Pera, J.; Weglarczyk, K.; Slowik, A.; Siedlar, M.; Dziedzic, T. The specific ex vivo released cytokine profile is associated with ischemic stroke outcome and improves its prediction. *J. Neuroinflamm.* **2020**, *17*, 7. [CrossRef] [PubMed]
164. Zhang, G.; Zhu, Z.; Wang, H.; Yu, Y.; Chen, W.; Waqas, A.; Wang, Y.; Chen, L. Exosomes derived from human neural stem cells stimulated by interferon gamma improve therapeutic ability in ischemic stroke model. *J. Adv. Res.* **2020**, *24*, 435–445. [CrossRef] [PubMed]
165. Chaudhuri, A.D.; Dastgheyb, R.M.; Yoo, S.-W.; Trout, A.; Talbot, C.C., Jr.; Hao, H.; Witwer, K.W.; Haughey, N.J. TNFα and IL-1β modify the miRNA cargo of astrocyte shed extracellular vesicles to regulate neurotrophic signaling in neurons. *Cell Death Dis.* **2018**, *9*, 363. [CrossRef] [PubMed]
166. Dickens, A.M.; Tovar-y-Romo, L.B.; Yoo, S.-W.; Trout, A.L.; Bae, M.; Kanmogne, M.; Megra, B.; Williams, D.W.; Witwer, K.W.; Gacias, M. Astrocyte-shed extracellular vesicles regulate the peripheral leukocyte response to inflammatory brain lesions. *Sci. Signal.* **2017**, *10*, eaai7696. [CrossRef]
167. Tian, Y.; Zhu, P.; Liu, S.; Jin, Z.; Li, D.; Zhao, H.; Zhu, X.; Shu, C.; Yan, D.; Dong, Z. IL-4-polarized BV2 microglia cells promote angiogenesis by secreting exosomes. *Adv. Clin. Exp. Med.* **2019**, *28*, 421–430. [CrossRef]
168. Zhu, Z.H.; Jia, F.; Ahmed, W.; Zhang, G.L.; Wang, H.; Lin, C.Q.; Chen, W.H.; Chen, L.K. Neural stem cell-derived exosome as a nano-sized carrier for BDNF delivery to a rat model of ischemic stroke. *Neural Regen. Res.* **2023**, *18*, 404–409. [CrossRef]
169. Attia, Z.I.; Kapa, S.; Lopez-Jimenez, F.; McKie, P.M.; Ladewig, D.J.; Satam, G.; Pellikka, P.A.; Enriquez-Sarano, M.; Noseworthy, P.A.; Munger, T.M. Screening for cardiac contractile dysfunction using an artificial intelligence–enabled electrocardiogram. *Nat. Med.* **2019**, *25*, 70–74. [CrossRef]
170. Su, Y.-L.; Kuo, L.-W.; Hsu, C.-H.; Chiang, C.-S.; Lu, Y.-J.; Chang, S.-J.; Hu, S.-H. Rabies virus glycoprotein-amplified hierarchical targeted hybrids capable of magneto-electric penetration delivery to orthotopic brain tumor. *J. Control. Release* **2020**, *321*, 159–173. [CrossRef]
171. Chivero, E.T.; Liao, K.; Niu, F.; Tripathi, A.; Tian, C.; Buch, S.; Hu, G. Engineered extracellular vesicles loaded with miR-124 attenuate cocaine-mediated activation of microglia. *Front. Cell Dev. Biol.* **2020**, *8*, 573. [CrossRef]
172. Yang, L.; Han, B.; Zhang, Z.; Wang, S.; Bai, Y.; Zhang, Y.; Tang, Y.; Du, L.; Xu, L.; Wu, F.; et al. Extracellular Vesicle-Mediated Delivery of Circular RNA SCMH1 Promotes Functional Recovery in Rodent and Nonhuman Primate Ischemic Stroke Models. *Circulation* **2020**, *142*, 556–574. [CrossRef] [PubMed]
173. Lindholm, P.; Saarma, M. Novel CDNF/MANF family of neurotrophic factors. *Dev. Neurobiol.* **2010**, *70*, 360–371. [CrossRef] [PubMed]
174. Houlton, J.; Abumaria, N.; Hinkley, S.F.; Clarkson, A.N. Therapeutic potential of neurotrophins for repair after brain injury: A helping hand from biomaterials. *Front. Neurosci.* **2019**, *13*, 790. [CrossRef]
175. Abe, K. Therapeutic potential of neurotrophic factors and neural stem cells against ischemic brain injury. *J. Cereb. Blood Flow Metab.* **2000**, *20*, 1393–1408. [CrossRef] [PubMed]
176. Khan, H.; Pan, J.-J.; Li, Y.; Zhang, Z.; Yang, G.-Y. Native and bioengineered exosomes for ischemic stroke therapy. *Front. Cell Dev. Biol.* **2021**, *9*, 619565. [CrossRef]
177. Ramos-Cejudo, J.; Gutiérrez-Fernández, M.; Otero-Ortega, L.; Rodríguez-Frutos, B.; Fuentes, B.; Vallejo-Cremades, M.T.; Hernanz, T.N.; Cerdán, S.; Díez-Tejedor, E. Brain-derived neurotrophic factor administration mediated oligodendrocyte differentiation and myelin formation in subcortical ischemic stroke. *Stroke* **2015**, *46*, 221–228. [CrossRef]
178. Lin, C.-Q.; Chen, L.-K. Cerebral dopamine neurotrophic factor promotes the proliferation and differentiation of neural stem cells in hypoxic environments. *Neural Regen. Res.* **2020**, *15*, 2057.
179. Donoso-Quezada, J.; Ayala-Mar, S.; González-Valdez, J. State-of-the-art exosome loading and functionalization techniques for enhanced therapeutics: A review. *Crit. Rev. Biotechnol.* **2020**, *40*, 804–820. [CrossRef]
180. Zhao, H.; Li, Y.; Chen, L.; Shen, C.; Xiao, Z.; Xu, R.; Wang, J.; Luo, Y. HucMSCs-derived miR-206-knockdown exosomes contribute to neuroprotection in subarachnoid hemorrhage induced early brain injury by targeting BDNF. *Neuroscience* **2019**, *417*, 11–23. [CrossRef]
181. Izadpanah, M.; Seddigh, A.; Ebrahimi Barough, S.; Fazeli, S.A.S.; Ai, J. Potential of Extracellular Vesicles in Neurodegenerative Diseases: Diagnostic and Therapeutic Indications. *J. Mol. Neurosci.* **2018**, *66*, 172–179. [CrossRef]
182. Morad, G.; Carman, C.V.; Hagedorn, E.J.; Perlin, J.R.; Zon, L.I.; Mustafaoglu, N.; Park, T.-E.; Ingber, D.E.; Daisy, C.C.; Moses, M.A. Tumor-derived extracellular vesicles breach the intact blood–brain barrier via transcytosis. *ACS Nano* **2019**, *13*, 13853–13865. [CrossRef] [PubMed]

pharmaceutics

MDPI

Article

Design of Dual-Targeted pH-Sensitive Hybrid Polymer Micelles for Breast Cancer Treatment: Three Birds with One Stone

Degong Yang [1,2], Ziqing Li [1], Yinghui Zhang [3], Xuejun Chen [1], Mingyuan Liu [3,*] and Chunrong Yang [1,*]

1 Department of Pharmacy, Shantou University Medical College, No. 22 Xinling Road, Shantou 515041, China
2 Guangdong Provincial Key Laboratory of Infectious Diseases and Molecular Immunopathology, Shantou University Medical College, No. 22 Xinling Road, Shantou 515041, China
3 Department of Pharmaceutical Sciences, Jiamusi University, 258 Xuefu Road, Jiamusi 154007, China
* Correspondence: yangchunrong@stu.edu.cn (M.L.); liumingyuan12@163.com (C.Y.)

Abstract: Breast cancer has a high prevalence in the world and creates a substantial socio-economic impact. Polymer micelles used as nano-sized polymer therapeutics have shown great advantages in treating breast cancer. Here, we aim to develop a dual-targeted pH-sensitive hybrid polymer (HPPF) micelles for improving the stability, controlled-release ability and targeting ability of the breast cancer treatment options. The HPPF micelles were constructed using the hyaluronic acid modified polyhistidine (HA-PHis) and folic acid modified Plannick (PF127-FA), which were characterized via ^{1}H NMR. The optimized mixing ratio (HA-PHis:PF127-FA) was 8:2 according to the change of particle size and zeta potential. The stability of HPPF micelles were enhanced with the higher zeta potential and lower critical micelle concentration compared with HA-PHis and PF127-FA. The drug release percents significantly increased from 45% to 90% with the decrease in pH, which illustrated that HPPF micelles were pH-sensitive owing to the protonation of PHis. The cytotoxicity, in vitro cellular uptake and in vivo fluorescence imaging experiments showed that HPPF micelles had the highest targeting ability utilizing FA and HA, compared with HA-PHis and PF127-FA. Thus, this study constructs an innovative nano-scaled drug delivery system, which provides a new strategy for the treatment of breast cancer.

Keywords: dual-targeted; pH-sensitive; hybrid polymer micelles; stability; breast cancer

Citation: Yang, D.; Li, Z.; Zhang, Y.; Chen, X.; Liu, M.; Yang, C. Design of Dual-Targeted pH-Sensitive Hybrid Polymer Micelles for Breast Cancer Treatment: Three Birds with One Stone. *Pharmaceutics* **2023**, *15*, 1580. https://doi.org/10.3390/pharmaceutics15061580

Academic Editor: Emanuela Fabiola Craparo

Received: 4 April 2023
Revised: 11 May 2023
Accepted: 19 May 2023
Published: 24 May 2023

1. Introduction

Breast cancer has become the most commonly diagnosed cancer in 2020, and the incidence is rising year after year. According to a report, the numbers of new breast cancer cases and deaths in the United States in 2021 were 284,200 and 43,600, respectively [1]. Breast cancer is mainly caused by malignant changes in the epithelium of breast ducts, which seriously affects the physical and mental health of female patients [2]. At present, there are a variety of treatment methods, such as surgery, radiotherapy, chemotherapy, and molecular targeted therapy. Among them, chemotherapy is an active treatment for all stages of breast cancer, which significantly prolongs the median survival of patients [3]. However, chemotherapeutic drugs along with killing the cancer cells, bring serious damages to the normal cells as well, thereby causing systemic toxicity [4]. Therefore, the development of a novel drug delivery system for targeted and controlled release of chemotherapeutic drugs to tumor sites has attracted widespread attention.

Nanocarriers are often applied for treating breast cancer [5]. An enzymatically transformable polymer-based nanotherapeutic approach containing colchicine and marimastat is developed to prevent malignant progression of metastatic breast cancer [6]. The exosome membrane coated nanoparticles containing cationic bovine serum albumin conjugated siS100A4 are designed, which significantly inhibits the growth of malignant breast cancer cells [7]. The active tumor targeting nanoparticles containing ferritin and a pH-sensitive molecular is developed to inhibit tumor cell growth and metastasis based on the combination of tumor immunity activation and ferritinophagy-cascade ferroptosis [8].

Polymer micelles are formed by the self-assembly of amphiphilic polymers, which have become one of the most attractive carriers of anticancer drugs [9] because polymeric micelles improve the solubility of insoluble drugs, reduce the toxicity of chemotherapeutic drugs, and improve the stability of drugs in biological media without losing activity [10,11]. However, maintaining the integrity of the polymer micelles in the circulation and for the drug release at the action site remain challenging [12]. The bloodstream causes the dilution of polymer micelles, thereby facilitating the premature release of the payload in the bloodstream [13]. When the temperature of the system is elevated above the glass transition temperature of the polymer micelles, the critical micelle concentration value is increased, which contributes to a liquid-like state of the micellar core and reduces stability [14]. Therefore, it is particularly important to design a safe and efficient polymer micelle for enhancing the stability, controlled release ability and targeting ability. A previous study showed that changing the surface charge of micelles with isomaltodextrin can improve stability [15]. Another study constructed the pH-sensitive polymeric micelles assembled for drug delivery by stereo complexation between PLLA-b-PLys and PDLA-b-mPEG [16]. To improve the targeting of micelles, yet another study devised a targeted polyelectrolyte complex micelle to deliver therapeutic nucleotides to inflamed endothelium in vitro by displaying the peptide VHPKQHR targeting VCAM-1 [17]. The obtained results highlight the urgent need to scientifically design efficient polymeric micelles for achieving the aforementioned three goals, that is, improved stability, controlled release ability and targeting ability.

This study aims to develop the dual-targeted pH-sensitive hybrid polymer micelles for improving the stability, controlled-release ability and targeting ability. A previous study demonstrated that hybrid micelles formed by mixing of two or more kinds of polymers exhibited higher stability than single-component polymer micelle [18,19]. Additionally, polyhistidine (PHis) was designed and synthesized for pH-sensitive controlled release [20]. In contrast, this study uses folic acid (FA) and hyaluronic acid (HA) to construct the dual-targeted polymer micelle. In a previous study, magnetic carbon nanospheres modified by FA were developed for the targeted delivery of adriamycin [21]. Sun constructed an HA-targeting drug delivery system based on a metal-organic skeleton for efficient antitumor therapy [22]. Taking these into account, this study prepared the mixed polymer micelles (HPPF) via HA-PHis and Plannick-FA (PF127-FA), which were shown in Figure 1. The anticancer activity of docetaxel (DTX) was five times higher than that of paclitaxel, but its water solubility was still poor, which did not achieve the concentration requirements of clinical application [23]. Therefore, it is expected to increase the solubility of DTX utilizing hybrid polymer micelles.

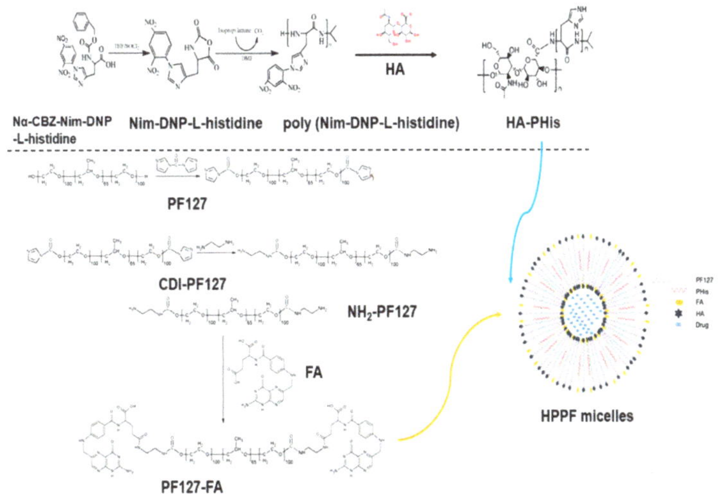

Figure 1. The structures of the mixed polymer micelles.

2. Materials and Methods

2.1. Materials, Cell Lines, and Animals

2.1.1. Materials

HA (*Mw* = 10,000), thionyl chloride, tetrahydrofuran, isopropylamine, N, N-Dimethy lformamide (DMF), N, N′-Carbonyldiimidazole (CDI), ethylenediamine and FA were obtained from Macklin Biochemical Co., Ltd. (Shanghai, China). N_{α}-CBZ-Nim-DNP-L-histidine, 1-Ethyl-3-(3-dimethylaminopropyl) carbodiimide (EDC), N-Hydroxysuccinimide (NHS) and N, N′-Dicyclohexylcarbodiimide (DCC) were obtained from GL Biochem Ltd. (Shanghai, China). PF127 was obtained from the BASF (Shanghai, China). DTX was obtained from the Jinhe Biotechnology Co., Ltd. (Shanghai, China). 3-(4,5-dimethyl-2-thiazolyl)-2,5-diphenyl tetrazolium bromide (MTT), coumarin 6 (Cou-6) and 4′,6-diamidino-2-phenylindole (DAPI) were obtained from Sigma (St. Louis, MO, USA).

2.1.2. Cell Lines and Animals

HepG2 (human liver cancer cells) and MCF-7 (human breast cancer cells) were purchased from the Cell Bank of the Chinese Academy of Sciences (Shanghai, China). All cells were cultured in DMEM medium (Gibco, Thermal Fisher, Lenexa, TX, USA) supplemented with 8% fetal bovine serum (Gibco, Thermal Fisher, Lenexa, TX, USA) and 1% penicillin-streptomycin in a humidified atmosphere of 95% air and 5% CO_2 at 37 °C, respectively.

Female BALB/c mice (18 ± 2 g) were purchased from the laboratory animal center of Shantou University Medical College (Shantou, China). All operational processes were carried out according to the NIH Guidelines for the Care and Use of Laboratory Animals and were approved by the Animal Ethics Committee of Shantou University Medical College (SUMC2022-152).

2.2. Synthesis and Characterization of HA-PHis

2.2.1. Synthesis and Characterization of Nim-DNP-L-Histidine

Briefly, Nα-CBZ-Nim-DNP-L-histidine was dissolved in anhydrous tetrahydrofuran, then thionyl chloride was added to react for 5 h. Finally, the products were obtained by filtration and recrystallization, and the structure was characterized using ^{1}H NMR.

2.2.2. Synthesis and Characterization of Poly (Nim-DNP-L-Histidine)

Nim-DNP-L-histidine was dissolved in DMF containing isopropylamine, and the solution was reacted under N_2 at room temperature for 4 days. Next, the solution precipitated in the cold diethyl ether. Finally, the poly (Nim-DNP-L-histidine) was obtained by solvent evaporation and characterized using ^{1}H NMR.

2.2.3. Synthesis and Characterization of HA-PHis

HA was dissolved in anhydrous formamide at 55 °C, then cooled to room temperature, then NHS and EDC were added to react for 2 h on ice. Subsequently, poly (Nim-DNP-L-histidine) was dissolved in DMF and added to HA solution to react for 48 h at room temperature. The mixture was dialyzed with distilled water for 3 days and lyophilized under vacuum. Next, the mixture was dissolved in anhydrous formamide containing mercaptoethanol to react for 48 h at room temperature for removing 2, 4-dinitrophenyl from poly (Nim-DNP-L-histidine). Finally, the HA-PHis were dialyzed with distilled water for 3 days and lyophilized. The structure of HA-PHis was characterized using ^{1}H NMR.

2.3. Synthesis and Characterization of PF127-FA

2.3.1. Synthesis and Characterization of CDI-PF127

An appropriate amount of PF127 was dissolved in acetone and precipitated by precooled n-hexane. The purified PF127 was obtained by vacuum drying, then dissolved in anhydrous acetonitrile. In addition, the CDI was dissolved in anhydrous acetonitrile, then slowly dripped into PF127 anhydrous acetonitrile solution within 2 h under nitrogen, for 4 h. Afterwards, it was concentrated by rotary evaporation and washed three times with precooled ether. The CDI-PF127 was collected by vacuum drying, and characterized using ^{1}H NMR.

2.3.2. Synthesis and Characterization of NH_2-PF127

CDI-PF127 was dissolved in anhydrous acetonitrile. The ethylenediamine was slowly dripped into the above solution within 3 h and stirred overnight at room temperature. The excess ethylenediamine was removed by rotary evaporation and washed with precooled ether three times. The white crystalline powder (NH_2-PF127) was obtained by vacuum drying, and characterized using ^{1}H NMR.

2.3.3. Synthesis and Characterization of PF127-FA

NH_2-PF127 was dissolved in anhydrous DMSO, then added to triethylamine as the liquid A. FA, NHS and DCC were dissolved in DMSO, and triethylamine was added and reacted for 10 h under magnetic stirring at room temperature (liquid B). Liquid B was slowly added to liquid A under the protection of nitrogen and stirred overnight at room temperature. The deionized water was slowly dripped into the reaction solution to remove the unreacted FA. The supernatant was dialyzed with deionized water for 3 days. The yellowish solid powder (PF127-FA) was obtained by freeze-drying, and characterized using ^{1}H NMR.

2.4. Preparation and Characterization of Micelles

HPPF micelles were prepared using the film dispersion method [24]. The copolymers were dissolved in acetonitrile, then dried. The mixing ratios of HA-PHis and PF127-FA were shown in Table 1. The optimized prescription of HPPF micelles was determined according to particle size and zeta potential. The particle size and zeta potential of HPPF micelles were determined via the Malvern particle size analyzer (Malvern, UK). The morphology of micelles was observed using transmission electron microscope (TEM).

Table 1. The mixing ratios of HA-PHis and PF127-FA.

Sample	HA-PHis:PF127-FA
A	9:1
B	8:2
C	7:3
D	6:4
E	5:5

The entrapment efficiency (*EE*%) and drug loading (*DL*%) of HPPF micelles were determined according to Formulas (1) and (2).

$$EE\% = (1 - \frac{C_{\text{free}}}{C_{\text{total}}}) \times 100\% \quad (1)$$

$$DL\% = \frac{W_{\text{drug}}}{W_{\text{lipid}}} \times 100\% \quad (2)$$

where, C_{free} was the concentration of free DTX (μg/mL); C_{total} was the total concentration of DTX in the suspension (μg/mL); W_{drug} was the amount of drugs encapsulated in HPPF micelles (mg); and W_{lipid} was the weight of mixed carrier material in the prescription (mg).

Pyrene was used to determine the critical micelle concentration (CMC) of HPPF micelles. When the polymer concentration was greater than a certain value, the excitation wavelength shifted from 334 nm to 336 nm. The different volumes of polymer solution were added to the pyrene, and the polymer concentration range was 10^{-4}–10^{-1} g/L.

2.5. In Vitro Drug Release

The drug-loaded micelles were added into the dialysis bag (interception of molecular weight: 12,000 Da), then placed in the PBS release medium. The medium was removed and the equal amount of fresh-release medium was replenished. The drug content in the release medium was determined via HPLC, and the cumulative release percent was calculated according to the Formula (3).

$$E_r = \frac{V_e \sum_{i-1}^{n-1} C_i + V_0 C_n}{m_{\text{drug}}} \quad (3)$$

where, E_r was cumulative drug release amount (%); V_e was replacement volume of PBS (mL); V_0 was total volume of release medium (mL); C_i was concentration of release solution during the *i* h displacement sampling (μg/mL); m_{drug} was total mass of drugs carried (mg); and *n* was number of replacement PBS.

2.6. Cytotoxicity

HepG2 and MCF-7 cells were chosen to evaluate cell cytotoxicity of blank HPPF and HPPF/DTX. The cell inoculation density was 6×10^4 cells·mL^{-1}, and the blank control group was the serum-containing medium group. The blank HA-PHis, blank PF127-FA, and blank HPPF (8:2) were added, and the concentration was 80, 40, 20, 10, and 5 μg·mL^{-1}, respectively. The HA-PHis/DTX, PF127-FA/DTX, and HPPF/DTX were added, and the concentration was 20, 15, 10, 5, 2, and 1 μg·mL^{-1}, respectively. The absorbance of wavelength 492 nm was determined using the enzyme-labeling instrument. The cell survival rate was calculated according to the Formula (4).

$$Cell\ survival\ rate\% = \frac{OD_{experimenta\ group}}{OD_{control\ group}} \quad (4)$$

where, *OD* was optical density.

2.7. *In Vitro Cellular Uptake*

HepG2 and MCF-7 cells in the logarithmic phase were inoculated at a concentration of 1×10^5 cells·mL^{-1}. Next, 100 μg·mL^{-1} of HA-PHis, PF127-FA, and HPPF containing coumarin-6 were added. DAPI was added for nucleus staining, and the cell uptake was observed using the laser confocal microscope.

2.8. *In Vivo Fluorescence Imaging and Tissue Distribution*

MCF-7/ADR tumor-bearing mice were injected with 200 μL HA-PHis, HPPF, and Dir fluorescence markers, respectively. At 0.5, 6, 12, 24, and 48 h, the fluorescence intensity of tumor site in mice was monitored using fluorescence imaging. After 48 h, the mice were killed and main organs (heart, liver, spleen, lung, kidney, and tumor) were washed with normal saline three times. Then, the fluorescence intensity of organ was measured.

2.9. *Statistical Analysis*

Results were expressed as mean ± S.D. The data were subjected to analysis of variance (ANOVA) using SPSS 21.0 software. $p < 0.05$ was taken as a significant level.

3. Results and Discussion

3.1. *Characterization of HA-PHis and PF127-FA*

According to the characteristic peaks in Figure 2a, δ_D = 9.18 ppm (-N=CH), δ_E = 7.71 ppm (-N-CH=C-), δ_G = 4.83 ppm (-CH-), and δ_F = 3.20 ppm (-CH_2-); thus indicating that NCA was synthesized successfully [25]. By comparing Figure 2a,b the appearance of isopropyl characteristic peak (δ_H = 0.79 ppm) indicated that PHis-DNP was formed [26]. The characteristic peaks in Figure 2c, δ_C 2.02 ppm (-$COCH_3$-), δ_D 1.30–1.39 ppm (-C-CH_3-), δ_B 7.34 ppm (-N-CH=C-) and δ_A 8.64 ppm (-N=CH-) indicated that HA-PHis was successfully synthesized [27].

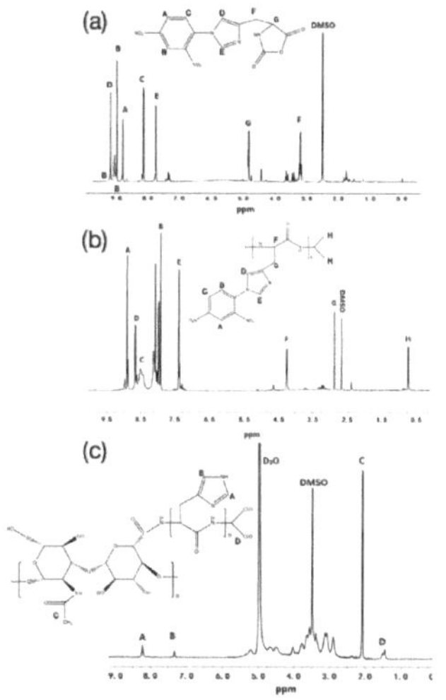

Figure 2. (**a**) ^{1}H-NMR spectrum of Nim-DNP-L-histidine, (**b**) ^{1}H-NMR spectrum of poly (Nim-DNP-L-histidine), (**c**) ^{1}H-NMR spectrum of HA-PHis.

The ^{1}H-NMR spectrum of PF127, FA, physical mixture of PF127 and FA, and PF127-FA were shown in Figure 3. The characteristic peaks of PF127 were δ_A 3.38 ppm ($CH_2CH(CH_3)O$), and δ_B 3.51 ppm ($CH_2CH(CH_3)O$). The characteristic peak shift of FA was δ_A 11.48 ppm (OH) [28]. The characteristic peak shift of physical mixture of PF127 and FA was 11.61 ppm, which illustrated that FA was covalently bound to PF127 [28]. In addition, the characteristic peak shift of OH (FA) disappeared, which proved that the COOH of FA interacted with the PF127 through the covalent bond. It proved that PF127-FA was synthesized.

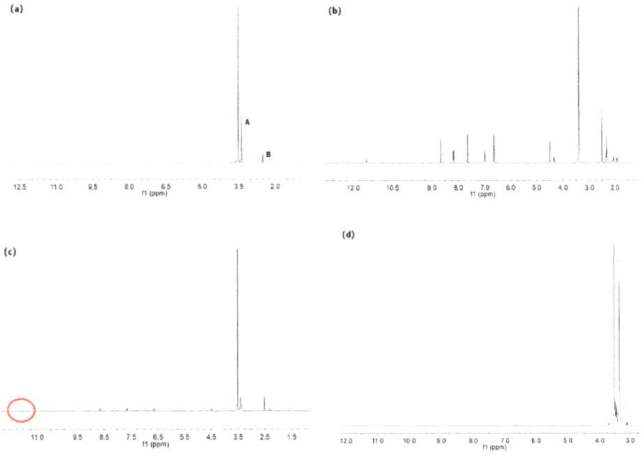

Figure 3. (**a**) ^{1}H-NMR spectrum of PF127, (**b**) ^{1}H-NMR spectrum of FA, (**c**) ^{1}H-NMR spectrum of physical mixture of PF127 and FA, (**d**) ^{1}H-NMR spectrum of PF127-FA.

3.2. *Characterization of Micelles*

3.2.1. Particle Size and Zeta Potential

The HPPF micelles were prepared using HA-PHis and PF127-FA, and particle size varied with the mass ratio of two block copolymers (Table 2). When the mass ratio was 5:5 and 6:4, two block polymers existed separately as single-component micelles. It demonstrated that they were not well assembled into hybrid polymer micelles [29]. When the mass ratio was 8:2 and 9:1, the hybrid polymer micelles with uniform particle size and good dispersion were formed. When the mass ratio was 9:1, the value of zeta potential was lower than that of 8:2. When the absolute value of zeta potential was higher, the electrostatic repulsive force between the particles was greater [30]. Therefore, the mixed micelles with a mass ratio of 8:2 was selected as the optimized prescription for next studies (PDI: 0.19 ± 0.06). In addition, the stability of HPPF (−17.4 ± 0.9 mV) was significantly enhanced compared with HA-PHis (−13.2 ± 7.8 mV) and PF127-FA (−8.5 ± 1.1 mV) ($p < 0.05$), which proved that the strategy using hybrid polymer micelles was successful.

Table 2. Particle size and zeta potential of polymer micelles ($n = 3$).

Sample	Particle Size (nm)	Zeta Potential (mV)	Single/Double Peak
HA-PHis	119.1 ± 7.7	−13.2 ± 7.8	Single peak
PF127-FA	40.0 ± 1.2	−8.5 ± 1.1	Single peak
A (9:1)	115.3 ± 6.1	−16.2 ± 0.8	Single peak
B (8:2)	119.6 ± 6.3	−17.4 ± 0.9	Single peak
C (7:3)	143.0 ± 6.3	−17.1 ± 3.2	Irregular single peak
D (6:4)	131.7 ± 7.0	−21.0 ± 2.5	Double peak
E (5:5)	122.3 ± 8.4	−19.2 ± 3.1	Double peak

3.2.2. Morphological Observation

The shape of HPPF/DTX and HA-PHis was observed using TEM and shown in Figure 4. The shape of HPPF/DTX was spherical and the distribution was uniform. The particle size of HPPF micelles was slightly larger than that of HA-PHis micelle. The reason was that PF127-FA and HA-PHis were self-assembled into HPPF micelles in an embedded form. The hydrophilic chain of HA-PHis was exposed owing to the long chain of PF127-FA, which caused the larger particle size [31].

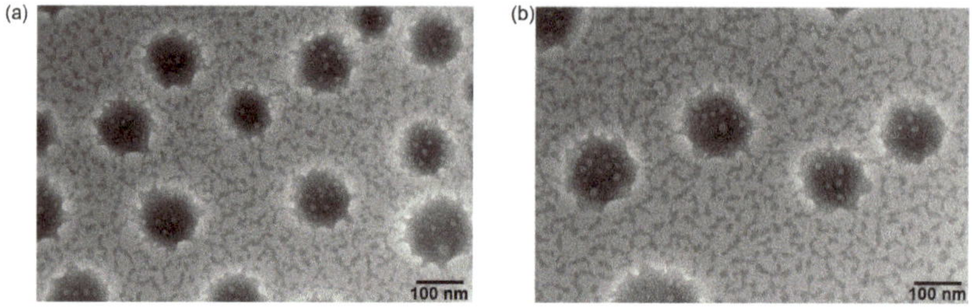

Figure 4. Morphological observation of HA-PHis (**a**) and HPPF/DTX (**b**) via TEM imaging.

3.2.3. Entrapment Efficiency and Drug Loading

The entrapment efficiency and drug loading of HPPF micelles were 87.2 ± 1.9% and 6.0 ± 0.1%, respectively, which were higher than HA-PHis (84.8 ± 2.1% and 4.2 ± 0.1%). The PF127-FA increased the proportion of hydrophobic blocks of the micelle core, which was beneficial to the loading of hydrophobic drugs (DTX). This study showed that the length of the hydrophobic blocks was closely related to drug loading [32]. Thus, HPPF micelles improved the poor solubility of DTX.

3.2.4. Determination of Critical Micelle Concentration

The aggregation behavior of HPPF micelles was investigated by measuring the fluorescence spectral curve of pyrene (Figure 5a). The critical micelle concentration of HPPF micelles was 0.04 mg·mL^{-1}. The lower critical micelle concentration was beneficial for the stability of micelles in vivo [33]. This study showed that the CMC value of micelles was an important factor that signified the stability, and that a lower CMC value provided greater solubilization of loaded payload [34].

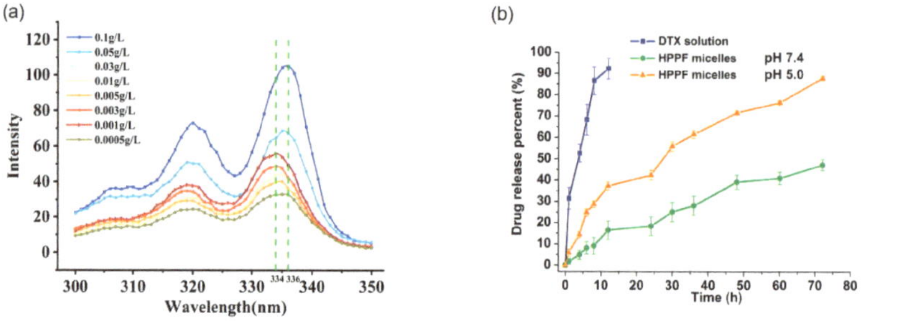

Figure 5. (**a**) The critical micelle concentration of HPPF micelles and (**b**) the drug release profiles from micelle.

3.2.5. In Vitro Drug Release

The in vitro drug release experiments were performed to investigate the pH-sensitive release of HPPF micelles in phosphate buffers with different pH values (7.4 and 5.0). As expected, more than 90% of the free drugs were released from DTX solution within 8 h at pH 7.4 (Figure 5b). However, within 72 h, only 45% of DTX was released from the HPPF micelles, which indicated that HPPF micelles ensured long-term stability in the bloodstream and prolonged the circulation time [35]. At pH 5.0, nearly 90% of DTX was liberated from the HPPF micelles within 8 h of incubation, which was in good agreement with previous studies [36]. The p*Ka* value of histidine was close to the tumor site acidic environment, which caused protonation and soluble transformation [37]. Hence, the pH sensitivity of PHis in HPPF micelles was confirmed. In addition, in vitro drug release behaviors were all consistent with the Higuchi model (r = 0.9545, r = 0.9573, and r = 0.9521), indicating that drugs were released through diffusion from the micelles [38]. In summary, the experiments proved the pH-sensitive behavior of the HPPF micelles.

3.3. *Cytotoxicity*

The effects of blank HA-PHis, PF127-FA and HPPF on the growth of HepG2 and MCF-7 cells were determined via MTT (Figure 6a,b). With the increase in the concentration, the survival rates of HepG2 and MCF-7 cells did not change significantly ($p > 0.05$), indicating that blank HA-PHis, PF127-FA and HPPF had no obvious cytotoxic effect on HepG2 and MCF-7 cells.

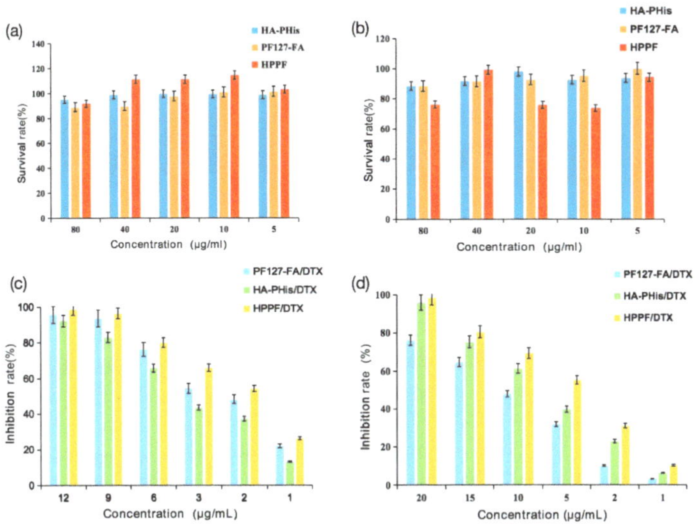

Figure 6. (**a**,**b**) Effects of concentration of blank carriers on HepG2 and MCF-7 cells survival rate ($n = 5$), (**c**,**d**) Effects of concentration of carriers containing DTX on cell survival rate in HepG2 and MCF-7 cells ($n = 5$).

Then, effects of micelles containing DTX on the cell survival rate in HepG2 and MCF-7 cells were evaluated and results were shown in Figure 6c,d. It was found that toxic effects were dependent on the concentration of micelles. For the HepG2 cells, the cytotoxicity of the micelles was ranked as follows: HPPF/DTX (IC_{50}: 1.7 μg/mL) > PF127-FA/DTX (IC_{50}: 2.5 μg/mL) > HA-PHis/DTX (IC_{50}: 4.6 μg/mL). This is because FA was specifically targeted on the surface of tumor cells, and FA receptor was highly expressed on the surface of tumor cells [39,40]. However, HA-PHis had no targeting ability to HepG2 cells owing to low expression of the CD44 receptor [41]. For the MCF-7 cells, the cytotoxicity of the micelles was ranked as follows: HPPF/DTX (IC_{50}: 4.2 μg/mL) > HA-PHis/DTX (IC_{50}: 7.7 μg/mL) > PF127-FA/DTX (IC_{50}: 10.3 μg/mL). HA-PHis had targeting ability to MCF-7 cells, because the CD44 receptor were overexpressed on the surface of the MCF-7 tumor [42]. Hence, the HPPF owned the highest targeting ability utilizing the FA and HA, which formed more DTX and killed tumor cells.

3.4. *In Vitro Cellular Uptake*

Cellular uptake of HPPF micelles were observed via laser confocal localization using HepG2 and MCF-7 cells. Coumarin-6 carrier was chosen as the probe. After incubation for 2 h, the fluorescence intensity of HepG2 cells was very dark, and the HPPF micelles were distributed in the cytoplasm of the cells, but not in the nucleus (Figure 7a). It was suggested that HPPF was swallowed into the cytoplasm by cells, but the uptake was very small [43]. The fluorescence intensity of MCF-7 cells was much stronger than that of HepG2 cells (Figure 7b). The HPPF micelles was mainly distributed in the cytoplasm, but not in the nucleus. The results showed that HPPF micelles were effectively swallowed endocytosis into the cytoplasm by MCF-7 cells. Additionally, the uptake was significantly higher than that of HepG2, which was in good agreement with the results of cytotoxicity. It also proved that only FA did not ensure that the prepared micelles were targeted to the tumor site. The previous study also proved that the conjugation of mesoporous silica nanoparticles with FA increased the efficiency of nanoparticles entering the cell and localization in the close vicinity of the nucleus [44]. The results of confocal microscopy proved that the HA-receptor mediated cellular uptake of redox-sensitive chitosan-based nanoparticle [45].

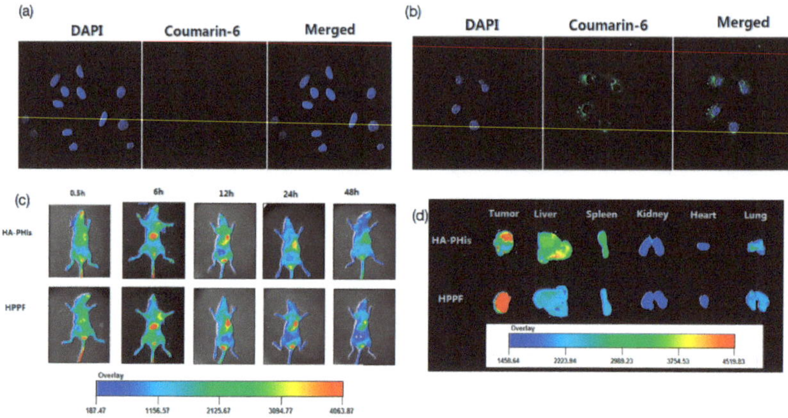

Figure 7. Cellular uptake of HPPF micelles using HepG2 (**a**) and MCF-7 cells (**b**), in vivo imaging results of HPPF micelles (**c**), the ex vivo images of organs (**d**).

3.5. In Vivo Fluorescence Imaging and Tissue Distribution

The targeting ability of HPPF micelles to tumors in mice was observed via in vivo fluorescence imaging. The HPPF micelles were distributed all over the body after injection for 0.5 h (Figure 7c). With the extension of time, the Dir fluorescence were transferred to the liver, spleen, and other organs. Additionally, the enhancement of fluorescence intensity indicated the accumulation of HPPF. After 12 h, the fluorescence intensity of tumor reached the peak, which was significantly higher than other tissues and organs. In addition, the HPPF fluorescence intensity of the tumor site was significantly higher than that in other organs, indicating good tumor targeting (Figure 7d). Compared with HPPF, the fluorescence intensity of HA-PHis was significantly weakened, indicating that HPPF increased the drug accumulation in tumor site and prolonged the accumulation time of drug in the tumor site. This is mainly attributed to the dual-targeted action of HA and FA, which effectively solved the off-target phenomenon. For example, the study developed high-efficiency dual-targeted nanoflowers containing ferroferric oxide and HA, which improved the specific uptake of drugs at tumor site by the dual action of CD44 ligand HA and magnetic nanoparticles guided by magnetic force [46].

4. Conclusions

In this study, a novel dual-target pH-sensitive HPPF hybrid micelle was successfully constructed. The optimal mixing ratio (HA-PHis: PF127-FA = 8:2) was obtained according to particle size and zeta potential. The HPPF micelles improved the stability with higher zeta potential and lower critical micelle concentration. The pH-sensitive release of HPPF micelles was demonstrated owing to histidine protonation. In vivo image demonstrated that the targeting ability of HPPF micelles was higher than FA and HA. In conclusion, this study provided a new strategy for the development of polymer micelle, which reduced the side effects of chemotherapeutic drugs and improved the treatment of breast cancer.

Author Contributions: Conceptualization, D.Y.; methodology, X.C. and Y.Z.; investigation, Z.L. and Y.Z.; writing—original draft preparation, D.Y.; writing—review and editing, C.Y.; project administration, C.Y.; funding acquisition, M.L. and C.Y. All authors have read and agreed to the published version of the manuscript.

Funding: This research was funded by the National Science Foundation of China (82273881 and 81874305, Chunrong Yang), Guangdong Basic and Applied Basic Research Foundation (2022A1515110476, Degong Yang), the Open Fund of Guangdong Provincial Key Laboratory of Infectious Diseases and Molecular Immunopathology (GDKL202214, Degong Yang) and SUMC Scientific Research Initiation Grant (510858046 and 510858056, Chunrong Yang and Degong Yang).

Institutional Review Board Statement: The animal study protocol was approved by the Animal Ethics Committee of Shantou University Medical College (protocol code SUMC2022-152 and 2022.08). for studies involving animals.

Informed Consent Statement: Not applicable.

Data Availability Statement: The data is unavailable due to privacy or ethical restrictions.

Conflicts of Interest: The authors declare no conflict of interest.

References

1. Siegel, R.L.; Miller, K.D.; Fuchs, H.E.; Jemal, A. Cancer statistics, 2021. *CA Cancer J. Clin.* **2021**, *71*, 7–33. [CrossRef]
2. Fujimoto, H.; Kazama, T.; Nagashima, T.; Sakakibara, M.; Suzuki, T.H.; Okubo, Y.; Shiina, N.; Fujisaki, K.; Ota, S.; Miyazaki, M. Diffusion-weighted imaging reflects pathological therapeutic response and relapse in breast cancer. *Breast Cancer* **2014**, *21*, 724–731. [CrossRef] [PubMed]
3. Early Breast Cancer Trialists' Collaborative Group (EBCTCG). Effects of chemotherapy and hormonal therapy for early breast cancer on recurrence and 15-year survival: An overview of the randomised trials. *Lancet* **2005**, *365*, 1687–1717. [CrossRef] [PubMed]
4. Truffi, M.; Mazzucchelli, S.; Bonizzi, A.; Sorrentino, L.; Allevi, R.; Vanna, R.; Morasso, C.; Corsi, F. Nano-strategies to target breast cancer-associated fibroblasts: Rearranging the tumor microenvironment to achieve antitumor efficacy. *Int. J. Mol. Sci.* **2019**, *20*, 1263. [CrossRef]
5. Rajana, N.; Mounika, A.; Chary, P.S.; Bhavana, V.; Urati, A.; Khatri, D.; Singh, S.B.; Mehra, N.K. Multifunctional hybrid nanoparticles in diagnosis and therapy of breast cancer. *J. Control. Release* **2022**, *352*, 1024–1047. [CrossRef] [PubMed]
6. Li, J.J.; Ge, Z.S.; Toh, K.; Liu, X.Y.; Dirisala, A.; Ke, W.D.; Wen, P.Y.; Zhou, H.; Wang, Z.; Xiao, S.Y.; et al. Enzymatically transformable polymersome-based nanotherapeutics to eliminate minimal relapsable cancer. *Adv. Mater.* **2021**, *33*, e2105254. [CrossRef]
7. Zhao, L.W.; Gu, C.Y.; Gan, Y.; Shao, L.L.; Chen, H.W.; Zhu, H.Y. Exosome-mediated siRNA delivery to suppress postoperative breast cancer metastasis. *J. Control. Release* **2020**, *318*, 1–15. [CrossRef] [PubMed]
8. Zuo, T.T.; Fang, T.X.; Zhang, J.; Yang, J.; Xu, R.; Wang, Z.H.; Deng, H.Z.; Shen, Q. pH-sensitive molecular-switch-containing polymer nanoparticle for breast cancer therapy with ferritinophagy-cascade ferroptosis and tumor immune activation. *Adv. Heal. Mater.* **2021**, *10*, e2100683. [CrossRef]
9. Tanner, P.; Baumann, P.; Enea, R.; Onaca, O.; Palivan, C.; Meier, W. Polymeric vesicles: From drug carriers to nanoreactors and artificial organelles. *Acc. Chem. Res.* **2011**, *44*, 1039–1049. [CrossRef]
10. Lee, S.W.; Yun, M.H.; Jeong, S.W.; In, C.H.; Kim, J.Y.; Seo, M.H.; Pai, C.M.; Kim, S.O. Development of docetaxel-loaded intravenous formulation, Nanoxel-PM™ using polymer-based delivery system. *J. Control. Release* **2011**, *155*, 262–271. [CrossRef]
11. Li, L.B.; Tan, Y.B. Preparation and properties of mixed micelles made of Pluronic polymer and PEG-PE. *Bioeng. J. Colloid. Interface Sci.* **2008**, *317*, 326–331. [CrossRef] [PubMed]
12. Biswas, S.; Kumari, P.; Lakhani, P.M.; Ghosh, B. Recent advances in polymeric micelles for anti-cancer drug delivery. *Eur. J. Pharm. Sci.* **2016**, *83*, 184–202. [CrossRef] [PubMed]
13. Hussein, Y.H.A.; Youssry, M. Polymeric micelles of biodegradable deblock copolymers: Enhanced encapsulation of hydrophobic drugs. *Materials* **2018**, *11*, 688. [CrossRef]
14. Kaur, j.; Mishra, V.; Singh, S.K.; Gulati, M.; Kapoor, B.; Chellappan, D.K.; Gupta, G.; Dureja, H.; Anand, K.; Dua, K.; et al. Harnessing amphiphilic polymeric micelles for diagnostic and therapeutic applications: Breakthroughs and bottlenecks. *J. Control. Release* **2021**, *334*, 64–95. [CrossRef] [PubMed]
15. Takagaki, R.; Ishida, Y.; Sadakiyo, T.; Taniguchi, Y.; Sakurai, T.; Mitsuzumi, H.; Watanabe, H.; Fukuda, S.; Ushio, S. Effects of isomaltodextrin in postprandial lipid kinetics: Rat study and human randomized crossover study. *PLoS ONE* **2018**, *13*, e0196802. [CrossRef] [PubMed]
16. Guo, Z.Y.; Zhao, K.; Liu, R.; Guo, X.L.; He, B.; Yan, J.Q.; Ren, J. pH-sensitive polymeric micelles assembled by stereocomplexation between PLLA-b-PLys and PDLA-b-mPEG for drug delivery. *J. Mater. Chem. B* **2019**, *7*, 334–345. [CrossRef]

17. Zhou, Z.J.; Yeh, C.F.; Mellas, M.; Oh, M.J.; Zhu, J.Y.; Li, J.; Huang, R.T.; Harrison, D.L.; Shentu, T.P.; Wu, D.; et al. Targeted polyelectrolyte complex micelles treat vascular complications in vivo. *Proc. Natl. Acad. Sci. USA* **2021**, *118*, e2114842118. [CrossRef]
18. Lin, M.H.; Dai, Y.; Xia, F.; Zhang, X.J. Advances in non-covalent crosslinked polymer micelles for biomedical applications. *Mater. Sci. Eng. C Mater. Biol. Appl.* **2021**, *119*, 111626. [CrossRef]
19. Luo, Y.L.; Yin, X.J.; Yin, X.; Chen, A.Q.; Zhao, L.L.; Zhang, G.; Liao, W.B.; Huang, X.X.; Li, J.; Zhang, C.Y. Dual pH/redox-responsive mixed polymeric micelles for anticancer drug delivery and controlled release. *Pharmaceutics* **2019**, *11*, 176. [CrossRef]
20. Tang, Q.; Zhao, D.L.; Yang, H.Y.; Wang, L.J.; Zhang, X.Y. A pH-responsive self-healing hydrogel based on multivalent coordination of $Ni2^{+}$ with polyhistidine-terminated PEG and IDA-modified oligochitosan. *J. Mater. Chem. B* **2019**, *7*, 30–42. [CrossRef]
21. Chen, L.; Zheng, J.; Du, J.L.; Yu, S.P.; Yang, Y.Z.; Liu, X.G. Folic acid-conjugated magnetic ordered mesoporous carbon nanospheres for doxorubicin targeting delivery. *Mater. Sci. Eng. C Mater. Biol. Appl.* **2019**, *104*, 109939. [CrossRef] [PubMed]
22. Sun, Q.Q.; Bi, H.T.; Wang, Z.; Li, C.X.; Wang, X.W.; Xu, J.T.; Zhu, H.; Zhao, R.X.; He, F.; Gai, S.L.; et al. Hyaluronic acid-targeted and pH-responsive drug delivery system based on metal-organic frameworks for efficient antitumor therapy. *Biomaterials* **2019**, *223*, 119473. [CrossRef]
23. Gao, K.; Sun, J.; Liu, K.; Liu, X.H.; He, Z.G. Preparation and characterization of a submicron lipid emulsion of docetaxel: Submicron lipid emulsion of docetaxel. *Drug Dev. Ind. Pharm.* **2008**, *34*, 1227–1237. [CrossRef] [PubMed]
24. Ghezzi, M.; Pescina, S.; Padula, C.; Santi, P.; Favero, E.D.; Cantù, L.; Nicoli, S. Polymeric micelles in drug delivery: An insight of the techniques for their characterization and assessment in biorelevant conditions. *J. Control. Release* **2021**, *332*, 312–336. [CrossRef] [PubMed]
25. Anson, C.E.; Briggs, J.C.; Haines, A.H.; Molinier, M. Synthesis of N-(2,4-dinitrophenyl) derivatives of D-ribosylamines; unexpected reaction and hydrolysis products. *Carbohydr. Res.* **2022**, *516*, 108564. [CrossRef]
26. Masila, V.M.; Ndakala, A.J.; Byamukama, R.; Midiwo, J.O.; Kamau, R.W.; Wang, M.; Kumarihamy, M.; Zhao, J.P.; Heydreich, M.; Muhammad, I. Synthesis, structural assignments and antiinfective activities of 3-O-benzyl-carvotacetone and 3-hydroxy-2-isopropyl-5-methyl- p-benzoquinone. *Nat. Prod. Res.* **2021**, *35*, 3599–3607. [CrossRef] [PubMed]
27. Chandrakala, M.; Gowda, N.M.N.; Murthy, K.G.S.; Nagasundara, K.R. Activation of -N=CH- bond in a Schiff base by divalent nickel monitored by NMR evidence. *Magn. Reason. Chem.* **2012**, *50*, 335–340. [CrossRef]
28. Rana, A.; Bhatnagar, S. Advancements in folate receptor targeting for anti-cancer therapy: A small molecule-drug conjugate approach. *Bioorg. Chem.* **2021**, *112*, 104946. [CrossRef]
29. Bae, Y.; Alani, A.W.G.; Rockich, N.C.; Chung Lai, T.S.Z.; Kwon, G.S. Mixed pH-sensitive polymeric micelles for combination drug delivery. *Pharm. Res.* **2010**, *27*, 2421–2432. [CrossRef]
30. Bhut, P.R.; Pal, N.; Mandal, A. Characterization of hydrophobically modified polyacrylamide in mixed polymer-gemini surfactant systems for enhanced oil recovery application. *ACS Omega* **2019**, *4*, 20164–20177. [CrossRef]
31. Naharros-Molinero, A.; Caballo-González, M.A.; de la Mata, F.J.; García-Gallego, S. Direct and reverse pluronic micelles: Design and characterization of promising drug delivery nanosystems. *Pharmaceutics* **2022**, *14*, 2628. [CrossRef] [PubMed]
32. Jia, L.; Wang, R.; Fan, Y. Encapsulation and release of drug nanoparticles in functional polymeric vesicles. *Soft Matter.* **2020**, *16*, 3088–3095. [CrossRef] [PubMed]
33. Lu, Y.; Yue, Z.G.; Xie, J.B.; Wang, W.; Zhu, H.; Zhang, E.; Cao, Z.Q. Micelles with ultralow critical micelle concentration as carriers for drug delivery. *Nat. Biomed. Eng.* **2018**, *2*, 318–325. [CrossRef]
34. Kaur, K.; Gulati, M.; Jha, N.K.; Disouza, J.; Patravale, V.; Dua, K.; Singh, S.K. Recent advances in developing polymeric micelles for treating cancer: Beakthroughs and bottlenecks in their clinical translation. *Drug Discov. Today* **2022**, *27*, 1495–1512. [CrossRef] [PubMed]
35. Xu, B.; Zhou, W.; Cheng, L.Z.; Zhou, Y.; Fang, A.P.; Jin, C.H.; Zeng, J.; Song, X.R.; Guo, X. Novel polymeric hybrid nanocarrier for curcumin and survivin shRNA co-delivery augments tumor penetration and promotes synergistic tumor suppression. *Front. Chem.* **2020**, *8*, 762. [CrossRef]
36. Di, Y.; Li, T.; Zhu, Z.H.; Chen, F.; Jia, L.Q.; Liu, W.B.; Gai, X.M.; Wang, Y.Y.; Pan, W.S.; Yang, X.G. pH-sensitive and folic acid-targeted MPeg-PhIs/Fa-Peg-Ve mixed micelles for the delivery of PTX-Ve and their antitumor activity. *Int. J. Nanomed.* **2017**, *12*, 5863–5877. [CrossRef]
37. Lee, E.S.; Na, K.; Bae, Y.H. Doxorubicin loaded pH-sensitive polymeric micelles for reversal of resistant MCF-7 tumor. *J. Control. Release* **2005**, *103*, 405–418. [CrossRef]
38. Khosroushahi, A.Y.; Naderi-Manesh, H.; Yeganeh, H.; Barar, J.; Omidi, Y. Novel water-soluble polyurethane nanomicelles for cancer chemotherapy: Physicochemical characterization and cellular activities. *J. Nanobiotechnology* **2012**, *10*, 2. [CrossRef]
39. Pan, Y.; Wang, Z.L.; Ma, J.L.; Zhou, T.P.; Wu, Z.; Ding, P.; Sun, N.; Liu, L.F.; Pei, R.J.; Zhu, W.P. Folic acid-modified fluorescent-magnetic nanoparticles for efficient isolation and identification of circulating tumor cells in ovarian cancer. *Biosensors* **2022**, *12*, 184. [CrossRef]
40. Al-Nemrawi, N.K.; Altawabeyeh, R.M.; Darweesh, R.S. Preparation and characterization of docetaxel-PLGA nanoparticles coated with folic acid-chitosan conjugate for cancer treatment. *J. Pharm Sci.* **2022**, *111*, 485–494. [CrossRef]
41. Yang, H.Y.; Du, J.M.; Jang, M.S.; Mo, X.W.; Sun, X.S.; Lee, D.S.; Lee, J.H.; Fu, Y. CD44-targeted and enzyme-responsive photo-cross-linked nanogels with enhanced stability for *in vivo* protein delivery. *Biomacromolecules* **2021**, *22*, 3590–3600. [CrossRef] [PubMed]

42. Hiscox, S.; Baruha, B.; Smith, C.; Bellerby, R.; Goddard, L.; Jordan, N.; Poghosyan, Z.; Nicholson, R.; Barrett-Lee, P.; Gee, J. Overexpression of CD44 accompanies acquired tamoxifen resistance in MCF7 cells and augments their sensitivity to the stromal factors, heregulin and hyaluronan. *BMC Cancer* **2012**, *12*, 458. [CrossRef]
43. Butt, A.M.; Abdullah, N.; Mat Rani, N.N.I.; Ahmad, N.; Mohd Amin, M.C.I. Endosomal escape of bioactives deployed via nanocarriers: Insights into the design of polymeric micelles. *Pharm. Res.* **2022**, *39*, 1047–1064. [CrossRef] [PubMed]
44. Miclea, L.C.; Mihailescu, M.; Tarba, N.; Brezoiu, A.M.; Sandu, A.M.; Mitran, R.A.; Berger, D.; Matei, C.; Moisescu, M.G.; Savopol, T. Evaluation of intracellular distribution of folate functionalized silica nanoparticles using fluorescence and hyperspectral enhanced dark field microscopy. *Nanoscale* **2022**, *14*, 12744–12756. [CrossRef] [PubMed]
45. Xu, W.; Wang, H.L.; Dong, L.H.; Zhang, P.; Mu, Y.; Cui, X.Y.; Zhou, J.P.; Huo, M.R.; Yin, T.J. Hyaluronic acid-decorated redox-sensitive chitosan micelles for tumor-specific intracellular delivery of gambogic acid. *Int. J. Nanomed.* **2019**, *14*, 4649–4666. [CrossRef]
46. Xiao, H.F.; Yu, H.; Wang, D.Q.; Liu, X.Z.; Sun, W.R.; Li, Y.J.; Sun, G.B.; Liang, Y.; Sun, H.F.; Wang, P.Y.; et al. Dual-Targeted Fe_3O_4@MnO_2 nanoflowers for magnetic resonance imaging-guided photothermal-enhanced chemodynamic/chemotherapy for tumor. *J. Biomed. Nanotechnol.* **2022**, *18*, 352–368. [CrossRef]

pharmaceutics

MDPI

Article

Influence of PEGDA Molecular Weight and Concentration on the In Vitro Release of the Model Protein BSA–FITC from Photo Crosslinked Systems

Natalia Rekowska [1], Katharina Wulf [1,2], Daniela Koper [1,3], Volkmar Senz [1], Hermann Seitz [4,5], Niels Grabow [1,5] and Michael Teske [1,*]

[1] Institute for Biomedical Engineering, University Medical Center Rostock, Friedrich-Barnewitz-Straße 4, 18119 Rostock, Germany
[2] Chair of Piston Machines and Internal Combustion Engines, University of Rostock, Albert-Einstein-Straße 2, 18059 Rostock, Germany
[3] Institute for Implant Technology and Biomaterials E.V., Friedrich-Barnewitz-Straße 4, 18119 Rostock, Germany
[4] Microfluidics, Faculty of Mechanical Engineering and Marine Technology, University of Rostock, Justus-von-Liebig-Weg 6, 18059 Rostock, Germany
[5] Department LL&M, Interdisciplinary Faculty, University of Rostock, Albert-Einstein-Str. 25, 18059 Rostock, Germany
* Correspondence: michael.teske@uni-rostock.de

Abstract: Novel 3D printing techniques enable the development of medical devices with drug delivery systems that are tailored to the patient in terms of scaffold shape and the desired pharmaceutically active substance release. Gentle curing methods such as photopolymerization are also relevant for the incorporation of potent and sensitive drugs including proteins. However, retaining the pharmaceutical functions of proteins remains challenging due to the possible crosslinking between the functional groups of proteins, and the used photopolymers such as acrylates. In this work, the in vitro release of the model protein drug, albumin–fluorescein isothiocyanate conjugate (BSA–FITC) from differently composed, photopolymerized poly(ethylene) glycol diacrylate (PEGDA), an often employed, nontoxic, easily curable resin, was investigated. Different PEGDA concentrations in water (20, 30, and 40 wt %) and their different molecular masses (4000, 10,000, and 20,000 g/mol) were used to prepare a protein carrier with photopolymerization and molding. The viscosity measurements of photomonomer solutions revealed exponentially increasing values with increasing PEGDA concentration and molecular mass. Polymerized samples showed increasing medium uptake with an increasing molecular mass and decreasing uptake with increasing PEGDA content. Therefore, the modification of the inner network resulted in the most swollen samples (20 wt %) also releasing the highest amount of incorporated BSA–FITC for all PEGDA molecular masses.

Keywords: drug delivery systems; 3D printing; photopolymerization; PEGDA; BSA–FITC; drug release

Citation: Rekowska, N.; Wulf, K.; Koper, D.; Senz, V.; Seitz, H.; Grabow, N.; Teske, M. Influence of PEGDA Molecular Weight and Concentration on the In Vitro Release of the Model Protein BSA–FITC from Photo Crosslinked Systems. *Pharmaceutics* **2023**, *15*, 1039. https://doi.org/10.3390/pharmaceutics15041039

Academic Editors: Ping Hu and Zheng Cai

Received: 17 February 2023
Revised: 20 March 2023
Accepted: 21 March 2023
Published: 23 March 2023

1. Introduction

Drug delivery systems (DDS) function as medical products that introduce a pharmaceutically active agent systemically or locally to the body in a highly controlled manner. In comparison with traditional enteral or parenteral routes of administration, they ensure the effectiveness and safety of the treatment with minor side effects. Furthermore, the application of DDS offers various possibilities regarding individual patient-tailored pharmaceutical therapies that are optimal for various persons and medical purposes. Although many approved DDSs have been successfully implemented as medications, recent advances in this research field reveal the great potential of this approach in the pharmaceutical sciences [1–4].

Among different techniques, 3D printing technologies enable the production of digitally designed, personalized, and complex DDS scaffolds that can also be precisely crafted as on-demand products [5–7]. In the future, these techniques should facilitate THE fabrication of numerous constructs with variable doses and release profiles specified for a particular person. They should also enable production of multidrug DDSs, which are difficult to achieve in traditional dosage formulations. Examples of such 3D-printed, multisubstance preparations can be found in the literature [8,9]. These flexible techniques are also studied as a tool for the preparation of medications for unique groups such as children [10] and patients requiring local treatment such as cancer therapy to avoid broad systemic side effects [11].

A common and promising 3D printing technique is stereolithography, employing photopolymerization in the manufacturing process, and it is versatile, cost-effective, and rapid [12–15]. In this method, drug carriers are hydrogels that are prepared via the solidification of photopolymers via free-radical-initiated chain polymerization reaction. Briefly, in the presence of a light source and a photoinitiator (PI), free radicals are formed. These excited molecules react with the acrylate or vinyl groups of the photopolymers, resulting in covalent crosslinking between polymer chains [16,17].

Stereolithography is a tool that allows for both the creation of personalized medication and the effective administration of very attractive and potent, but also challenging therapeutic agents such as proteins. Proteins are susceptible to protease degradation and other inactivating factors under physiological conditions. This is why alternatives to traditional routes of administration, enhancing their bioavailability, such as drug delivery systems are intensively investigated [18–20]. Stereolithography is also a gentle and accurate curing technique for DDSs releasing thermolabile substances such as proteins and should be thoroughly investigated in this context [21]. Understanding the factors influencing the photopolymerization process and the characteristics of a polymer material is crucial for the design of novel, patient-tailored, highly controllable DDS devices [19]. Most of the studies employing stereolithography as a DDS preparation method focused on the incorporation of small, synthetic molecules without photo-cross-linkable groups such as ibuprofen, paracetamol, aspirin, ketoprofen, caffeine, or prednisolone [22–24].

In this study, we investigate the well-established photopolymerizable poly(ethylene) glycol diacrylate (PEGDA), differing in molecular mass (4000, 10,000, and 20,000 g/mol), as a carrier for model protein drug albumin–fluorescein isothiocyanate conjugate (BSA–FITC). BSA–FITC was used as the model drug because it has a similar molecular mass and structure to those of bone morphogenetic protein (BMP-2), and exhibits similar binding affinity to collagen type as that of some other growth factors [25,26]. PEGDA, as a biocompatible and hydrophilic compound, is often studied for different biomedical applications such as 3D printing techniques [25–28]. Moreover, examples of PEGDA scaffolds as DDS incorporating peptide active agents were reported [29,30]. Loading a protein through matrix swelling is a gentle process that does not affect the protein structure. Preparing protein-releasing DDSs with methods employing photopolymerization remains challenging due to the possible crosslinking between the reactive groups of the polymer, such as acrylate and vinyl groups, and proteins, such as amino and sulfhydryl groups [31,32]. Previous studies showed that the modulation of the inner structure of the PEGDA network via the combination of different monomer masses fundamentally impacts the biophysical properties of the scaffold and could crucially influence water diffusion rates [27,33]. This indicates that altering the molecular mass and polymer concentration in the matrix determines the mechanical hydrogel properties such as softness and protein drug release via diffusion through the scaffolds [34]. Therefore, here, we investigate the in vitro BSA–FITC release to present the drug release profiles of differently composed matrices. BSA–FITC was chosen as a model drug due to the high sensitivity of fluorescent quantification [35,36]. The intramolecular quenching effect that alters the fluorescent emission and is characteristic for fluorescently labeled ligands can be overcome with a simple proteolytic procedure [37]. We also analyzed other important hydrogel characteristics such as the swelling ratio and thermal behavior of the prepared DDS. Additionally, the rheological behavior of the unpolymerized photopolymers was examined. Such considerations are essential to recognize the potential of the generated biomaterial for particular medical applications, and are necessary to predict their compatibility with 3D printing devices.

2. Materials and Methods

2.1. Materials

Poly(ethyleneglycol) diacrylate M_w = 4000 g/mol ($PEGDA_{4000}$), poly(ethyleneglycol) diacrylate M_w = 10,000 g/mol ($PEGDA_{10000}$), poly(ethyleneglycol) diacrylate M_w = 20,000 g/mol ($PEGDA_{20000}$), pronase from *Streptomyces griseus*, albumin–fluorescein isothiocyanate conjugate (BSA–FITC), photoinitiator (PI) lithium phenyl-2,4,6-trimethylbenzoylphosphinate (LAP), and buffer components N-[tris(hydroxymethyl)methyl]-2-aminoethansulfonsäure (TES), NaCl, KCl, and CaCl2 were all purchased from Merck KGaA (Darmstadt, Germany).

2.2. TES Buffer Preparation

The TES buffer was prepared by dissolving 30 mM TES, 140 mM NaCl, 4 mM KCl, and 10 mM $CaCl_2$ in purified water, and adjusting the pH to 7.5.

2.3. PEGDA Polymerization

Samples were prepared from 20, 30, or 40 wt % of $PEGDA_{4000}$, $PEGDA_{10000}$, or $PEGDA_{20000}$ in water/methanol (1:2) (*w/w*) solutions. Each sample contained 0.5% (*w/w*) LAP as PI and 0.075% (*w/w*) of BSA–FITC as the model drug (both referring to PEGDA amount).

Samples were prepared in a silicone holder that we produced to form cylinder samples (Ø = 6 mm, h = 1 mm). The solutions were carefully pipetted into the wells of the silicone holder on the laboratory scales (KERN 770, Frommern, Germany) to ensure the same polymer amount in each sample. The samples were polymerized in the UV chamber (CL-1000L, UVP, Upland, CA, USA) at λ = 365 nm for 10 min, and dried for 24 h in the vacuum chamber.

2.4. Morphology Analysis

Scanning electron microscopy (SEM) images were obtained with the use of Quanta FEG 250 (FEI GmbH, Dreieich, Germany) under 50 Pa and 3 kV. A secondary Everhart–Thornley electron detector (ETD) was used. Image magnification ranged from 50× to 1000×.

2.5. Differential Scanning Calorimetry

Thermal analysis was carried out with a DSC1 (Mettler Toledo GmbH, Greifensee, Switzerland) under a nitrogen purge. High-purity indium and zinc were used for temperature calibration, and an indium standard was used to calibrate the fusion heat (ΔH). The weights of the samples ranged from 10 to 20 mg. We used the $-50 \rightarrow 200 \rightarrow -50 \rightarrow 250$ °C temperature profile for the measurements with a heating rate of q = 10 K/min (n = 3). The data were analyzed with respect to melting temperature (T_m). Due to the focus on the drug release properties of the generated systems, we used the first heating cycle for analysis.

2.6. Swelling Behavior Evaluation

The swelling behavior of the hydrogels was studied in the TES buffer at 37 °C. Disk samples (Ø = 6 mm) were weighed before and after 24 h of swelling. The swelling behavior was tested separately 3 times for each hydrogel (n = 3).

2.7. Rheological Measurements

The viscosity of 20, 30, and 40 wt % of $PEGDA_{4000}$, $PEGDA_{10000}$ and $PEGDA_{20000}$ dissolved in water/methanol (1:2) without the addition of the model drug and PI was characterized using rotary rheometer Haake Rheostress 1 (Thermo Scientific, Karlsruhe,

Germany) and a 1° cone with plate geometry. For the applied shear rates, a gradient from 100 to 300 s^{-1} shear stress of each PEGDA solution was measured at 15 °C (n = 3), and the viscosity values were calculated from the Newtonian conditional equation by dividing shear stress τ by the corresponding shear rate γ.

2.8. In Vitro Release of BSA–FITC

The in vitro drug release of BSA–FITC was separately conducted for each sample (Ø = 6 mm, h = 1 mm) in 1 mL TES at 37 °C and shaking with 100 rpm in the dark. The release was performed for over 1032 h (43 days) with complete medium exchange at particular time points. In order to avoid the quenching effect of FITC, the release was followed by the digestive procedure with pronase described by Breen et al. [37]. Briefly, each medium sample was treated with pronase from Streptomyces griseus (100 µg per sample) and incubated in the dark for 72 h before fluorescent determination at 37 °C. The residual release of BSA–FITC was determined by solving the sample in formic acid, followed by freeze-drying to remove the acid and the uptake of the residues in TES and the described digestion by pronase procedure. Standard calibration solutions of BSA–FITC were prepared in TES.

The fluorescent BSA–FITC determination was performed in black 96-well plates (Greiner Bio-One 655086, Frickenhausen, Germany) with Fluostar Optima (BMG LABTECH, Ortenberg, Germany), with excitation at 485 nm and emission at 520 nm. Mean values (MVs) and standard deviations (SDs) were calculated from n = 5 samples.

2.9. Statistical Analysis

Statistical differences were determined with one-way analysis of variance (ANOVA) that was followed by multiple-comparison procedures (Holm Sidak method) provided by SigmaPlot (Systat Software Inc., San Jose, CA, USA). p values < 0.05 indicated significant differences.

3. Results

3.1. Rheological Behavior

The rheological behavior of unpolymerized pure PEGDA water/methanol (1:2) solutions was measured. The relationship between the shear stress and the shear rate is illustrated in Figure 1. A linear increase in shear stress with increasing shear rate was observed for all of polymer concentrations, meaning that all materials exhibited Newtonian behavior. This behavior was also observed for $PEGDA_{10000}$ and $PEGDA_{20000}$ (Supplementary Figures S1 and S2).

The average dynamic viscosity for each PEGDA solution was calculated and is presented in Figure 2. The viscosity of the samples increased with the increasing concentration of the polymer in the sample. This trend is remarkable, especially in the case of $PEGDA_{20000}$, where viscosity increased from 64 mPa·s for the 20 wt % solution to 576 mPa·s for the 40 wt % solution, which corresponds a 900% increase in viscosity. In the case of $PEGDA_{10000,}$ it was a 679% increase, and a 409% increase for $PEGDA_{4000}$. Significantly increased values of the viscosity were also observed for samples with a higher molecular mass. Here, the highest discrepancies were observed for the 40 wt % samples: 64 s, 179, and 575 mPa·s for $PEGDA_{4000}$, $PEGDA_{10000}$ and $PEGDA_{20000}$, respectively.

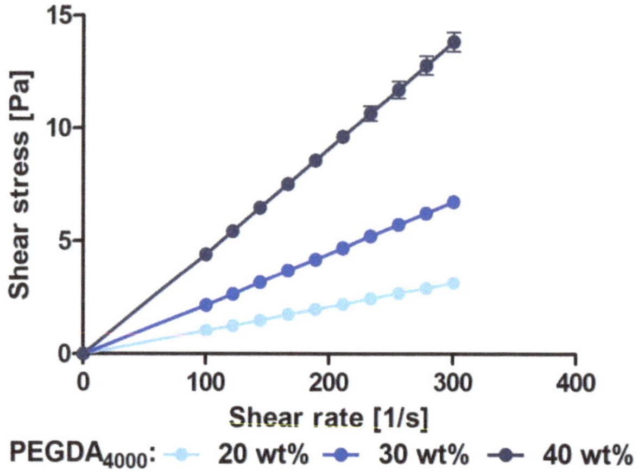

Figure 1. Exemplary shear stress/shear rate representation of $PEGDA_{4000}$ solutions in H_2O/MeOH (1:2) with different concentrations of the polymer at 15 °C (n = 3).

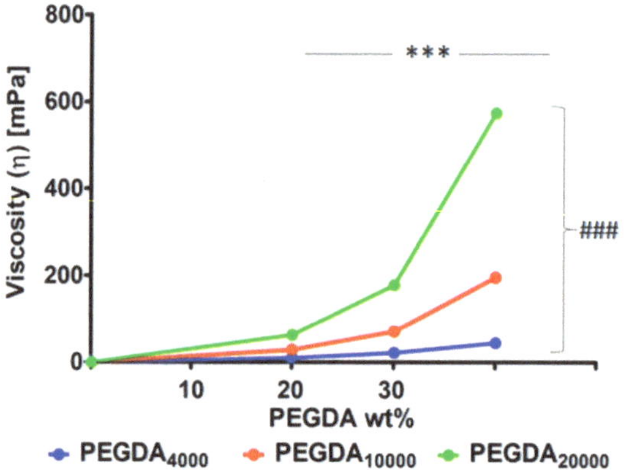

Figure 2. Average viscosity (mPa·s) for unpolymerized PEGDA solutions with different concentrations of the polymer in H_2O/MeOH (1:2) at 15 °C (n = 3). There were significant differences for all of the samples, marked with *** for differences between different wt % of the same polymer, and with ### for differences between the same wt % of the same polymer ($p < 0.001$).

3.2. Surface Morphology

The surface morphology of all investigated samples (PEGDAs 4000, 10,000, and 20,000 g/mol) was characterized with SEM. The PEGDA sample surfaces showed no visible changes by changing the molecular mass of the polymer (Figure 3). Increasing the polymer concentration in the sample (20, 30, and 40 wt %) also did not introduce any changes in the surface morphology, with the only exception of the $PEGDA_{4000}$ 40 wt % samples, of which the surface was more structured (Figure S3). Moreover, the PEGDA surface morphology was unaffected by the incorporation of BSA–FITC as the model drug (Figure S4).

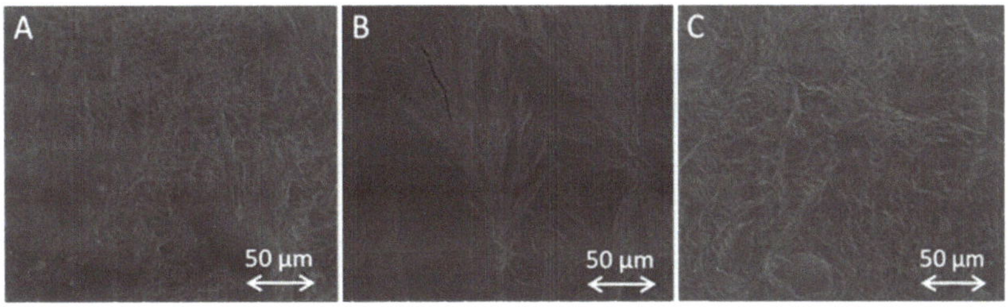

Figure 3. Comparison of representative SEM images for PEGDA samples (20 wt %) with different molecular masses of (**A**) 4000, (**B**) 10,000, or (**C**) 20,000 g/mol containing BSA–FITC.

3.3. Thermal Properties

Figure 4 shows the melting temperature *Tm* of the PEGDA hydrogels with various molecular masses in different concentrations. The tested samples showed no trends in *Tm* with increasing polymer concentration. In contrast, increasing the molecular weight of the monomers increased *Tm* for the same polymer concentrations. However, these differences were not significant, and only a tendency was detected. Thermal behavior was unaffected by the addition of model drug BSA–FITC (Figure S5).

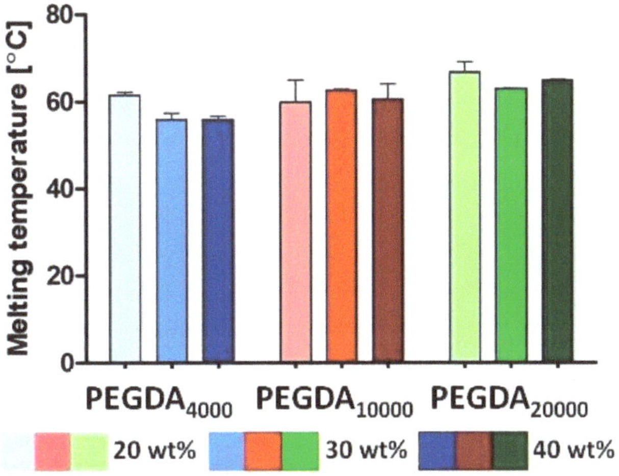

Figure 4. Mean melting temperature (°C) ± SD for $PEGDA_{4000}$, $PEGDA_{10000}$, and $PEGDA_{20000}$ samples containing 20, 30, or 40 wt % of the polymer and loaded with 0.075 wt % BSA–FITC (referring to PEGDA amount, n = 3).

3.4. Swelling Behavior

The swelling behavior of PEGDA hydrogels with different molecular masses and their concentration are shown in Figure 5. The increase in the molecular mass of PEGDA resulted in a significantly increased amount of the absorbed medium ($p < 0.001$). This trend was especially distinct in the 20 wt % samples. After 24 h of swelling in the TES buffer, the mass of the samples containing 20 wt % of $PEGDA_{4000}$ increased by about 6 times; in the case of $PEGDA_{10000}$, it was over 8 times, and for $PEGDA_{20000}$, it was about 12 times. A similar tendency with a slightly lower absorbed medium amount, but with significant differences, was observed for the samples containing 30 and 40 wt % of the polymer. Here, only the 30 wt % $PEGDA_{4000}$ samples exhibited a discrepancy and took up less of the medium than the $PEGDA_{4000}$ 40 wt % samples did; this difference was not significant.

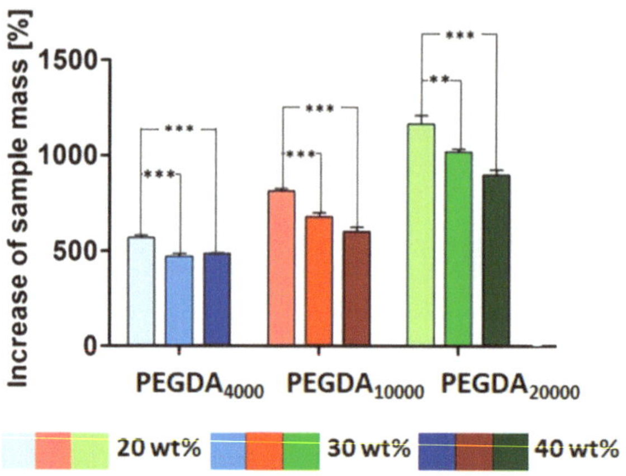

Figure 5. Increase in sample weight (samples with BSA–FITC) in percentages after 24 h swelling in a TES buffer at 37 °C (n = 3). Significant decreases in weight growth between the 20 wt % samples and higher concentrations are marked with ** for $p < 0.01$ and *** for $p < 0.001$. Significant differences in weight between the same concentration of different molecular masses of PEGDA occurred for all of the samples ($p < 0.001$) and are not marked on the graph.

Exemplary samples containing 40 wt % of PEGDA before and after the test are illustrated in Figure 6. The depicted results refer to samples containing BSA–FITC as the model drug. Results for the pure PEGDA samples were similar and can be found in Supplementary Figure S6.

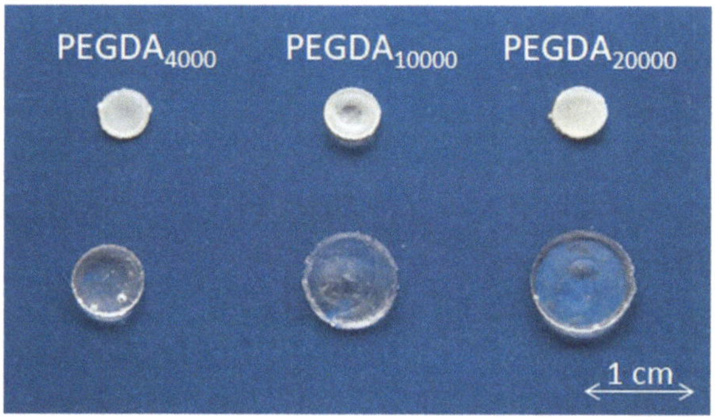

Figure 6. Macrophoto of exemplary samples $PEGDA_{4000}$, $PEGDA_{10000}$, and $PEGDA_{20000}$ with 40 wt % polymer content before (**top**) and after (**bottom**) 24 h of swelling in a TES buffer at 37 °C.

3.5. In Vitro Drug Release

The release of model drug BSA–FITC from the PEGDA samples is shown in Figure 7. In order to compare the release curves regarding PEGDAs with a different molecular mass (Figure 7A,C,E) and polymer weight (Figure 7B,D,F), polymer and BSA–FITC concentrations were kept constant for all samples. The total release of BSA–FITC was normalized to 1 mg of PEGDA in the samples to compensate for the differences in sample weight. $PEGDA_{4000}$ samples released the most BSA–FITC within 43 days of the experiment: on average, 0.58 µg BSA–FITC/mg $PEGDA_{4000}$ (C and E). In the case of $PEGDA_{10000}$, it was 0.48 µg/mg PEGDA, and for $PEGDA_{20000}$, it was 0.53 µg/mg PEGDA. Only samples containing 20 wt % of the $PEGDA_{20000}$ polymer demonstrated a higher release than that of the other specimens with 20 wt %.

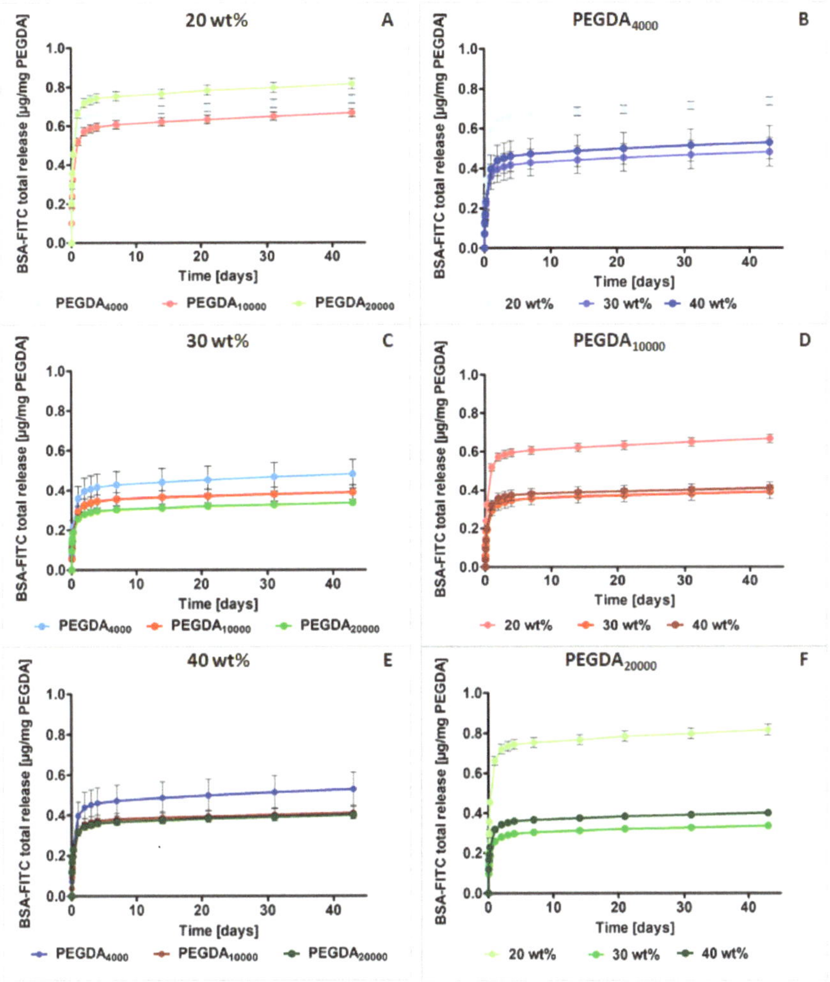

Figure 7. Total quantitative release of BSA–FITC within 43 days normalized to 1 mg PEGDA in mean ± SD. (**left**) Different PEGDA concentrations: (**A**) 20 wt %; (**C**) 30 wt %; (**E**) 40 wt %. (**right**) PEGDAs with different molecular mass: (**B**) PEGDA 4000 g/mol; (**D**) PEGDA 10,000 g/mol; (**F**) PEGDA 20,000 g/mol. Each sample contained 0.075 wt % of BSA–FITC (referring to PEGDA amount). Release occurred in 1 mL of a TES buffer at 37 °C by shaking at 100 rpm in the dark (n = 5).

For all analyzed molecular masses, 20 wt % of PEGDA samples had the highest BSA–FITC release in comparison with that of other concentrations. Differences between the 30 and 40 wt % samples for all of PEGDAs were rather negligible, ranging between 0.02 and 0.06 µg of the released BSA–FITC/mg PEGDA. All BSA–FITC release profiles were comparable in shape, with an initial burst release within the first 2 days.

4. Discussion

Our investigation, characterizing PEGDA as a potential material for 3D photochemical DDS applications, was designed to keep the wt % of all of the components (polymer and BSA–FITC) in the samples equal for all compared specimens in order to analyze the influence of the polymer concentration (20, 30 and 40 wt %) and molecular mass of the used PEGDA (4000, 10,000, and 20,000 g/mol).

The possible reasons and explanations for the in vitro BSA–FITC release presented here are summarized in Figure 8, which shows the hydrogel network formed with the photopolymerization of differently concentrated $PEGDA_{4000}$, $PEGDA_{10000}$, and $PEGDA_{20000}$ solutions, and the possible resulting differences.

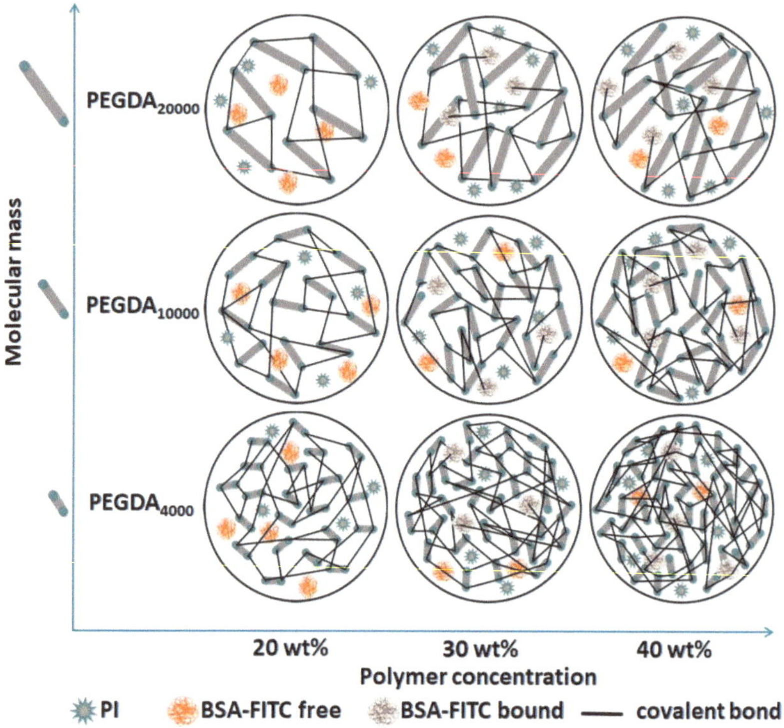

Figure 8. Schematic illustration of hydrogel network formed with the photopolymerization of differently concentrated $PEGDA_{4000}$, $PEGDA_{10000}$, and $PEGDA_{20000}$ solutions with PI (stars) and BSA–FITC (balls). PEGDA is represented as sticks connected into longer chains with covalent bonds.

Studies on the mechanics of the analyzed systems were published [38]. In summary, the samples' elongation capacity (range: ~8 to ~958%) clearly increased with increasing molecular mass, whereas increasing the PEGDA concentration resulted in significantly higher tensile strength (range: ~0.2 to ~13 MPa). The mechanical properties could lead to applications as a drug delivery system for soft tissue with low mechanical stress, tissue engineering, or as coatings due to their swelling behavior, discussed later.

In addition to focusing on the release of model protein BSA–FITC, our earlier studies also considered the biocompatibility of similar PEGDA material systems [28]. As a result, thorough rinsing to remove water-soluble toxic photoinitiators or low-molecular-weight residues is mandatory. The swelling of PEGDA facilitates rinsing with aqueous solutions. The loss of covalently bound active agent BSA–FITC during rinsing is unlikely, but possible changes in mechanics must be taken into account.

4.1. Swelling Behavior

Many factors, including different physical and chemical forces, influence the water uptake and swelling behavior of hydrogels [28]. For instance, entanglements, the presence of crystallites, and crosslinks significantly hinder water absorption [39]. Samples prepared from PEGDA with a higher molecular mass absorbed more of the medium (4000 < 10,000 < 20,000). Similar observations were reported before [40,41]. Most likely, the increased molecular mass clearly decreased the number of free acrylate groups, which are able to form covalent crosslinks (Figure S7). This resulted in a lower crosslinking degree (Figure 8) and higher elastic response of the PEGDA chains, and a higher amount of water that could be absorbed [41,42]. The molecular weight, length, and mobility of the monomer chains is an important factor affecting photopolymerization and thereby the resulting crosslinking degree [43]. The longer the chains are, the more restricted their mobility is. Mobility decreases even more during the photopolymerization process and hinders the chains' migration towards the radical groups [44]. This is another factor that can lead to fewer covalent crosslinks and greater mesh size, which increases the uptake of water [42]. A significantly decreased amount of the absorbed medium in samples containing more polymers can be explained by the fact that the higher density of the polymer chains in the matrix reduced the diameter of the pores between them (smaller mesh, schematically shown in Figure 8), which decreases the water uptake in hydrogels [45]. The exceptions were the $PEGDA_{4000}$ 30 and 40 wt % samples, where no difference was observed. We assumed that, although there were more available acrylate groups (Figure S7) in the $PEGDA_{4000}$ 40 wt % solution, the fast process of photopolymerization led to a rapid decrease in PEGDA chain mobility and the termination of the reaction [44,45].

4.2. *Viscosity of PEGDA Solutions*

The viscosity characterization of biomaterials employed in stereolithography is largely studied as one of the crucial factors in choosing the resin for a 3D printing process [46]. The high viscosity of the material negatively affects the polymerization and conversion rates of reactive C=C double bonds due to the decreased mobility of the monomer molecules in the reacting solution [47,48]. In addition, processability in various lithographic 3D printing processes significantly depends on the viscosity of the resins. In general, low viscosity is advantageous in laser-based stereolithography and digital light processing (DLP). In laser-based stereolithography, high viscosities can lead to problems during recoating, as the generation of thin resin layers becomes increasingly difficult due to poor flowability [49]. A limit of 3 Pa·s viscosity was reported in the literature in the context of ceramic slurries [50]. In a typical DLP process, the build surface is illuminated from below via a glass window, eliminating the recoating step. The increase in viscosity alters the flow dynamics of the resin, and affects the wetting mechanism of the build window, increasing the mechanical force required to lift the build platform [51]. In the DLP process, a viscosity limit of 3 Pa·s was mentioned in the literature in connection with ceramic-loaded slurries [52]. In the literature, fixed viscosity limits are rarely mentioned, since the limit value, especially for particle-laden slurries, must be determined individually for each material, and depends on the specific stereolithography or DLP equipment and the tolerable loss of component quality caused by increased viscosity.

Among the investigated materials in this study, the polymer with the highest molecular mass, $PEGDA_{20000}$, showed the highest viscosity of all used concentrations (Figure 2). These observations are consistent with the existing literature reporting that higher molecular mass results in impaired chain mobility. This, in turn, increases flow resistance. The relatively small differences between the 20 wt % solutions drastically grew with the increasing concentration of the polymer in the solution. This means that, for PEGDA, the viscosity increased exponentially with increasing molecular mass. This also indicates that PEGDA's molecular mass and concentration both increased the viscosity of the solution, the former by decreasing chain mobility through the higher chain length, and the latter because of the increasing number of particles in the solution. However, since the viscosity values of all investigated PEGDA compositions were far from the limit of 3 Pa·s, it could be assumed that the material could be processed on many common laser-based stereolithography and DLP systems [50,52]. Should there still be problems with 3D printing due to high viscosity, resins could be processed at elevated temperatures. Alternatively, infrared (IR) lamps can be used as a heat source [53].

4.3. Surface Morphology

Analysis of the sample surface did not reveal any clear variations between the drug-loaded and pure PEGDA samples. All of the investigated specimens had a slightly structured and nonuniform appearance. Therefore, the addition of low concentrations of model protein BSA–FITC did not strongly impact the morphology during photopolymerization.

4.4. Thermal Properties

Drug incorporation did not have a significant influence on the *Tm* of the investigated polymerized samples. The increase in the PEGDA's molecular mass slightly increased *Tm*. The phenomenon of an increased *Tm* via increasing the molecular mass of the used monomers was described in the literature [54,55]. This is explained by the fact that an increase in chain length results in fewer free acrylate end groups; therefore, the mobility of the end (acrylate) groups is also limited, which increases *Tm* values [56,57]. Therefore, the high differences in the molecular weight of the monomers had negligible influence on the Tm of the generated networks.

4.5. In Vitro Drug Release

All of the samples showed similar curves, with an initial burst release within the first 2 days followed by a slower release of the last 10–15% of BSA–FITC within the next 40 days (Figure 7).

The highest absolute release of BSA–FITC could be observed for all 20 wt % samples. In these samples, as described in Section 4.1, the highest uptake of the medium was also observed. These observations are consistent with the existing literature where the material degree of the swelling was reported as one of the factors significantly influencing the in vitro drug release, and higher water absorption was related to higher drug release [58]. Consequently, water diffusion and the elution of the model drug were facilitated.

However, next to water diffusion, the formation of covalent bounds between BSA–FITC and PEGDA during the photopolymerization process may be an important aspect in the release of proteins from polymer matrices. PEGDA particles, instead of reacting only with each other, also covalently bound the incorporated BSA–FITC under formation of hydrolysable ester bonds with functional groups such as –NH2 or –SH [59]. A lower PEGDA concentration most probably results in less crosslinked BSA–FITC and more unbound BSA–FITC. Thus, from the samples containing higher PEGDA, substantially lower amounts of unbound BSA–FITC per 1 mg PEGDA could be released (Figure 7). This explanation was confirmed via the released BSA–FITC amounts from all 30 and 40 wt % PEGDAs, which were lower than those for the 20 wt % PEGDA. The reduction in released BSA–FITC amounts between the 20 and 30 or 40 wt % samples of PEGDA increased with increasing molecular mass. Compared to the 20 wt % PEGDA, 30 wt % $PEGDA_{4000}$ released 35% less BSA–FITC; for $PEGDA_{10000}$, it was 42% less, and for $PEGDA_{20000}$, it was 61 wt % less (Figure S8). Furthermore, this effect could possibly be related to the higher viscosity of the 30 and 40 wt % PEGDA solutions, which resulted in the reduced movability of PEGDA monomer chains and the hindered crosslinking.

Surprisingly, the released amount of BSA–FITC from all 30 and 40 wt % PEGDAs was relatively similar. Thus, for 30 and 40 wt % PEGDAs, no significant reduction in the released BSA–FITC amounts was detected for the different molecular masses and consequently the different viscosities (Figure 7). This happened even though the higher concentration of the polymer was equivalent with an increased number of reactive acrylate groups (Supplementary Figure S7). In the case of concentrations up from around 30 wt % of PEGDA, the amount of the bound or trapped BSA–FITC did not clearly change, even though the differences in viscosity drastically increased for the 30 and 40 wt % samples, so viscosity up from 30 wt % probably did not influence the formation of crosslinks during the curing any more (Figure S9). In addition to the influence of crosslinking on the release and stability of BSA–FITC, UV light irradiation must also be taken into account. We assumed that its influence was small, since the sample polymerized quickly and a UV light-absorbing polymer was thereby formed at the surface. The choice of PI and light source also needs to be further optimized and tested for applications in stereolithography.

Apart from crosslinking, the release behavior could be affected by generating copolymers or blend compositions (not used in this work), or the degradation rate of the matrix [60]. Nevertheless, PEGDA is a slow degrading polymer; thus, the influence of degradation on drug release is probably negligible [61].

5. Conclusions

There has been much attention focused on achieving the sustained release of a drug, and thereby a better and more controlled therapeutic effect [62]. Photoresins such as PEGDA could be taken into consideration as protein carriers for the development of DDS resins for novel 3D printing techniques. Knowledge about its properties, such as viscosity and the resulting crosslinking structure, is crucial in choosing the best printable composition of the resins to possibly crosslink and release the drug as desired.

In this work, the influence of the PEGDA composition on the release of model protein drug BSA–FITC was studied. This systematic study revealed that PEGDA concentration and molecular mass have an unambiguous influence on its viscosity. These affect the mechanism of photopolymerization and the formation of covalent bonds between reacting photomonomers and protein drugs, and the swelling behavior of the resulting 3D print. The analysis of the release outcomes showed that the factors influencing drug release are complex, and at the higher concentrations of PEGDA, no simple correlations among viscosity, water uptake, and the released protein could be found, which leaves room for interpretation and needs further study. However, between 20 and 30 wt %, factors such as swelling behavior and viscosity had the highest impact on the crosslinking between the different components in the system and on the in vitro BSA–FITC release. Within this range, drug release may be highly tunable, which indicates that accurate investigations such as ours are challenging, but also essential and required in understanding designing drug depots in 3D printing such as stereolithography. Further investigations of crosslinking and the adjustment of resin properties for inkjet use and exposure parameters are necessary.

Supplementary Materials: The following supporting information can be downloaded at: https://www.mdpi.com/article/10.3390/pharmaceutics15041039/s1. Figure S1: exemplary shear stress/shear rate representation of $PEGDA_{10000}$ solutions in H_2O/MeOH (1:2) with different concentrations of the polymer at 15 °C (n = 3); Figure S2: exemplary shear stress/shear rate representation of $PEGDA_{20000}$ solutions in H2O/MeOH (1:2) with different concentrations of the polymer at 15 °C (n = 3); Figure S3: comparison of SEM images of the surface of PEGDA samples with different molecular masses (4000 g/mol, 10,000 g/mol and 20,000 g/mol) and their concentrations with BSA–FITC; Figure S4: comparison of SEM images of the surface of PEGDA samples with different molecular masses (4000 g/mol, 10,000 g/mol and 20,000 g/mol) and their concentrations without BSA–FITC; Figure S5: mean melting temperature (°C) with SD for $PEGDA_{4000}$, $PEGDA_{10000}$, and $PEGDA_{20000}$ samples containing 20, 30, or 40 wt % of the polymer without BSA–FITC (n = 3); Figure S6: increase in sample (Ø = 6 mm, thickness = 1 mm) weight (pure PEGDA without BSA–FITC) in percentages with SD after 24 h swelling in a TES buffer at 37 °C (n = 3); Figure S7: theoretical number of free acrylate groups in 1 mL of unpolymerized of different PEGDA solutions; Figure S8: differences in percentage between the 20–30 and 20–40 wt % PEGDA samples in the released amount of BSA–FITC; Figure S9: relationship between total BSA–FITC release and PEGDA viscosity (4000, 10,000, and 20,000 g/mol) solutions (20, 30, and 40 wt %).

Author Contributions: Conceptualization, M.T. and K.W.; methodology, N.R., D.K., K.W. and M.T.; formal analysis, N.R.; investigation, N.R.; resources, V.S. and N.G.; data curation, N.R., K.W., D.K. and M.T.; writing—original draft preparation, N.R., K.W. and M.T.; writing—review and editing, V.S., N.G. and H.S.; visualization, N.R. and K.W.; supervision, N.G., V.S. and H.S.; project administration, M.T.; funding acquisition, M.T., H.S. and N.G. All authors have read and agreed to the published version of the manuscript.

Funding: The financial support from the Federal Ministry of Education and Research (BMBF) within RESPONSE "Partnership for Innovation in Implant Technology", the German Research Foundation

(DFG) within the "3D printed drug delivery systems with the ability of the time controlled drug release" project (grant numbers TE1233/1-1 and SE 1807/6-1) and the Federal Ministry for Economic Affairs and Climate Action (grant numbers KK5364801RU1 and KK5037210RU1) is gratefully acknowledged.

Data Availability Statement: Not applicable.

Acknowledgments: The authors would like to thank Babette Hummel, Katja Hahn, and Jan Oldenburg for their practical assistance.

Conflicts of Interest: The authors declare no conflict of interest. Furthermore, the funders had no role in the design of the study; in the collection, analyses, or interpretation of data; in the writing of the manuscript; or in the decision to publish the results.

References

1. Seyfoddin, A.; Dezfooli, S.M.; Greene, C.A. *Engineering Drug Delivery Systems*; Woodhead Publishing: Duxford, UK, 2020; ISBN 0081025483.
2. Indurkhya, A. Influence of Drug Properties and Routes of Drug Administration on the Design of Controlled Release System. In *Dosage Form Design Considerations*; Tekade, R.K., Ed.; Academic Press: London, UK; San Diego, CA, USA; Cambridge, UK; Oxford, UK, 2018; Chapter 6; ISBN 9780128144237.
3. Li, C.; Wang, J.; Wang, Y.; Gao, H.; Wei, G.; Huang, Y.; Yu, H.; Gan, Y.; Wang, Y.; Mei, L.; et al. Recent progress in drug delivery. *Acta Pharm. Sin. B* **2019**, *9*, 1145–1162. [CrossRef] [PubMed]
4. Sandler, N.; Preis, M. Printed Drug-Delivery Systems for Improved Patient Treatment. *Trends Pharmacol. Sci.* **2016**, *37*, 1070–1080. [CrossRef]
5. Domsta, V.; Seidlitz, A. 3D-Printing of Drug-Eluting Implants: An Overview of the Current Developments Described in the Literature. *Molecules* **2021**, *26*, 4066. [CrossRef]
6. Elkasabgy, N.A.; Mahmoud, A.A.; Maged, A. 3D printing: An appealing route for customized drug delivery systems. *Int. J. Pharm.* **2020**, *588*, 119732. [CrossRef]
7. Auriemma, G.; Tommasino, C.; Falcone, G.; Esposito, T.; Sardo, C.; Aquino, R.P. Additive Manufacturing Strategies for Personalized Drug Delivery Systems and Medical Devices: Fused Filament Fabrication and Semi Solid Extrusion. *Molecules* **2022**, *27*, 2784. [CrossRef] [PubMed]
8. Khaled, S.A.; Burley, J.C.; Alexander, M.R.; Yang, J.; Roberts, C.J. 3D printing of five-in-one dose combination polypill with defined immediate and sustained release profiles. *J. Control. Release* **2015**, *217*, 308–314. [CrossRef]
9. Robles-Martinez, P.; Xu, X.; Trenfield, S.J.; Awad, A.; Goyanes, A.; Telford, R.; Basit, A.W.; Gaisford, S. 3D Printing of a Multi-Layered Polypill Containing Six Drugs Using a Novel Stereolithographic Method. *Pharmaceutics* **2019**, *11*, 274. [CrossRef] [PubMed]
10. Januskaite, P.; Xu, X.; Ranmal, S.R.; Gaisford, S.; Basit, A.W.; Tuleu, C.; Goyanes, A. I Spy with My Little Eye: A Paediatric Visual Preferences Survey of 3D Printed Tablets. *Pharmaceutics* **2020**, *12*, 1100. [CrossRef] [PubMed]
11. Wang, Y.; Sun, L.; Mei, Z.; Zhang, F.; He, M.; Fletcher, C.; Wang, F.; Yang, J.; Bi, D.; Jiang, Y.; et al. 3D printed biodegradable implants as an individualized drug delivery system for local chemotherapy of osteosarcoma. *Mater. Des.* **2020**, *186*, 108336. [CrossRef]
12. Palo, M.; Holländer, J.; Suominen, J.; Yliruusi, J.; Sandler, N. 3D printed drug delivery devices: Perspectives and technical challenges. *Expert Rev. Med. Devices* **2017**, *14*, 685–696. [CrossRef]
13. Pandey, M.; Choudhury, H.; Fern, J.L.C.; Kee, A.T.K.; Kou, J.; Jing, J.L.J.; Her, H.C.; Yong, H.S.; Ming, H.C.; Bhattamisra, S.K.; et al. 3D printing for oral drug delivery: A new tool to customize drug delivery. *Drug Deliv. Transl. Res.* **2020**, *10*, 986–1001. [CrossRef] [PubMed]
14. Fazel-Rezai, R. *Biomedical Engineering—Frontiers and Challenges*; IntechOpen: Rijeka, Croatia, 2011; ISBN 978-953-307-309-5.
15. Konasch, J.; Riess, A.; Mau, R.; Teske, M.; Rekowska, N.; Eickner, T.; Grabow, N.; Seitz, H. A Novel Hybrid Additive Manufacturing Process for Drug Delivery Systems with Locally Incorporated Drug Depots. *Pharmaceutics* **2019**, *11*, 661. [CrossRef] [PubMed]
16. Choi, J.R.; Yong, K.W.; Choi, J.Y.; Cowie, A.C. Recent advances in photo-crosslinkable hydrogels for biomedical applications. *Biotechniques* **2019**, *66*, 40–53. [CrossRef]
17. Ito, Y. *Photochemistry for Biomedical Applications: From Device Fabrication to Diagnosis and Therapy*; Springer: Singapore, 2018; ISBN 978-981-13-0151-3.
18. Jain, A.; Jain, A.; Gulbake, A.; Shilpi, S.; Hurkat, P.; Jain, S.K. Peptide and protein delivery using new drug delivery systems. *Crit. Rev. Ther. Drug Carr. Syst.* **2013**, *30*, 293–329. [CrossRef] [PubMed]
19. Tekade, R.K. *Basic Fundamentals of Drug Delivery*; Academic Press: London, UK; San Diego, CA, USA, 2019; ISBN 0128179090.
20. Morishita, M.; Goto, T.; Nakamura, K.; Lowman, A.M.; Takayama, K.; Peppas, N.A. Novel oral insulin delivery systems based on complexation polymer hydrogels: Single and multiple administration studies in type 1 and 2 diabetic rats. *J. Control. Release* **2006**, *110*, 587–594. [CrossRef] [PubMed]

21. Abdella, S.; Youssef, S.H.; Afinjuomo, F.; Song, Y.; Fouladian, P.; Upton, R.; Garg, S. 3D Printing of Thermo-Sensitive Drugs. *Pharmaceutics* **2021**, *13*, 1524. [CrossRef]
22. Martinez, P.R.; Goyanes, A.; Basit, A.W.; Gaisford, S. Fabrication of drug-loaded hydrogels with stereolithographic 3D printing. *Int. J. Pharm.* **2017**, *532*, 313–317. [CrossRef]
23. Madzarevic, M.; Medarevic, D.; Vulovic, A.; Sustersic, T.; Djuris, J.; Filipovic, N.; Ibric, S. Optimization and Prediction of Ibuprofen Release from 3D DLP Printlets Using Artificial Neural Networks. *Pharmaceutics* **2019**, *11*, 544. [CrossRef]
24. Healy, A.V.; Fuenmayor, E.; Doran, P.; Geever, L.M.; Higginbotham, C.L.; Lyons, J.G. Additive Manufacturing of Personalized Pharmaceutical Dosage Forms via Stereolithography. *Pharmaceutics* **2019**, *11*, 645. [CrossRef] [PubMed]
25. Hanna, K.; Yasar-Inceoglu, O.; Yasar, O. Drug Delivered Poly(ethylene glycol) Diacrylate (PEGDA) Hydrogels and Their Mechanical Characterization Tests for Tissue Engineering Applications. *MRS Adv.* **2018**, *3*, 1697–1702. [CrossRef]
26. Warr, C.; Valdoz, J.C.; Bickham, B.P.; Knight, C.J.; Franks, N.A.; Chartrand, N.; van Ry, P.M.; Christensen, K.A.; Nordin, G.P.; Cook, A.D. Biocompatible PEGDA Resin for 3D Printing. *ACS Appl. Bio Mater.* **2020**, *3*, 2239–2244. [CrossRef] [PubMed]
27. O'Donnell, K.; Boyd, A.; Meenan, B.J. Controlling Fluid Diffusion and Release through Mixed-Molecular-Weight Poly(ethylene) Glycol Diacrylate (PEGDA) Hydrogels. *Materials* **2019**, *12*, 3381. [CrossRef] [PubMed]
28. Rekowska, N.; Huling, J.; Brietzke, A.; Arbeiter, D.; Eickner, T.; Konasch, J.; Riess, A.; Mau, R.; Seitz, H.; Grabow, N.; et al. Thermal, Mechanical and Biocompatibility Analyses of Photochemically Polymerized PEGDA250 for Photopolymerization-Based Manufacturing Processes. *Pharmaceutics* **2022**, *14*, 628. [CrossRef]
29. Liu, S.; Yeo, D.C.; Wiraja, C.; Tey, H.L.; Mrksich, M.; Xu, C. Peptide delivery with poly(ethylene glycol) diacrylate microneedles through swelling effect. *Bioeng. Transl. Med.* **2017**, *2*, 258–267. [CrossRef] [PubMed]
30. Gao, Y.; Hou, M.; Yang, R.; Zhang, L.; Xu, Z.; Kang, Y.; Xue, P. PEGDA/PVP Microneedles with Tailorable Matrix Constitutions for Controllable Transdermal Drug Delivery. *Macromol. Mater. Eng.* **2018**, *303*, 1800233. [CrossRef]
31. Shadish, J.A.; DeForest, C.A. Site-Selective Protein Modification: From Functionalized Proteins to Functional Biomaterials. *Matter* **2020**, *2*, 50–77. [CrossRef]
32. Davidovich-Pinhas, M.; Bianco-Peled, H. Novel mucoadhesive system based on sulfhydryl-acrylate interactions. *J. Mater. Sci. Mater. Med.* **2010**, *21*, 2027–2034. [CrossRef]
33. Mazzoccoli, J.P.; Feke, D.L.; Baskaran, H.; Pintauro, P.N. Mechanical and cell viability properties of crosslinked low- and high-molecular weight poly(ethylene glycol) diacrylate blends. *J. Biomed. Mater. Res. A* **2010**, *93*, 558–566. [CrossRef]
34. Lee, S.; Tong, X.; Yang, F. The effects of varying poly(ethylene glycol) hydrogel crosslinking density and the crosslinking mechanism on protein accumulation in three-dimensional hydrogels. *Acta Biomater.* **2014**, *10*, 4167–4174. [CrossRef]
35. Qiao, X.; Wang, L.; Ma, J.; Deng, Q.; Liang, Z.; Zhang, L.; Peng, X.; Zhang, Y. High sensitivity analysis of water-soluble, cyanine dye labeled proteins by high-performance liquid chromatography with fluorescence detection. *Anal. Chim. Acta* **2009**, *640*, 114–120. [CrossRef]
36. Hungerford, G.; Benesch, J.; Mano, J.F.; Reis, R.L. Effect of the labelling ratio on the photophysics of fluorescein isothiocyanate (FITC) conjugated to bovine serum albumin. *Photochem. Photobiol. Sci.* **2007**, *6*, 152–158. [CrossRef] [PubMed]
37. Breen, C.J.; Raverdeau, M.; Voorheis, H.P. Development of a quantitative fluorescence-based ligand-binding assay. *Sci. Rep.* **2016**, *6*, 25769. [CrossRef] [PubMed]
38. Rekowska, N.; Arbeiter, D.; Seitz, H.; Mau, R.; Riess, A.; Eickner, T.; Grabow, N.; Teske, M. The influence of PEGDA's molecular weight on its mechanical properties in the context of biomedical applications. *Curr. Dir. Biomed. Eng.* **2022**, *8*, 181–184. [CrossRef]
39. Anthony, M. Lowman and Nikolaos, A. Peppas. Analysis of the Complexation/Decomplexation Phenomena in Graft Copolymer Networks. *Macromolecules* **1997**, *30*, 4959–4965. [CrossRef]
40. Yang, X.; Dargaville, B.L.; Hutmacher, D.W. Elucidating the Molecular Mechanisms for the Interaction of Water with Polyethylene Glycol-Based Hydrogels: Influence of Ionic Strength and Gel Network Structure. *Polymers* **2021**, *13*, 845. [CrossRef]
41. Della Sala, F.; Biondi, M.; Guarnieri, D.; Borzacchiello, A.; Ambrosio, L.; Mayol, L. Mechanical behavior of bioactive poly(ethylene glycol) diacrylate matrices for biomedical application. *J. Mech. Behav. Biomed. Mater.* **2020**, *110*, 103885. [CrossRef]
42. Karoyo, A.H.; Wilson, L.D. A Review on the Design and Hydration Properties of Natural Polymer-Based Hydrogels. *Materials* **2021**, *14*, 1095. [CrossRef]
43. Ju, H.; McCloskey, B.D.; Sagle, A.C.; Kusuma, V.A.; Freeman, B.D. Preparation and characterization of crosslinked poly(ethylene glycol) diacrylate hydrogels as fouling-resistant membrane coating materials. *J. Membr. Sci.* **2009**, *330*, 180–188. [CrossRef]
44. Peris, E.; Bañuls, M.-J.; Maquieira, Á.; Puchades, R. Photopolymerization as a promising method to sense biorecognition events. *Trends Analyt. Chem.* **2012**, *41*, 86–104. [CrossRef]
45. Karamchand, L.; Makeiff, D.; Gao, Y.; Azyat, K.; Serpe, M.J.; Kulka, M. Biomaterial inks and bioinks for fabricating 3D biomimetic lung tissue: A delicate balancing act between biocompatibility and mechanical printability. *Bioprinting* **2023**, *29*, e00255. [CrossRef]
46. Zandrini, T.; Liaros, N.; Jiang, L.J.; Lu, Y.F.; Fourkas, J.T.; Osellame, R.; Baldacchini, T. Effect of the resin viscosity on the writing properties of two-photon polymerization. *Opt. Mater. Express* **2019**, *9*, 2601. [CrossRef]
47. Marcinkowska, A.; Andrzejewska, E. Viscosity effects in the photopolymerization of two-monomer systems. *J. Appl. Polym. Sci.* **2010**, *116*, 280–287. [CrossRef]
48. Lin, J.-T.; Liu, H.-W.; Chen, K.-T.; Cheng, D.-C. Modeling the Kinetics, Curing Depth, and Efficacy of Radical-Mediated Photopolymerization: The Role of Oxygen Inhibition, Viscosity, and Dynamic Light Intensity. *Front. Chem.* **2019**, *7*, 760. [CrossRef] [PubMed]

49. Wozniak, M.; de Hazan, Y.; Graule, T.; Kata, D. Rheology of UV curable colloidal silica dispersions for rapid prototyping applications. *J. Eur. Ceram. Soc.* **2011**, *31*, 2221–2229. [CrossRef]
50. Hinczewski, C.; Corbel, S.; Chartier, T. Ceramic suspensions suitable for stereolithography. *J. Eur. Ceram. Soc.* **1998**, *18*, 583–590. [CrossRef]
51. Shahzadi, L.; Li, F.; Alejandro, F.; Breadmore, M.; Thickett, S. Chapter 4 Resin design in stereolithography 3D printing for microfluidic applications. In *3D Printing with Light*; Xiao, P., Zhang, J., Eds.; De Gruyter: Berlin, Germany; Boston, MA, USA, 2021. [CrossRef]
52. Komissarenko, D.A.; Sokolov, P.S.; Evstigneeva, A.D.; Shmeleva, I.A.; Dosovitsky, A.E. Rheological and Curing Behavior of Acrylate-Based Suspensions for the DLP 3D Printing of Complex Zirconia Parts. *Materials* **2018**, *11*, 2350. [CrossRef] [PubMed]
53. Li, X.; Xie, B.; Jin, J.; Chai, Y.; Chen, Y. 3D printing temporary crown and bridge by temperature controlled mask image projection stereolithography. *Procedia Manuf.* **2018**, *26*, 1023–1033. [CrossRef]
54. Omelczuk, M.O.; McGinity, J.W. The influence of polymer glass transition temperature and molecular weight on drug release from tablets containing poly(DL-lactic acid). *Pharm. Res.* **1992**, *9*, 26–32. [CrossRef]
55. Chen, J.; Yuan, T.; Liu, Z. Supramolecular medical antibacterial tissue adhesive prepared based on natural small molecules. *Biomater. Sci.* **2020**, *8*, 6235–6245. [CrossRef] [PubMed]
56. Jadhav, N.; Gaikwad, V.; Nair, K.; Kadam, H. Glass transition temperature: Basics and application in pharmaceutical sector. *Asian J. Pharm.* **2009**, *3*, 82. [CrossRef]
57. Comyn, J. What are adhesives and sealants and how do they work? In *Adhesive Bonding: Science, Technology and Applications*; Adams, R.D., Ed.; Woodhead Publishing an Imprint of Elsevier: Duxford, UK; Cambridge, MA, USA; Kidlington, UK, 2021; pp. 41–78. ISBN 9780128199541.
58. Guo, F.; Zhang, W.; Pei, X.; Shen, X.; Yan, Q.; Li, H.; Yun, J.; Yang, G. Biodegradable star-shaped polycyclic ester elastomers: Preparation, degradability, protein release, and biocompatibility in vitro. *J. Bioact. Compat. Polym.* **2017**, *32*, 178–195. [CrossRef]
59. Li, Z.; Jiang, Y.; Wüst, K.; Callari, M.; Stenzel, M.H. Crosslinking of Self-Assembled Protein–Polymer Conjugates with Divanillin. *Aust. J. Chem.* **2020**, *73*, 1034–1041. [CrossRef]
60. Bao, W.; Zhang, X.; Wu, H.; Chen, R.; Guo, S. Synergistic Effect of Ultrasound and Polyethylene Glycol on the Mechanism of the Controlled Drug Release from Polylactide Matrices. *Polymers* **2019**, *11*, 880. [CrossRef] [PubMed]
61. Browning, M.B.; Cereceres, S.N.; Luong, P.T.; Cosgriff-Hernandez, E.M. Determination of the in vivo degradation mechanism of PEGDA hydrogels. *J. Biomed. Mater. Res. A* **2014**, *102*, 4244–4251. [CrossRef] [PubMed]
62. Yoo, J.; Won, Y.-Y. Phenomenology of the Initial Burst Release of Drugs from PLGA Microparticles. *ACS Biomater. Sci. Eng.* **2020**, *6*, 6053–6062. [CrossRef] [PubMed]

pharmaceutics

Article

A Pilot Study Exploiting the Industrialization Potential of Solid Lipid Nanoparticle-Based Metered-Dose Inhalers

Lei Shu [1,†], Wenhua Wang [2,†], Chon-iong Ng [1], Xuejuan Zhang [1,*], Ying Huang [1], Chuanbin Wu [1], Xin Pan [2] and Zhengwei Huang [1,*]

1 College of Pharmacy, Jinan University, Guangzhou 510006, China
2 School of Pharmaceutical Sciences, Sun Yat-sen University, Guangzhou 510275, China
* Correspondence: zhangxj02230223@jnu.edu.cn (X.Z.); huangzhengw@jnu.edu.cn (Z.H.); Tel.: +86-020-39943117 (Z.H.)
† These authors contributed equally to this work.

Abstract: Background: Delivery of inhalable nanoparticles through metered-dose inhalers (MDI) is a promising approach to treat lung disease such as asthma and chronic obstructive pulmonary disease. Nanocoating of the inhalable nanoparticles helps in stability and cellular uptake enhancement but complicates the production process. Thus, it is meaningful to accelerate the translation process of MDI encapsulating inhalable nanoparticles with nanocoating structure. Methods: In this study, solid lipid nanoparticles (SLN) are selected as a model inhalable nanoparticle system. An established reverse microemulsion strategy was utilized to explore the industrialization potential of SLN-based MDI. Three categories of nanocoating with the functions of stabilization (by Poloxamer 188, encoded as SLN(0)), cellular uptake enhancement (by cetyltrimethylammonium bromide, encoded as SLN(+)), and targetability (by hyaluronic acid, encoded as SLN(−)) were constructed upon SLN, whose particle size distribution and zeta-potential were characterized. Subsequently, SLN were loaded into MDI, and evaluated for the processing reliability, physicochemical nature, formulation stability, and biocompatibility. Results: The results elucidated that three types of SLN-based MDI were successfully fabricated with good reproducibility and stability. Regarding safety, SLN(0) and SLN(−) showed negligible cytotoxicity on cellular level. Conclusions: This work serves as a pilot study for the scale-up of SLN-based MDI, and could be useful for the future development of inhalable nanoparticles.

Keywords: inhalation; solid lipid nanoparticle; metered-dose inhaler; pilot study; nanocoating

Citation: Shu, L.; Wang, W.; Ng, C.-i.; Zhang, X.; Huang, Y.; Wu, C.; Pan, X.; Huang, Z. A Pilot Study Exploiting the Industrialization Potential of Solid Lipid Nanoparticle-Based Metered-Dose Inhalers. *Pharmaceutics* **2023**, *15*, 866. https://doi.org/10.3390/pharmaceutics15030866

Academic Editor: Luigi Battaglia

Received: 28 January 2023
Revised: 1 March 2023
Accepted: 2 March 2023
Published: 7 March 2023

1. Introduction

Inhalable nanoparticles have been widely reported in the literature to treat lung diseases such as lung carcinoma [1], systemic diseases such as diabetes [2], and to act as vaccine carriers [3]. A literature survey via PubMed suggested that 2760 relevant papers were published since 1998 (searching date: 11 January 2023). Their pharmacodynamic effects are demonstrated in animal models and have shown good therapeutic efficacies in patients. Clinical translation of inhalable nanoparticles may provide promising solutions to serious chronic illness such as respiratory diseases.

It should be noted that the prerequisite for the clinical pulmonary delivery of inhalable nanoparticles is a satisfactory deposition outcome. According to the previous study, transforming nanoparticles into micro-sized aerosols with appropriate aerodynamic attributes can achieve satisfactory deposition [4]. As inhalable nanoparticles are generally fabricated in liquid state, encapsulating into nebulizers and metered-dose inhalers (MDI) that can transform individual nanoparticles into micro-sized aerosols with proper aerodynamic characteristics is a promising settlement. Compared to nebulizers, MDI are portable and easy to use [5]. Hence, developing a nanoparticles-containing MDI is of great significance.

However, there are no inhalable nanoparticles in MDI forms currently available in the market. The nanocoating structure of inhalable nanoparticles is a major obstacle for its industrialization. The term nanocoating refers to the surface modification layer on the nanoparticles for the stabilization [6], cellular uptake enhancement [7], and to achieve the targetability [8]. A range of synthetic polymers such as poloxamer, [poly(ethylene oxide)-poly(propylene oxide)-poly(ethylene oxide) block copolymer [9], surfactants such as Tween [10] and cetyltrimethylammonium bromide (CTAB) [11], and natural substances such as chitosan [12], hyaluronic acid (HA) [13], and folate [14] have been used for nanocoating. The loading of inhalable nanoparticles into MDI includes a high-pressure propellant filling process [15], which may compromise the nanocoating functions. A multilayer nanocoating with different materials further complicate the design and development process. Hence, although the nanocoating endows inhalable nanoparticles with aforementioned properties, the difficulty in industrialization for inhalable nanoparticles-based MDI is substantially increased. It is urgent to exploit new strategies to facilitate the industrialization of related products.

A reverse microemulsion technology [16] to produce nanoparticles-incorporated MDI has been reported by our group [17]. The emulsification layer of reverse microemulsion system consist of surfactant and co-surfactant that can sterically refrain the nanocoating and protect it from collapse during MDI filling process. By exploiting the applicability of this strategy on a larger scale, the industrialization progress of inhalable nanoparticles-based MDI may be triggered.

In this study, the industrialization potential of MDI loading nanoparticles with different nanocoating was preliminarily investigated. A multilayer nanocoating was introduced to scrutinize the robustness of production. A typical lipid-based nanomedicine, solid lipid nanoparticles (SLN) was selected as the model inhalable nanoparticles and coated rationally with Poloxamer 188 (representing the stabilization function), Poloxamer 188 plus CTAB (positive surface charge, representing the cellular uptake enhancement function), and Poloxamer 188 plus CTAB plus HA (negative surface charge, representing the targetability function). The involved nanoparticles and the nanoarchitecture thereof were summarized in Figure 1. The nanostructure design was partly referred to the literature [13].

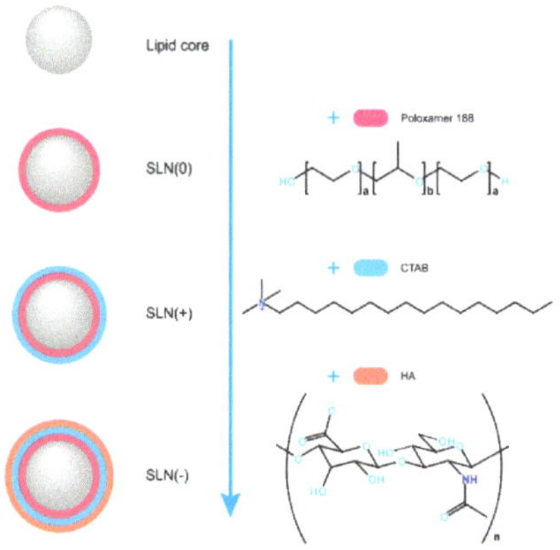

Figure 1. Scheme for the involved nanoparticles. Abbreviations in the figure: SLN- solid lipid nanoparticles; CTAB- cetyltrimethylammonium bromide; HA- hyaluronic acid.

2. Materials and Methods

2.1. Materials

Palmityl palmitate and absolute ethanol were purchased from Aladdin Industrial, Inc. (Shanghai, China). Poloxamer 188 was supplied by BASF SE (Ludwigshafen, Germany). CTAB was obtained from Sinopharm Chemical Reagent Co., Ltd. (Shanghai, China). HA (average molecular weight: 1 MDa) and dimethyl sulfoxide (DMSO) were purchased from Macklin Inc. (Shanghai, China). Pluronic L64 was supplied by Wengjiang Chemical Inc.

(Shaoguan, China). Methylthiazolyldiphenyl-tetrazolium bromide (MTT) was obtained from Merck KGaA (Darmstadt, Germany). Phosphate buffer saline (PBS), DMEM media, fetal bovine serum, and trypsin were purchased from Thermo Fisher Scientific Inc. (Waltham, MA, USA). Propellant HFA 134a (chemically 1, 1, 1, 2-tetrafluoroethane) was supplied by Kemu Chemical Inc. (Shanghai, China). A549 cells (ATCC code: CCL-185) were purchased from National Collection of Authenticated Cell Cultures (Shanghai, China). Ultra-pure water provided by PureLAB Option system (ELGA Lab Water, Inc., High Wycombe, UK) was used throughout this study.

2.2. *SLN Preparation*

SLN were prepared according to the documented method [13]. Palmityl palmitate (150 mg) and Poloxamer 188 (25 mg) were placed in a vessel and melted at 80 °C. Then, 5 mL of water was added dropwise into the melted mixture and the system was stirred for 5 min at an oscillator. Ultrasonication (BILON-650Y, BiLon Instrument Co., Ltd., Shanghai, China) in an ice bath was applied with a 20% power and 2 s/2 s working/rest cycling. This formulation was encoded as SLN(0) (undecorated SLN).

CTAB solution with a concentration of 3.75 $mg{\cdot}mL^{-1}$ was prepared by dissolving 3.75 g CTAB solid in 1 L water. Then, 100 μL of CTAB solution was diluted by 5 mL water. The rest procedures were as described above and this formulation was named as SLN(+) (positive charge decorated SLN). SLN(+) was mixed with HA solution (0.625 $mg{\cdot}mL^{-1}$) at a volume ratio of 5:4, and the system was stirred at ambient temperature for 30 min to produce SLN(−) (negative charge decorated SLN).

2.3. *Particle Size Distribution and Zeta-Potential Characterization*

2.3.1. Particle Size

SLN(0), SLN(+), and SLN(−) were diluted 120 times and 1 mL of the samples was equilibrated for 2 min and subjected to particle size measurement via Nano ZS90 (Malvern Instruments Ltd., Malvern, UK). Average size and polydispersity index (PDI) were measured using Nano ZS90 and were referred to prior to data analysis.

2.3.2. Autocorrelation Function Curve

The change of autocorrelation function along with time was recorded during particle size determination, within 10^8 μs. The function value was normalized by setting the initial value as 1, and an average of three functions was plotted as a curve. The quality reports by Nano ZS90 were referred to prior to data analysis.

2.3.3. Zeta-Potential

The samples in Section 2.3.1 were also subjected to zeta-potential determination, through the corresponding module of Nano ZS90. Each sample was determined in triplicates. The quality reports by Nano ZS90 were referred to prior to data analysis.

2.4. *MDI Filling*

Before formal filling procedure, the pipeline of type 15 filling machine (Zhihua Aerosol Equipment Ltd., Zhongshan, China) was washed by HFA 134a and the vacuum pump of the filling machine was allowed for equilibrium.

The filling process of MDI had been reported elsewhere [18], and the content of components could be referred to the literature [17]. Pluronic L64, ethanol, and SLN (SLN(0), SLN(+) and SLN(−)) were added successively into the aerosol container, which was sealed by a 50-μL metered-dose valve. It was noticed that the fresh prepared SLN systems were used. The mixture was vortexed for 1 min, and HFA 134a were filled through the filling machine. The MDI products were allowed to stand for 10 min to recover to room temperature. MDI was manufactured continuously for at least three batches. A batch consisted of 15 MDI products.

2.5. MDI Evaluations

2.5.1. Appearance

A laser pen (Deli Group Co., Ltd., Shanghai, China) was used to lignite the MDI products at a distance of 5 cm, and the photographs representing Tyndall's effect were taken.

2.5.2. Filling Reproducibility

Using the method in Section 2.4, ten products were prepared. The aerosol container and the MDI products were accurately weighed and recorded as W_0 and W', respectively. The weight of filled HFA 134a (ΔW) was calculated as follows:

$$\Delta W = W_0 - W' \quad (1)$$

The relative standard deviation (RSD) values of ΔW were calculated to evaluate the filling reproducibility.

2.5.3. Total Shots

The MDI products were fired into a 500 mL beaker containing approximately 50 mL of water, until the formulations were aerosolized completely. The interval between shots were 5 s. The number of total shots was examined.

2.5.4. Valve Precision

After discarding the first three shots, the MDI products were fired according to Section 2.5.3. Before and after each shot, the MDI products were weighted. The reducing weight per press was recorded to evaluate the valve precision.

2.5.5. Leak Detection

The MDI products were stored in dark condition at 20 ± 2 °C temperature and $60 \pm 5\%$ relative humidity, for 15 d. On day 0, 3, 5, 10, and 15, the weight of MDI products was recorded to detect the possible leakage.

2.5.6. Re-Dispersity

On day 0, 3, 5, and 10 of storage under the conditions described in Section 2.5.5, the MDI products were carefully retrieved and shaken manually for 30 s. The dispersity and suspending stability were inspected visually.

2.5.7. Stability of Particle Size

The MDI products were stored according to Section 2.5.5, and the evolution of average size and PDI within 10 d was determined to assess the stability. Alongside with the test, instability phenomena such as flocculation, sedimentation, and layering were monitored visually.

2.6. Cytotoxicity Studies

A549 cells were cultivated using DMEM media and fetal bovine serum. They were cultivated to a confluence of 90% and processed by trypsin. The cells were transferred to 96-well plates at a density of 1×10^4 mL^{-1}. SLN-based MDI products were aerosolized and the residues were reconstructed with culture media adding into A549 cells at concentrations of 0.50, 0.75, 1.00, 1.50, 2.00, and 3.00 μg·mL^{-1}. After incubation for 24 h and 72 h, the media was discarded and replaced by MTT solution (5 mg·mL^{-1}) before incubating it for another 4 h. MTT solution was replaced by DMSO and the optical density (OD) was determined at 570 nm (OD_{570}) and 630 nm (OD_{630}) using a plate reader (Synergy H1, BioTek Instruments, Inc., Winooski, VT). The cell viability was calculated using the following Equation (2):

$$\text{Cell viability (\%)} = (OD_{570,sample} - OD_{630,sample})/(OD_{570,blank} - OD_{630,blank}) \times 100\% \quad (2)$$

2.7. Statistics

The acquired data were expressed as mean ± standard deviation, wherever applicable, and then processed by statistical analysis via *t*-test or one-way analysis of variance (ANOVA). $p < 0.05$ was considered as a significant difference.

3. Results

This study exploited the industrialization potential of MDI based on a series of SLN with increasing layers of nanocoating. The model SLN were evaluated and then SLN-based MDI were produced and characterized to ensure the quality and reproducibility of the prepared formulation. Cytotoxicity of SLN-based MDI was tested to preliminarily highlight the administration safety.

3.1. Evaluations of SLN

SLN(0) with nanocoating of Poloxamer 188, SLN(+) with nanocoating of Poloxamer 188 + CTAB, and SLN(−) with nanocoating of Poloxamer 188 + CTAB + HA were prepared through sonification method envisioning to achieve the stabilization, cellular uptake enhancement, and targetability, respectively. The particle size distribution and zeta-potential are shown in Figure 2.

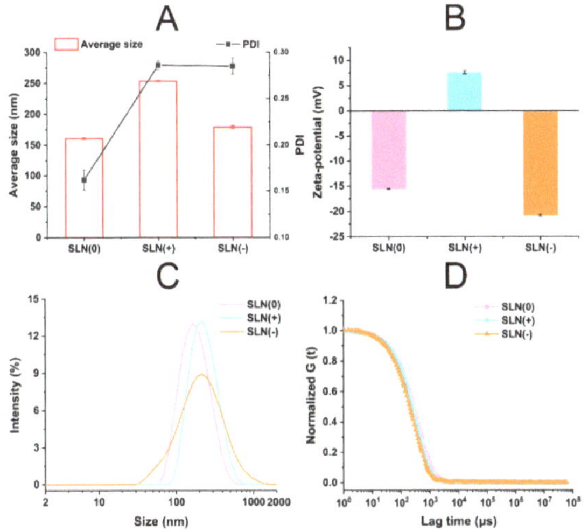

Figure 2. Characterizations. Average size and PDI (**A**), zeta-potential (**B**), particle size distribution curves (**C**), and autocorrelation function curves (**D**) ($n = 3$).

The average size of SLN(0), SLN(+), and SLN(−) was measured to be ~160 nm, ~250 nm, and ~180 nm, respectively. And the PDI values were all recorded below 0.3, suggesting a relatively homogeneous nanoparticle distribution (Figure 2A). The low PDI values also indicated good storage stability. The average size of SLN(+) and SLN (−) was higher than that of SLN(0) ($p < 0.05$) due to the thickness of nanocoating. The markedly large size of SLN(+) was probably because of the large hydrolyzed diameter of CTAB nanocoating [19].

As shown in Figure 2B, SLN(+) and SLN(−) exhibited positive charge and negative charge, respectively, which was resulted from the natural charge of corresponding nanocoating. SLN(0) revealed a ~−15 mV zeta-potential might be due to adsorption of anions by Poloxamer 188 in the Stern layer [20]. SLN(−) possessed significantly higher negative charge than SLN(0) ($p < 0.05$), suggesting that the natural charge of HA was more intense than the absorbed anions.

The particle size distribution curve verified the homogeneity in Figure 2C and all the formulations were in monodisperse phase with only one peak. For the distribution curves, no frontal peak or tailed peak was found. The autocorrelation function curves representing the signal decay profile of all the formulations were similar (Figure 2D), indicating that the nanocoating did not induce the aggregation.

SLN with three types of nanocoating were successfully fabricated and characterized, viz., SLN(0), SLN(+), and SLN(−). The size distribution was homogeneous, which was favorable for subsequent scale-up studies.

3.2. *Evaluations of SLN-Based MDI*

SLN(0), SLN(+), and SLN(−) were produced into MDI through previously reported reverse microemulsion strategy. A series of characterizations was performed on the produced samples. Before reporting the results, it was worth mentioning that the lipid material of SLN, palmityl palmitate had negligible solubility in ethanol at ambient temperature (see Table S1 and the literature [21]) and therefore, addition of ethanol in the MDI filling process would not exert dissolution effect upon the SLN.

The photographs of MDI products displaying the Tyndall's effect are provided in Figure S1. All the products were transparent with a pale gray color and a red laser beam was observed. The colloidal physicochemical nature of MDI products was demonstrated. No effect of the nanocoating was observed on the produce appearance.

The propellant filling reproducibility was tested and the average filling amount of HFA 134a was measured ~7.8 g (Figure 3A) with no statistical difference ($p > 0.05$). Reproducibility was confirmed with low RSD (<1%). The numbers of total shots were around 140 (Figure 3B) suggesting that the products might be suitable for long-term usage. The total shots of SLN(+) was circa 135, lower than SLN(0) and SLN(−). The positive charge on SLN(+), might have contributed toward the physical interactions with glass container which led to enhanced stability of the formulation. The average weight per press was c.a. 58 mg with uniform and acceptable standard deviation values (Figure 3C). Valve precision was validated with low statistical difference ($p > 0.05$). The weight of MDI tested after 15 days of storage ($p > 0.05$) (Figure 3D) remained constant, elucidating no leakage. Additionally, during storage, after manual shaking, the MDI products could maintain stable dispersion for at least 5 min, facilitating the clinical administration. It was worth noticing that filling reproducibility and valve precision of all SLN systems had similar performance. We could infer that the performance of MDI filling process was reproducible in various formulations. Actually, filling reproducibility and valve precision were determined by the filling machine and had insignificant effect on the formulations.

The change in particle size distribution of MDI products was evaluated for 10 days (Figure 4). After encapsulation, the average size of different groups tuned to be approximately 175 nm (Figure 4A). The difference in the particle size of Figure 4A with Figure 2A might be due to the presence of Pluronic L64 in MDI formulations. With diverse size range of SLN, the reverse microemulsion system seemed to exhibit particle confinement capacity (probably endowed by Pluronic L64). All PDI values were lower than 0.25 elaborating a sharp distribution of particle size (Figure 4B). Within 10 d, the average size and PDI did not change significantly ($p > 0.05$), suggesting stable particle size distribution. Moreover, no flocculation, sedimentation, and layering phenomenon were observed during the 10 d storage, strengthening the fact of satisfactory stability.

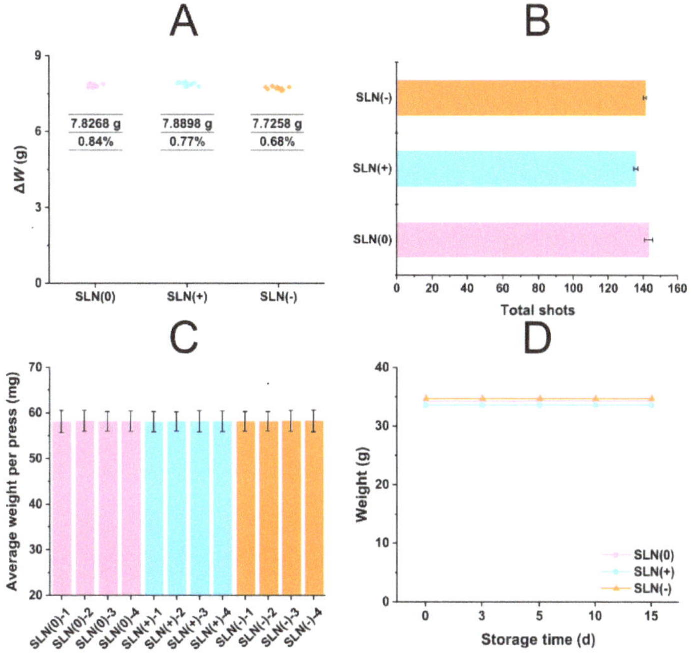

Figure 3. Evaluations of SLN-based MDI: Filling reproducibility (**A**), total shots (**B**), valve precision (**C**), and leak detection (**D**) (n = 10).

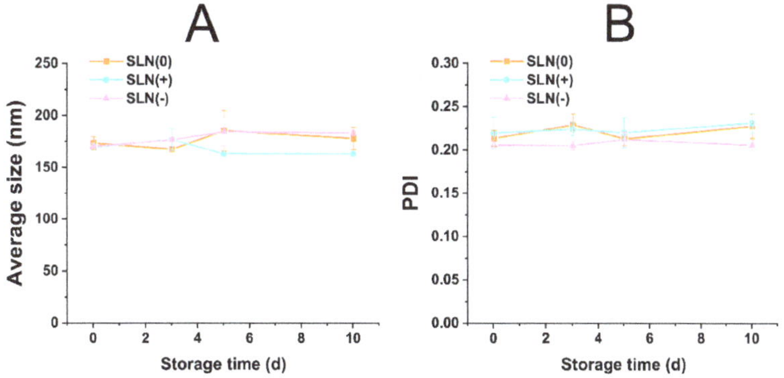

Figure 4. Evaluations of SLN-based MDI: evolution of average size (**A**) and PDI (**B**) versus time (n = 10).

3.3. Safety Evaluation

The biocompatibility of MDI products l was assessed through MTT assay. The results are presented in Figure 5. At 24 h (Figure 5A), the viability of A549 cells (human lung carcinoma cell line) was higher than 80% at 0.50~3.00 μg·mL^{-1} concentrations, suggesting good biocompatibility of all the MDI formulations prepared from SLN(0) and SLN(+) and SLN(−). The cell viability of SLN(+) dropped below 80% at 0.75 μg·mL^{-1} or higher concentrations after 72 h, whereas no change was recorded in case of SLN(0) and SLN(−). This phenomenon could be explained by the contribution of inherent cytotoxicity of CTAB [22]. CTAB is absent in SLN(0) whereas, it was veiled by HA layer in SLN(−) and therefore effect was minimized. It could also be conjectured that Poloxamer 188 and HA nanocoating had neglectable cytotoxicity. In summary, the MDI products, SLN(0) and SLN(−) might have acceptable safety in pulmonary delivery. As the volume of lung lining fluid was about 25 mL and given the maximum concentration in this work (3.00 μg·mL^{-1}), it could be roughly calculated that SLN(0) and SLN(−) dose up to 75 μg was tolerable after administration.

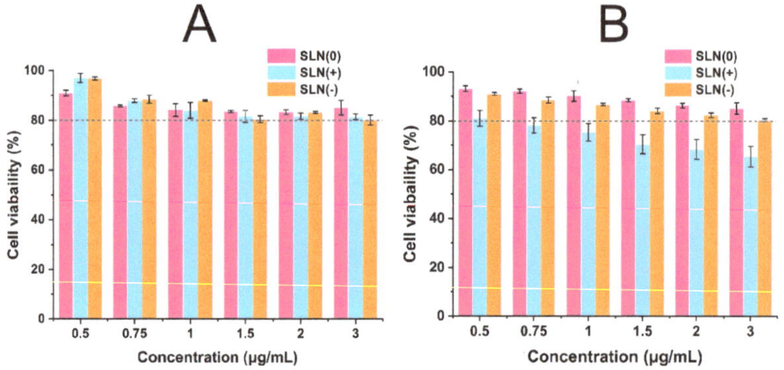

Figure 5. Safety evaluation: cell viability at 24 h (**A**) and 72 h (**B**) of MDI products prepared by SLN(0), SLN(+), and SLN(−) (n = 4).

Above-mentioned results elaborated the feasibility and reproducibility of the proposed production strategy of SLN-based MDI products and suggested that SLN(0) and SLN(−) could be exploited for their industrialization potential.

4. Discussion

4.1. Study-Design Aspect

The industrialization of inhalable nanoparticles is always a difficult task for the academia and industry. The main problems are: (1) How to obtain nanoparticle with reproducibility on a large scale? (2) How to transform nanoparticle into MDI with reproducibility on a large scale? Answering these two questions stepwise, will help in resolving the industrialization dilemma.

For question (1), since most nanoparticle systems under development were of sophisticated design, it was typically hard to produce those nanoparticles with reproducibility. It was worth noticing that lipid-based nanoparticle was an inspiring exception with great scale-up potential [23]. Therefore, we selected SLN, a representative lipid-based nanoparticle for subsequent study. As shown by the results in Section 3.1, the prepared SLN including SLN(0), SLN(+), and SLN(−), were of reproducible quality and potentially answering the question (1).

The transformation of SLN into MDI is more complicated than the transformation of pure drug into MDI. Physical stability of SLN (mainly mirrored by the particle size [24]) is critical which has no relevance in the case of pure drug. Pluronic L64 was added during the MDI filling process to enhance the physical stability. It could serve as an emulsifier for suspending SLN in the propellant of MDI formulation [17]. Demonstrated in the results Section 3.2, SLN-based MDI with good reproducibility and physical stability could be obtained. As a consequence, question (2) could be addressed.

We must notice that in addition to the formulation design, the credibility of SLN sonication instrument and MDI filling machine played an unneglectable role in addressing questions (1) and (2), respectively. Attention must be paid to the instrument configuration and functions during the development of SLN-based MDI.

The scale-up potential of MDI products of three SLN systems, namely SLN(0), SLN(+), and SLN(−), was demonstrated. The above workflow might also be applicable for the development of other similar systems, most probable for lipid-based nanomedicines, e.g., liposomes, cubosomes, or exosomes. We perceived that this work could act as a precedent for further attempts for inhalable nanoparticle industrialization.

4.2. Cytotoxicity Aspect

SLN(0) and SLN(−) showed good biocompatibility in comparison to SLN(+). The reason is the presence of CTAB in SLN(+). Various cationic materials has been reported to be toxic, even including the most commonly used cationic lecithin for cationic liposome preparation, i.e., 1,2-dioleoyl-3-trimethylammonium-propane (DOTAP) [25]. The underlying mechanism was the strong interaction between cationic materials and anionic cell membrane which disturbs the physiological structure and function of the latter [26]. In this work, CTAB was preliminarily chosen because it was involved in the established method by our group [27]; we also expected to accelerate the scale-up of that previously developed inhalable nanoparticle. We perceived that a mere modification of outer layer of SLN with CTAB or similar cationic materials was inappropriate for clinical use. Considering that the CTAB nanocoating was intended for cellular uptake enhancement, we inferred that SLN(+) might be used for the establishment of respiratory injury laboratory models [28] especially after loading with positive inducing agents such as lipopolysaccharides (LPS). We might witness clinical translation of systems such as SLN(0) and SLN(−) in the near future. SLN(0) could be used to deliver a wide range of therapeutic drugs and due to the recognition of HA toward CD44 receptors on tumor cell membrane [29], SLN(−) are prospective in targeted cancer therapy.

Noticeably, a single pilot cytotoxicity examination was insufficient to confer the clinical safety. The cytotoxicity effect on multiple cell lines (Calu-3, Beas-2b, etc.) and safety test on animal models (mouse, rat, dog, etc.) will be reported in due course.

4.3. Limitation Aspect

Although this work put forward a strategy to boost the industrial translation of SLN-based MDI by addressing the abovementioned two main questions related to stability of the formulation, there are still some limitations. For instance, SLN carriers without cargoes were employed in the tests. We elucidated the feasibility and reproducibility of SLN (carrier only)-based MDI and planning to examine the scenario of SLN (drugs encapsulated)-based MDI. Based on the A549 (lung cancer cells) model employed in this study, we will first incorporate anticancer drugs such as cisplatin, paclitaxel, and sorafenib.

5. Conclusions

In this study, a proof-of-concept of the industrialization of inhalable nanoparticles was conducted. SLN with different nanocoatings, SLN(0), SLN(+), and SLN(−) were prepared and encapsulated into MDI. The MDI products possessed homogeneous particle size distribution and good stability and performed well in evaluations which include appearance, filling reproducibility, valve precision, leak detection, and re-dispersity. SLN(0) and SLN(−) showed good biocompatibility tested against A549 cells (with >80% at XX), while SLN(+) exerted observable cytotoxicity. We suggested to pay more attention to the scale-up for MDI products based on SLN(0) and SLN(−) in the current stage.

Supplementary Materials: The following supporting information can be downloaded at: https://www.mdpi.com/article/10.3390/pharmaceutics15030866/s1, Figure S1: Evaluations of SLN-based MDI: Photographs of MDI products based on SLN(0) (A), SLN(+) (B) and SLN(−) (C); Table S1: Qualitative solubility test of palmityl palmitate at room temperature.

Author Contributions: Data analysis and manuscript writing, L.S.; illustration and formulation design, W.W.; preparation and particle size measurement, C.-i.N.; else evaluations and manuscript polishing, X.Z. and Y.H.; conceptualization and proof-reading, X.P. and C.W.; cytotoxicity tests, supervision, and fund-seeking, Z.H. All authors have read and agreed to the published version of the manuscript.

Funding: This research was funded by National Natural Science Foundation of China grant number 82104070.

Institutional Review Board Statement: Not applicable.

Informed Consent Statement: Not applicable.

Data Availability Statement: The data presented in this study are available on request from the corresponding author.

Acknowledgments: The authors would like to thank Vikramjeet Singh from University College London (UCL) for his help in language polishing. We also thanked Disang Feng and Xiao Yue from Guangzhou Novaken Pharmaceutical Co., Ltd. (Guangzhou, China) for their help in configuring and debugging the MDI filling machine.

Conflicts of Interest: The authors declare no conflict of interest.

References

1. Elbatanony, R.S.; Parvathaneni, V.; Kulkarni, N.S.; Shukla, S.K.; Chauhan, G.; Kunda, N.K.; Gupta, V. Afatinib-loaded inhalable PLGA nanoparticles for localized therapy of non-small cell lung cancer (NSCLC)—Development and in-vitro efficacy. *Drug Deliv. Transl. Res.* **2021**, *11*, 927–943. [CrossRef] [PubMed]
2. Li, H.-Y.; Xu, E.-Y. Innovative pMDI formulations of spray-dried nanoparticles for efficient pulmonary drug delivery. *Int. J. Pharm.* **2017**, *530*, 12–20. [CrossRef] [PubMed]
3. Alfagih, I.M.; Kaneko, K.; Kunda, N.K.; Alanazi, F.; Dennison, S.R.; Tawfeek, H.M.; Saleem, I.Y. In vitro characterization of inhalable cationic hybrid nanoparticles as potential vaccine carriers. *Pharmaceuticals* **2021**, *14*, 164. [CrossRef] [PubMed]
4. Ali, M.E.; Lamprecht, A. Spray freeze drying for dry powder inhalation of nanoparticles. *Eur. J. Pharm. Biopharm.* **2014**, *87*, 510–517. [CrossRef] [PubMed]
5. Ari, A.; Fink, J.B. Recent advances in aerosol devices for the delivery of inhaled medications. *Expert Opin. Drug Deliv.* **2020**, *17*, 133–144. [CrossRef]
6. Gagliardi, A.; Voci, S.; Salvatici, M.C.; Fresta, M.; Cosco, D. Brij-stabilized zein nanoparticles as potential drug carriers. *Colloids Surf. B Biointerfaces* **2021**, *201*, 111647. [CrossRef]
7. Shaabani, E.; Sharifiaghdam, M.; De Keersmaecker, H.; De Rycke, R.; De Smedt, S.; Faridi-Majidi, R.; Braeckmans, K.; Fraire, J.C. Layer by layer assembled chitosan-coated gold nanoparticles for enhanced siRNA delivery and silencing. *Int. J. Mol. Sci.* **2021**, *22*, 831. [CrossRef]
8. Luo, Z.; Dai, Y.; Gao, H. Development and application of hyaluronic acid in tumor targeting drug delivery. *Acta Pharm. Sin. B* **2019**, *9*, 1099–1112. [CrossRef]
9. Li, X.; Ma, Y.; Zhong, X.-L.; Wang, L.-S. Silver sulfide nanoparticles on MWCNTs stabilized by poloxamer: An enhanced electrochemical sensor for high sensitivity detection of 2, 4, 6-trinitrotoluene. *Microchem. J.* **2020**, *159*, 105488. [CrossRef]
10. Wang, X.; Wei, Y.; Wang, S.; Chen, L. Red-to-blue colorimetric detection of chromium via Cr (III)-citrate chelating based on Tween 20-stabilized gold nanoparticles. *Colloids Surf. A Physicochem. Eng. Asp.* **2015**, *472*, 57–62. [CrossRef]
11. Alkilany, A.M.; Nagaria, P.K.; Hexel, C.R.; Shaw, T.J.; Murphy, C.J.; Wyatt, M.D. Cellular uptake and cytotoxicity of gold nanorods: Molecular origin of cytotoxicity and surface effects. *Small* **2009**, *5*, 701–708. [CrossRef]
12. Alshehri, S.; Imam, S.S.; Rizwanullah, M.; Fakhri, K.U.; Rizvi, M.M.A.; Mahdi, W.; Kazi, M. Effect of chitosan coating on PLGA nanoparticles for oral delivery of thymoquinone: In vitro, ex vivo, and cancer cell line assessments. *Coatings* **2020**, *11*, 6. [CrossRef]
13. Lee, S.-E.; Lee, C.D.; Ahn, J.B.; Kim, D.-H.; Lee, J.K.; Lee, J.-Y.; Choi, J.-S.; Park, J.-S. Hyaluronic acid-coated solid lipid nanoparticles to overcome drug-resistance in tumor cells. *J. Drug Deliv. Sci. Technol.* **2019**, *50*, 365–371. [CrossRef]
14. Al-Musawi, S.; Albukhaty, S.; Al-Karagoly, H.; Almalki, F. Design and synthesis of multi-functional superparamagnetic core-gold shell nanoparticles coated with chitosan and folate for targeted antitumor therapy. *Nanomaterials* **2020**, *11*, 32. [CrossRef]
15. Vallorz, E.; Sheth, P.; Myrdal, P. Pressurized metered dose inhaler technology: Manufacturing. *AAPS PharmSciTech* **2019**, *20*, 177. [CrossRef]
16. Shan, Z.; Tan, Y.; Qin, L.; Li, G.; Pan, X.; Wang, Z.; Yu, X.; Wang, Q.; Wu, C. Formulation and evaluation of novel reverse microemulsions containing salmon calcitonin in hydrofluoroalkane propellants. *Int. J. Pharm.* **2014**, *466*, 390–399. [CrossRef]
17. Wang, W.; Huang, Z.; Xue, K.; Li, J.; Wang, W.; Ma, J.; Ma, C.; Bai, X.; Huang, Y.; Pan, X. Development of aggregation-caused quenching probe-loaded pressurized metered-dose inhalers with fluorescence tracking potentials. *AAPS PharmSciTech* **2020**, *21*, 296. [CrossRef]
18. Li, X.; Huang, Y.; Huang, Z.; Ma, X.; Dong, N.; Chen, W.; Pan, X.; Wu, C. Enhancing stability of exenatide-containing pressurized metered-dose inhaler via reverse microemulsion system. *AAPS PharmSciTech* **2018**, *19*, 2499–2508. [CrossRef]
19. Pastoriza-Santos, I.; Pérez-Juste, J.; Liz-Marzán, L.M. Silica-coating and hydrophobation of CTAB-stabilized gold nanorods. *Chem. Mater.* **2006**, *18*, 2465–2467. [CrossRef]
20. Honary, S.; Zahir, F. Effect of zeta potential on the properties of nano-drug delivery systems-a review (Part 1). *Trop. J. Pharm. Res.* **2013**, *12*, 255–264.
21. Lester, D.; Bergmann, W. Contributions to the study of marine products. VI. The occurrence of cetyl palmitate in corals. *J. Org. Chem.* **1941**, *6*, 120–122. [CrossRef]
22. Ozcicek, I.; Aysit, N.; Cakici, C.; Ayturk, N.U.; Aydeger, A.; Erim, U.C. The Effects of Various Surface Coatings of Gold Nanorods on Toxicity, Neuronal Localization, Microstructural Alterations, and In vitro/In vivo Biodistribution. *Adv. Mater. Interfaces* **2022**, *9*, 2101369. [CrossRef]

23. Khairnar, S.V.; Pagare, P.; Thakre, A.; Nambiar, A.R.; Junnuthula, V.; Abraham, M.C.; Kolimi, P.; Nyavanandi, D.; Dyawanapelly, S. Review on the Scale-Up Methods for the Preparation of Solid Lipid Nanoparticles. *Pharmaceutics* **2022**, *14*, 1886. [CrossRef] [PubMed]
24. Chunhachaichana, C.; Sawatdee, S.; Rugmai, S.; Srichana, T. Development and characterization of nanodispersion-based sildenafil pressurized metered-dose inhaler using combined small-angle X-ray scattering, dynamic light scattering, and impactors. *J. Drug Deliv. Sci. Technol.* **2022**, *76*, 103749. [CrossRef]
25. Sun, M.W.; Dang, U.J.; Yuan, Y.H.; Psaras, A.M.; Osipitan, O.; Brooks, T.A.; Lu, F.K.; Di Pasqua, A.J. Optimization of DOTAP/chol Cationic Lipid Nanoparticles for mRNA, pDNA, and Oligonucleotide Delivery. *AAPS PharmSciTech* **2022**, *23*, 135. [CrossRef]
26. Ivask, A.; Suarez, E.; Patel, T.; Boren, D.; Ji, Z.X.; Holden, P.; Telesca, D.; Damoiseaux, R.; Bradley, K.A.; Godwin, H. Genome-Wide Bacterial Toxicity Screening Uncovers the Mechanisms of Toxicity of a Cationic Polystyrene Nanomaterial. *Environ. Sci. Technol.* **2012**, *46*, 2398–2405. [CrossRef]
27. Wang, W.; Wang, W.; Jin, S.; Fu, F.; Huang, Z.; Huang, Y.; Wu, C.; Pan, X. Open Pocket and Tighten Holes: Inhalable Lung Cancer-Targeted Nanocomposite for Enhanced Ferroptosis-Apoptosis Synergetic Therapy. *Chem. Eng. J.* **2023**, *458*, 141487. [CrossRef]
28. Sun, Y.; Guo, F.; Zou, Z.; Li, C.G.; Hong, X.X.; Zhao, Y.; Wang, C.X.; Wang, H.L.; Liu, H.L.; Yang, P.; et al. Cationic nanoparticles directly bind angiotensin-converting enzyme 2 and induce acute lung injury in mice. *Part. Fibre Toxicol.* **2015**, *12*, 4. [CrossRef]
29. Weng, X.; Maxwell-Warburton, S.; Hasib, A.; Ma, L.F.; Kang, L. The membrane receptor CD44: Novel insights into metabolism. *Trends Endocrinol. Metab.* **2022**, *33*, 318–332. [CrossRef]

pharmaceutics MDPI

Article

Coatings of Cyclodextrin/Citric-Acid Biopolymer as Drug Delivery Systems: A Review

Karen Escobar [1], Karla A. Garrido-Miranda [2], Ruth Pulido [3,4,5], Nelson Naveas [3,4,5], Miguel Manso-Silván [4,5,*] and Jacobo Hernandez-Montelongo [1,*]

1 Departamento de Ciencias Matemáticas y Físicas, Universidad Católica de Temuco, Temuco 4813302, Chile
2 Agriaquaculture Nutritional Genomic Center, CGNA, Temuco 4780000, Chile
3 Departamento de Ingeniería Química y Procesos de Minerales, Universidad de Antofagasta, Antofagasta 1270300, Chile
4 Departamento de Física Aplicada and Instituto Universitario de Ciencia de Materiales Nicolás Cabrera, Universidad Autónoma de Madrid, 28049 Madrid, Spain
5 Instituto Universitario de Ciencias de Materiales Nicolás Cabrera, Universidad Autónoma de Madrid, 28049 Madrid, Spain
* Correspondence: miguel.manso@uam.es (M.M.-S.); jacobo.hernandez@uct.cl (J.H.-M.)

Abstract: In the early 2000s, a method for cross-linking cyclodextrins (CDs) with citric acid (CTR) was developed. This method was nontoxic, environmentally friendly, and inexpensive compared to the others previously proposed in the literature. Since then, the CD/CTR biopolymers have been widely used as a coating on implants and other materials for biomedical applications. The present review aims to cover the chemical properties of CDs, the synthesis routes of CD/CTR, and their applications as drug-delivery systems when coated on different substrates. Likewise, the molecules released and other pharmaceutical aspects involved are addressed. Moreover, the different methods of pretreatment applied on the substrates before the in situ polymerization of CD/CTR are also reviewed as a key element in the final functionality. This process is not trivial because it depends on the surface chemistry, geometry, and physical properties of the material to be coated. The biocompatibility of the polymer was also highlighted. Finally, the mechanisms of release generated in the CD/CTR coatings were analyzed, including the mathematical model of Korsmeyer–Peppas, which has been dominantly used to explain the release kinetics of drug-delivery systems based on these biopolymers. The flexibility of CD/CTR to host a wide variety of drugs, of the in situ polymerization to integrate with diverse implantable materials, and the controllable release kinetics provide a set of advantages, thereby ensuring a wide range of future uses.

Keywords: cyclodextrins; cyclodextrin polymers; implant coating; drug delivery

check for updates

Citation: Escobar, K.; Garrido-Miranda, K.A.; Pulido, R.; Naveas, N.; Manso-Silván, M.; Hernandez-Montelongo, J. Coatings of Cyclodextrin/Citric-Acid Biopolymer as Drug Delivery Systems: A Review. *Pharmaceutics* **2023**, *15*, 296. https://doi.org/10.3390/pharmaceutics15010296

Academic Editors: Ping Hu, Zheng Cai and Francesca Maestrelli

Received: 25 November 2022
Revised: 23 December 2022
Accepted: 12 January 2023
Published: 16 January 2023

1. Introduction

Medical implant surgery involves inherent risks, such as infections, local swelling and induration, inadequate healing, and others, which become more complicated in cases of immunosuppression caused by several diseases or conditions [1]. A very effective strategy to reduce these postoperative risks is to coat the implants with polymeric drug-delivery systems [2]. One of the most versatile drug-delivery systems is the cyclodextrin/citric-acid biopolymer (CD/CTR), which has been successfully used in the last years as a coating on different materials and implants for the local controlled release of several molecules. The synthesis of this biopolymer was developed by Martel et al. (2002) [3] and consists of the use of CTR, a polycarboxylic acid, as the cross-linking agent of CDs.

CDs are cyclic oligosaccharides with hydrophilic outer surfaces and a lipophilic central cavity, which allows the formation of reversible complexes with drugs and thus used as efficient delivery carriers [4]. CDs, as building blocks, are easily cross-linked with CTR, yielding a three-dimensional polymer network suitable for enhanced drug-delivery applications. Such volume structure presents extended interactions with drugs, prolonging residence time in the medium and/or increasing efficiency and specificity toward targeted sites [5].

The success of using CD/CTR on a wide range of surfaces is due to its cost-effectiveness and ease of in situ polymerization, which can be tuned by the reaction time at low temperatures. However, a pretreatment on the substrate surface is mandatory prior to performing the CD/CTR polymerization. This process is not trivial because it depends on the surface chemistry, geometry, and physical properties of the material to treat. Another important aspect of CD/CTR is the high capacity and diversity of molecules that can be loaded in its matrix, its biocompatibility [6,7], and biodegradability [8,9].

The most common mechanism of release of drug-delivery systems based on CD/CTR is the Fickian diffusion [10], which is a process in which the transport of the penetrant (water, PBS, or corporal fluids) is a diffusion process driven by the penetrant concentration gradient [11]. Usually, this phenomenon in CD/CTR systems is modeled by the semiempirical mathematical model of Korsmeyer–Peppas [12,13]. Although this tool is very useful for predicting the release kinetics before the release systems are realized, they must be used with criteria because they do not provide further insights into complex systems [14].

This review aims to cover the chemical properties of CDs, the syntheses of CD/CTR, and its applications as drug-delivery systems when coated on medical implants and other materials. The molecules released and other pharmaceutical aspects involved are discussed. Moreover, the different routes of the performed pretreatments on the substrates before the in situ polymerization of CD/CTR are also reviewed. The biocompatibility of the polymer was also highlighted. Finally, the mechanisms of release generated in the CD/CTR coatings were analyzed, including the Korsmeyer–Peppas model, which has been the most successfully semiempirical mathematical model to explain the release kinetics of drug-delivery systems based on these biopolymers.

2. Cyclodextrins

CDs are low molecular-weight cyclic oligosaccharides synthesized from the enzymatic degradation of starch. There are three main families of native cyclodextrins comprising six to eight ($\alpha = 6, \beta = 7, \gamma = 8$) D-glucopyranose units linked through glycosidic bonds between carbon 1 and 4 by a covalent bond [15]. Cyclodextrins have the advantages of being nontoxic, soluble in water, easily modifiable, and highly bioavailable. In addition, they are accessible and very useful in the industry [16,17]. The main physical properties of native CDs are presented in Table 1.

Table 1. Characteristics of native cyclodextrins.

Property	α-CD	β-CD	γ-CD
D-glucopyranose units	6	7	8
Molecular weight (g/mol)	972	1135	1297
Solubility in water at 25 °C (% w/v)	14.5	1.85	23.2
Outer diameter (Å)	14.6	15.4	17.5
Cavity diameter (Å)	4.7–5.3	6.0–6.5	7.5–8.3
Height (Å)	7.9	7.9	7.9

CDs are characterized by having a hydrophilic outer surface and a hydrophobic cavity (Figure 1) that allows them to form a rigid, cone-shaped cavity, where it can accept host molecules [18]. In this way, they form inclusion complexes by noncovalent interactions, and without complex chemical reactions [19]. Because each host molecule is individually surrounded by a CD, advantageous qualities can be provided in the chemical composition and in the physical properties of the host [4], such as stabilization of substances sensitive to light or to oxygen [20], modification of the chemical reactivity of host molecules [21], fixation of highly volatile substances, improvement of the solubility of substances [22], and protection against the degradation of substances by microorganisms [23], among others.

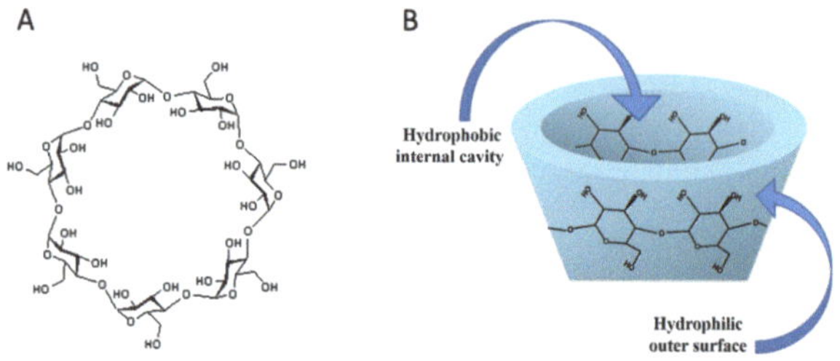

Figure 1. β-CD molecule: (**A**) chemical structure, and (**B**) toroidal shape.

As α-CD presents the smaller internal cavity, its structure is the most rigid and stable of native CDs [24]. This makes it resistant to enzymatic hydrolysis, so it has several applications in the food industry. Unlike to γ-CD, which has a wider cavity, this is the most flexible and less stable CD [25]. In fact, in some conditions can collapse and not maintain its toroidal shape. From a pharmaceutical point of view, β-CD presents the best-balanced characteristics to obtain the higher inclusion-complexing capacity. For example, the values of inclusion-complex formation constants for α-CD, β-CD and γ-CD with salicylic acid is 11, 65, and 13 M^{-1}, respectively. When the complex is formed with ibuprofen, this tendency is sharper: 55, 2600, and 59 M^{-1} for α-CD, β-CD and γ-CD, respectively [25].

On the other hand, native CDs present a variable number of hydroxyl groups capable of chemically reacting to incorporate different functional groups, which makes the formation of a great variety of derivatives possible [26]. The substituents can advantageously contribute to the inclusion of some specific host molecules and improve the ability to solubilize and stabilize the molecules in comparison with native CDs [27]. However, derivative CDs tend to be significantly more expansive than native CDs. Some examples of derivative β-CDs are the (2- hydroxypropyl)-β-cyclodextrin (HP-β-CD), random methylated β-cyclodextrin (RM-β-CD) and sulfobutyl ether-β-cyclodextrin (SBE-β-CD) (Table 2) [28].

Table 2. Characteristics of some derivative β-cyclodextrins.

Property	β-CD	HP-β-CD	RM-β-CD	SBE-β-CD
Number of substituted units	0	0.65	1.8	0.9
Molecular weight (g/mol)	1135	1400	1312	2163
Solubility in water at 25 °C (% w/v)	1.85	>600	>500	>500

CDs and their derivatives can be used as controlled drug release systems due to their characteristic cavity and their ability to form reversible complexes with drugs (Figure 2). In this way, the host molecule is slowly released from the cavity without altering the physical, chemical and biological properties of the drugs. In addition, CDs prolong the residence time of the molecules in the diffusion medium and increase the efficiency and specificity toward the target tissues [8,29]. Being considered biologically inert, CDs have been applied as pharmaceutical excipients for numerous drug formulations. Cyclodextrins α, β, γ and the derivative HP-β-CD are currently recognized as safe by the FDA, and by the European Pharmacopoeia [28].

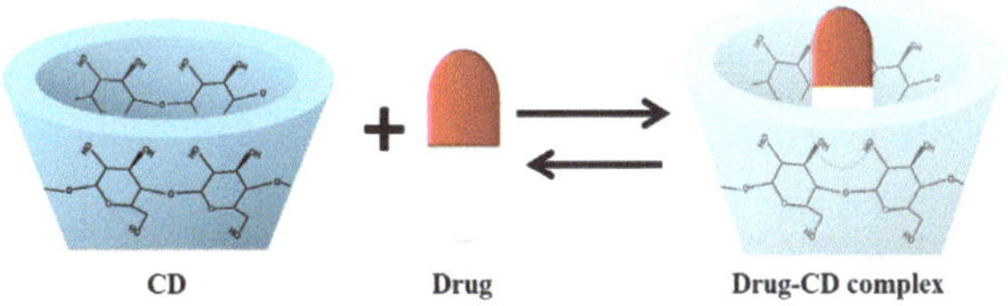

Figure 2. Dynamic equilibrium for drug-cyclodextrin complex.

3. Cyclodextrin/Citric Acid Biopolymer

In some cases, monomer units of CDs cannot form inclusion complexes with certain hydrophilic or high molecular mass drugs. Therefore, to increase this interaction, CDs and their derivatives have been used as building blocks for the development of a wide variety of networks, and polymer assemblies [18]. The main strategies applied to develop polymers of CDs can be classified into three large groups: (i) grafting of CDs to preformed polymers, (ii) polymerization with acrylic groups, and (iii) cross-linking with bi- or multifunctional agents, such as epichlorohydrin, biepoxides, and diisocyanates [30]. In the latter, the resulting polymer consists of a three-dimensional network that is suitable for drug-delivery applications. Figure 3 shows some types of polymers containing CDs. These CDs polymers are usually employed for drug-delivery applications; however, when they include molecules as quaternized amines they also present antibacterial effect [17]. The use of epichlorohydrin as a cross-linking agent of CDs has been the most widely used method. However, it has the drawbacks of taking place in concentrated basic media, in addition to the cross-linking agent being a toxic and carcinogenic reagent. As a result, the polymers obtained according to this route are not compatible with pharmaceutical or food uses [31]. Concerns about sustainability and human and environmental toxicity are driving the application of green chemistry principles to polymer synthesis. In this context, notable efforts are being made to select safe cross-linking agents and solvents [32]. In that sense, CTR is an effective multifunctional monomer for diverse syntheses; it is a nontoxic cross-linking agent, which is a natural organic acid with a multicarboxylic structure [33]. Moreover, CTR is very versatile because, under the defined conditions, it leads to soluble and insoluble polymers [31]. It plays roles in coforming ester cross-linking to improve compatibility coordination, balance the hydrophobicity of the polymer network, and provide other hydrogen bonding and binding sites for biocompatibility [34].

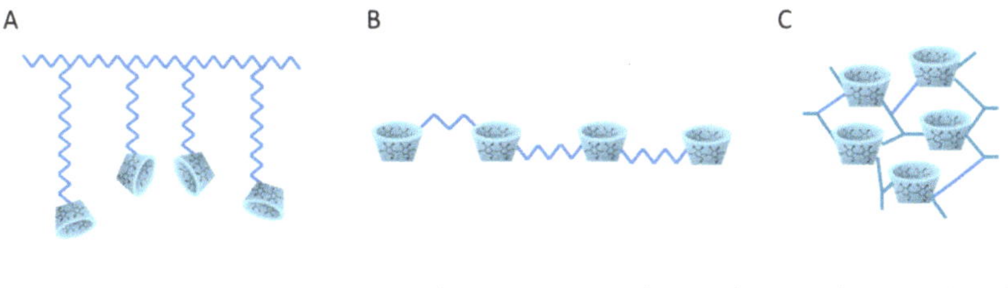

Figure 3. Types of polymers containing cyclodextrins: (**A**) pendent, (**B**) linear, and (**C**) cross-linked.

The origin of CD/CTR dates back to 1988 when Welch reported that the 1,2,3,4-butanetetracarboxylic acid (BTCA), a polycarboxylic acid (PCA), was able to provide effective cross-linking for cotton cellulose for a durable press finishing [35]. Later, in 1996, Yang and Wang studied the mechanism of this reaction and showed that the esterification between PCAs and cellulose occurred with the intermediate of a five- or six-membered cyclic anhydrides [36]. Then, in 2002, Martel et al. developed a cross-linking method that, compared to the others previously proposed in the literature, exclusively used nontoxic and environmentally friendly reagents [37]. This method consists of crosslinking CDs with biocompatible PCAs, like CTR, in the presence of phosphorus catalysts. The reaction begins with the dehydration of the PCAs, which generates a cyclic anhydride intermediate that easily reacts with the hydroxyl groups of the CDs through an esterification reaction. Then, two of the remaining carboxylic groups of the reacted PCAs can form a second anhydride that also reacts with another CD molecule. This reaction was made possible when PCAs contained at least three neighbouring carboxylic groups, like CTR [37]. In this reaction, sodium hypophosphite monohydrate ($NaH_2PO_2 \cdot H_2O$) is used as catalyst. Figure 4 shows the cross-linking mechanism between CTR and CD [10]. CD can be one of the three native CD forms or HPβ-CD [31,37].

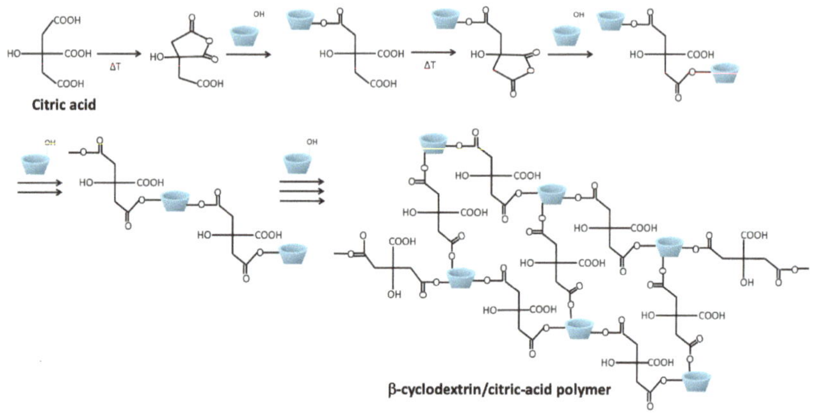

Figure 4. Polyesterification reaction between citric acid and β-cyclodextrin for the formation of the cross-linked polymer.

To incorporate the CD/CTR on implant surfaces or other materials, the copolymer is covalently grafted onto the medical device (for example, on cellulose surfaces), or fixed by physical interactions around fibres (for example, based on polyester or polypropylene) or is mechanically locked within biomaterial pores (for example, within porous polyvinylidene difluoride membranes) [38]. On the other hand, the performance of the polymerization on a sample depends on the curing temperature, the reaction time, and the CD/CTR ratio. For example, the solubility of the polymer decreases with increasing temperature and reaction time, and the swellability decreases with an increasing temperature and a decreasing CD/CTR molar ratio [31,37].

In the case of the polymerization yield, it can be obtained from the mass increase or by determining the amount of carboxylic groups present in the polymer [29,37]. In this way, the coating process can be optimized to achieve maximum polymerization performance at a given temperature and time [39].

4. Coatings of Cyclodextrin/Citric Acid Biopolymer as Drug-Delivery Systems

The properties of a material are often determined by its surface rather than its bulk composition. In fact, surfaces are technologically significant in several areas, such as catalysis, biomedicine, environmental remediation, etc., because they play a critical role in the performance and success of materials' applications [40]. In recent years, the functionalization or coating of surfaces has become an essential topic in materials science and engineering. Here, the coating aims at improving the material's performance or making it more suitable for a specific application [41].

Several studies have reported applications of CD-based coatings both in biomedical [42–46] and nonbiomedical applications [16,37,39,47–50]. On the one hand, in the context of nonbiomedical applications, CD-based coatings have been used to prevent corrosion problems and to remediate pollutants or dyes. On the other hand, for biomedical applications, the importance of CD-based surface coatings has increased, in terms of both biocompatibility and drug delivery [51–53], mainly intended as molecular delivery systems, such as the delivery of antibiotics [42,43] and drugs [44–46], among others.

The CD/CTR biopolymers have been widely used as drug-delivery systems when they are incorporated as coatings on different medical implants and other materials. The mechanisms involved in loading molecules consist of an inclusion of the drugs inside the CDs cavity, as well as less specific interactions with the cross-linked polymer network and its carboxylic groups available for supplementary interactions with the drug through hydrogen bonds [44]. Tables 3–5 present the most highlighted works performed during the last two decades, regarding the applications of coatings of cyclodextrin/citric-acid biopolymers as drug-delivery systems.

Table 3. Applications of coatings of cyclodextrin/citric-acid biopolymers as drug-delivery systems (Part 1).

Coating	Substrate	Drug	Application	Key Results	Ref.
β-CD/CTR	Polyvinylidene difluoride (PVDF) membranes for periodontology	Doxycyclin (DOX) and chlorhexidine (CHX), antimicrobial agents	A membrane for guided tissue regeneration applicable in periodontology	Grafted membranes, delivered DOX and CHX in larger quantities within 24 h and 10 days, respectively, in comparison with raw membranes than delivered low amounts of both molecules within the first few hours of tests; treated membranes showed biocompatibility to L132 cells	[54], 2006
β-CD/CTR, HP-β-CD/CTR, γ-CD/CTR and HP-γ-CD/CTR	Polyvinylidene difluoride (PVDF) membranes for periodontology	Chlorhexidine diacetate (CHX), an antiseptic	To cure periodontal lesions	Grafted membranes released CHX during 60–80 days, more than tenfold of raw membranes	[55], 2007
HP-β-CD/CTR	Polyester vascular prostheses	Ciprofloxacin, vancomycin, rifampicin; antibiotics	To minimize the risk of infection of arteries replacement surgeries	Higher amounts of the antibiotics were absorbed in the coated prostheses compared to the pristine ones, which was reflected in the microbiological tests (*S. aureus*, *E. coli* and *Enteroccocus* sp.); coated samples showed proliferation of HPMEC cells	[56], 2008
β-CD/CTR, HP-β-CD/CTR, γ-CD/CTR and HP-γ-CD/CTR	Polyamide inguinal meshes	Ciprofloxacin (CFX), an antibiotic	To avoid bacterial contamination of inguinal wounds	Meshes grafted with HP-γ-CD/CTR presented a 10-fold CFX absorption than raw samples, and also showed a longer antimicrobial effect (*S. aureus*, *S. epidermidis*, *E. coli*); fibroblastic cells proliferated on grafted samples	[57], 2008

Table 3. *Cont.*

Coating	Substrate	Drug	Application	Key Results	Ref.
HP-β-CD/CTR	Microporous hydro-xyapatite (HA)	Ciprofloxacin (CFX) and vancomycin (VCM), antibiotics	To prevent preoperative infection in bone-graft surgeries	Functionalized HA showed prolonged antibiotics release and higher antibacterial activity against *S. aureus* than pristine HA; treated samples presented cytocompatibility to osteoblasts	[58], 2009
HP-γ-CD/CTR	Polypropylene (PP) meshes for the treatment of hernias	Ciprofloxacin (CFX), an antibiotic	To prevent abdominal postoperative wound infections	Microbiological tests using *S. aureus, S. epidermidis, E. coli* confirmed the higher sustained antibacterial activity of the coated meshes than uncoated samples; treated samples did not affect fibroblast proliferation	[59], 2011
β-CD/CTR	Three papers used for sterilization: noncoated paper, a 10% cotton-based medical bandage, and a medical crepe paper	Chlorhexidine digluconate (digCHX), an antiseptic agent	To provide bactericidal properties to cellulose-based materials of medical use	All functionalized papers maintained the release for periods up to 20 days	[60], 2013
α-CD/CTR, β-CD/CTR, γ-CD/CTR and HP-β-CD/CTR	Poly(2-hydroxyethyl methacrylate)-based contact lenses	Ethoxzolamide (ETOX), a carbonic anhydrase inhibitor	An ocular treatment for glaucoma	Ionic interactions between CD polymers and contact lenses sustained the ETOX release for several weeks	[32], 2013
LbL of chitosan and β-CD/CTR	Nonwoven polyethylene terephthalate (PET) textile	4-*tert*-butyl benzoic acid (TBBA), an antimicrobial agent	The release of antimicrobial agents and antiproliferative drugs in cancer therapies	TBBA release kinetics was controlled by the number of layers in the LbL system	[61], 2013

Table 4. Applications of coatings of cyclodextrin/citric-acid biopolymers as drug-delivery systems (Part 2).

Coating	Substrate	Drug	Application	Key Results	Ref.
LbL of chitosan and β-CD/CTR	Nonwoven polyethylene terephthalate (PET) textile	Methylene blue (MB), a cationic dye with antimicrobial properties	To design biomaterials to trap and release therapeutic molecules directly to targeted areas	LbL systems displayed sustained antibacterial effects against *S. epidermidis* of the textile through the MB prolonged release; samples were cytocompatible to human epithelial embryonic cells	[62], 2013

Table 4. *Cont.*

Coating	Substrate	Drug	Application	Key Results	Ref.
β-CD/CTR	Layers of nanoporous and macroporous silicon (nPSi and mPSi)	Ciprofloxacin (CFX), an antibiotic; and prednisolone (PDN), an antiinflammatory	Intraocular drug delivery system for postophthalmic surgery	Both functionalized samples controlled released therapy concentrations of CFX and PDN required for an adult human eye. Treated samples presented cytocompatibility to L132 cells	[10], 2014
A bilayer of β-CD/CTR and microfibrillated cellulose (MFC)	Food packaging paper	Carvacrol, an antibacterial molecule	A strategy to prolong food shelf-life	Treated paper sustained four times the drug than raw paper, and were antibacterial for 14 h against *B. subtilis*	[63], 2014
Me-β-CD/CTR	CoCr vascular stents	Paclitaxel (PTX), a highly hydrophobic anticancer agent	To obtain commercial stents that promote arterial wall healing	Coated stents held more PTX over time compared to the uncoated samples in human plasma, and were cytocompatible to HPMEC cells	[64], 2014
β-CD/CTR	Paper points (PP) for endodontic therapies	Chlorhexidine digluconate (digCHX), an antiseptic agent for periodontal therapies	A treatment of the periodontal pocket by preventing its recolonization by the subgingival microflora	Coated PP showed a prolonged release of digCHX in human plasma and sustained antibacterial activity against four periodontal pathogens: *F. nucleatum, P. melaninogenica, A. actinomycetemcomitans* and *P. gingivalis*	[65], 2014
HP-β-CD/CTR	Visceral mesh of (polyethylene terephthalate, PET fibres	Ropivacaine, an anaesthetic	To reduce postoperatory pain	The coated meshes impregnated in 10 mg/mL ropivacaine solution adsorbed up to 17.7 mg/g of drug, with a prolonged release of 100 min; coated samples loaded with ropivacaine showed cytocompatibility with NIH3T3 cells (fibroblasts)	[44], 2014
LbL of chitosan and β-CD/CTR	Titanium disks	Gentamicin, an antibiotic	To address perioperative infections	The amount of loaded drug was easily controlled by modulating the number of layers involved in the LbL system; coated disks exhibited microbial activity up to 6 days against *S. aureus*	[8], 2015
LbL of epichlorohydrin-glycidyltrimethyl-ammoniumchloride-β-CD and β-CD/CTR	Non-woven polyethylene terephthalate (PET) textile	4-*tert*-butyl benzoic acid (TBBA), an antimicrobial agent	To reduce the risk of infection in implantable PET biomaterials	Thermal cross-linking of the LbL system enhanced the stability and TBBA release kinetics, which was reflected in its high antibacterial effect against *S. aureus*, and *E. coli*; samples were noncytotoxic to L132 epithelial cells	[9], 2016
HP-β-CD/CTR	Poly-L-lactic acid (PLLA) parietal reinforcement	Ciprofloxacin (CFX), an antibiotic	To prevent bacterial infections in surgeries of hernias of the abdominal wall	The cytocompatibility with fibroblasts of meshes, and the antibacterial effect of CFX against *S. aureus* and *E. coli.*, were found to be dependent on the degree of functionalization	[66], 2017

Table 5. Applications of coatings of cyclodextrin/citric-acid biopolymers as drug-delivery systems (Part 3).

Coating	Substrate	Drug	Application	Key Results	Ref.
β-CD/CTR	Nanoporous microparticles (nPSi)	Florfenicol (FF), the most important antibiotic employed in aquaculture	To efficientize the medical effect of ingested antimicrobials in salmon aquacultures	Treated samples allowed a major control in the drug time release kinetics compared to raw samples, in both distilled water and simulated seawater	[67], 2018
Me-β-CD/CTR	Woven polyethylene terephthalate (PET) vascular prostheses	Ciprofloxacin (CFX), an antibiotic	To reduce the risk of synthetic vascular graft infection (SVGI), a postoperative infection	CFX release from virgin prostheses was faster than from functionalized prostheses	[68], 2019
β-CD/CTR	Nanoporous microparticles (nPSi)	Caffeic acid (CA) and pinocembrin (Pin), polyphenols	A safe alternative system for oral administration of polyphenols	Coated microparticles loaded higher amounts of both polyphenols, which also showed a better-controlled release than uncoated samples; treated microparticles presented cytocompatibility to HUVEC cells	[69], 2019
LbL of epichlorohydrin-glycidyltrimethyl-ammoniumchloride-β-CD and β-CD/CTR	Nonwoven polyethylene terephthalate (PET) textile	Triclosan (TCS), a broad spectrum antimicrobial agent	To reduce the risk of infection in implantable PET biomaterials	Treated textile loaded TCS four times than control and displayed a high and constant level over at least 28 days that pristine textile; treated samples showed intrinsic contact killing property and also extrinsic release killing against *S. aureus* and *E. coli*	[70], 2020
Nanofibers (NFs) of chitosan and HP-β-CD/CTR produced by electrospinning	Auto-expansible NiTiNOL stents	Simvastatin (SV), a lipid-lowering medication	To prevent restenosis	The extension of the release time of SV depended on the duration of electrospinning and on the presence of HP-β-CD/CTR in the NFs matrix	[71], 2020
β-CD/CTR	Polytrimethylene terephthalate (PTT) textiles	Zn^{2+} and Cu^{2+} as antibacterial metal ions	To obtain an ecofriendly biobased antibacterial system for PTT fabrics	Coated textile showed an antibacterial effect to *S. aureus* and *E. coli*; Cu^{2+} displayed a stronger antibacterial ability	[72], 2021
β-CD/CTR	Nanoporous microparticles (nPSi)	Caffeic acid (CA) and pinocembrin (Pin), polyphenols	To improve the antiangiogenic and antioxidant activity of CA and Pin for the treatment of atherosclerosis	Coated microparticles showed higher antiangiogenic activity of CA and Pin than both in solution to treat HUVEC cells; in addition, coated microparticles presented a more time controlled antioxidant effect than uncoated samples	[73], 2022
β-CD/CTR	Nanozeolite	Ibuprofen (IB), a nonsteroidal antiinflammatory drug	An ecofriendly platform for IB delivery	β-CD/CTR-nanozeolite containing IB (30 wt%) showed the highest release at pH = 3.6 within the first 3–48 h of release time	[34], 2022

The most used CD/CTR polymer has been the β-CD/CTR due to the high capacity of loading and releasing diverse drugs of β-CD when cross-linked. In addition, β-CD is an accessible low-cost molecule [74]. Other CD/CTR polymers that have been tested include native and derivative CDs, such as α-CD/CTR, γ-CD/CTR, HP-β-CD/CTR, and Me-β-CD/CTR. The most frequent technique is to add β-CD/CTR to the surface of the substrate as a single coating by an in situ polymerization. However, due to the anionic characteristic of β-CD/CTR, it has been also used in layer-by-layer assemblies (LbL) in combination with cationic polymers [8,9,62,70]. Another frequently used CD/CTR polymer is the HP-β-CD/CTR, which due to its extra hydroxypropyl groups of HP-β-CD allows the inclusion of specific guest molecules, and ameliorates the ability to solubilize and stabilize drugs [66]. This polymer has been used as a single coating and combined with chitosan to produce nanofibers by electrospinning [71]. Nevertheless, HP-β-CD is a more expensive CD in comparison with its native version.

The fan of coated medical implants and materials with CD/CTR polymers is diverse. Among implants are several plastic devices like PVDF membranes for periodontology [54,55], polyester vascular prostheses [56], polyamide inguinal meshes [57], polypropylene meshes for the treatment of hernias [59], poly(2-hydroxyethyl methacrylate) contact lenses [32], PET textiles [9,61,62,70], meshes [44], and vascular prostheses [68], PLLA parietal reinforcement [66], and PTT textiles [72]. Organic and inorganic materials have been used as substrates for the CD/CTR coatings, such as cellulose papers [60,63,65], hydroxyapatite [58], porous silicon [10,67,69,73], and zeolite [34]. Metal medical devices include titanium disks [8], CoCr [64], and NiTiNOL stents [71].

The thickness of this type of coating is in the order of microns. This is going to depend on the CD/CTR polymer, substrate, and coating technique. Moreover, the homogeneity of the coating is going to be strongly influenced by the geometry of the substrate. For example, 2.5 µm-thickness of a homogeneous β-CD/CTR coating was achieved on nanoporous silicon (nPSi) and macroporous silicon (mPSi) (Figure 5(A1–A4)) [10]. In a contrasting way, a coating of HP-β-CD/CTR applied to PET visceral mesh was heterogeneous with polymer structures of tens of microns added to the mesh fibres (Figure 5(B1,B2)) [44].

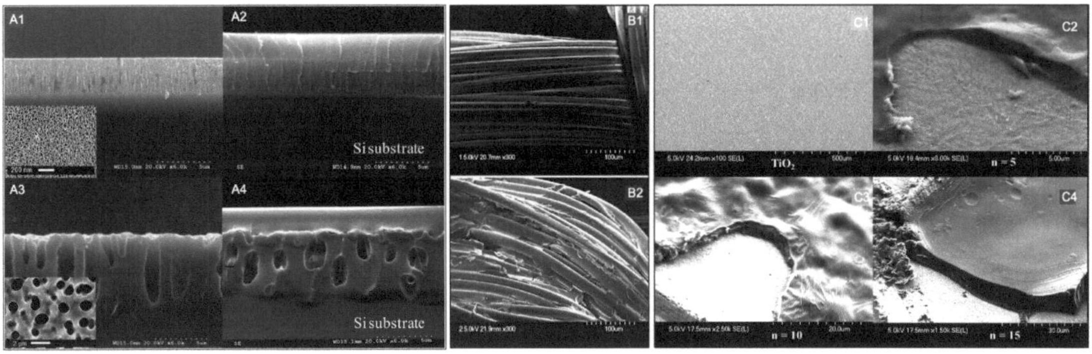

Figure 5. SEM images of: (**A1**) nPSi, (**A2**) nPSi-β-CD/CTR, (**A3**) mPSi, (**A4**) mPSi-β-CD/CTR; (**B1**) PET visceral mesh, (**B2**) PET-HP-β-CD/CTR, (**C1**) Ti, (**C2**) Ti-LbL of 5 bilayers, (**C3**)Ti-LbL of 10 bilayers, and (**C4**) Ti-LbL of 15 bilayers. Bilayers are chitosan and β-CD/CTR. Adapted from [8,10,44], with permission from Elsevier and ACS.

On the other hand, when the LbL technique is used to assemble a CD/CTR polymer, its thickness could be controlled according to the number of bilayers. Figure 5(C1–C4) shows the increase of thickness of the chitosan-β-CD/CTR assembling on titanium disks: 5, 10, and 15 bilayers were 6, 8, and 10 µm, respectively [8]. However, it should be mentioned that the most recent work of Jahangard et al. (2022) reported a β-CD/CTR layer, on the order of nanometers, for the functionalization of nanozeolite [34].

The principal application of the developed systems has been the prevention of preoperative and postoperative risks in implant surgeries, mainly focused on minimizing the risk of bacterial infections. Thereby, the most used drugs in the systems have been antibiotics, with ciprofloxacin being the most common. Other antibiotics have been also used, depending on the system (CD/CTR-implant) and application, even alternative antimicrobial agents such as the dye methylene blue [62] and the metal ions Zn^{2+} and Cu^{2+} [72].

As systems evolved, new prominent medical applications were explored like ocular treatments [10,32], arterial wall healing [64], and treatments for restenosis [71] and atherosclerosis [73]. Regarding veterinary applications, Hernandez–Montelongo et al. (2014) [67] proposed a system to improve the effect of ingested antimicrobials in salmon aquaculture. In the case of industrial uses, Lavoine et al. (2014) [63] explored a strategy to prolong food shelf life.

In general, all the works reported that coated samples with CD/CTR polymers showed a higher capacity to load drugs than uncoated samples. In the same sense, the treated substrates displayed more prolonged and sustained release than the untreated substrates. For example, Lepretre et al. (2007) [55] reported that PVDF membranes for periodontology coated with various CD/CTR polymers released considerably higher amounts of antibiotic chlorhexidine than raw membranes. Untreated samples released only 1 mg/g in a few hours, whereas membranes grafted with β-CD/CTR, γ-CD/CTR and HP-β-CD/CTR released up to 12 mg/g of drug within 55, 65, and 80 days, respectively.

As most of the CD/CTR-implant systems were loaded with antibiotics to prevent bacterial infections, they were mainly tested with bacteria *S. aureus*, *S. epidermidis* (both Gram-positive) and *E. coli* (Gram-negative). Other tested bacterial strains were *Enteroccocus* sp., *B. subtilis*, *F. nucleatum*, *P. melaninogenica*, *A. actinomycetemcomitans* and *P. gingivalis*. For example, Figure 6A shows the antibacterial property of a PET textile coated with an LbL assembling of a cationic and anionic β-CD/CTR polymers, this system released the antimicrobial triclosan for 24 h [70], and coated textiles displayed the double of inhibition zone than uncoated samples.

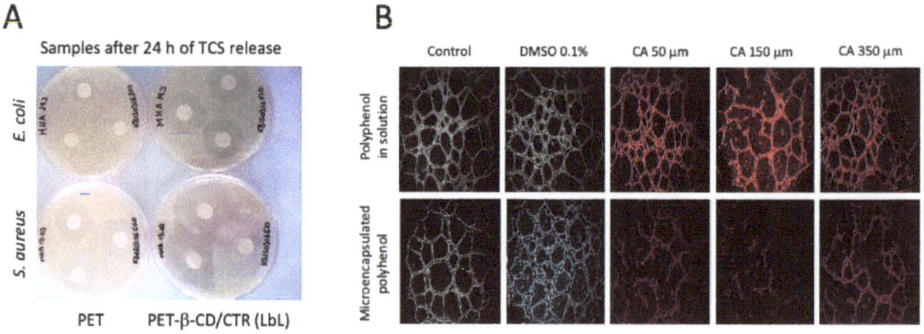

Figure 6. (**A**) Representative images of Kirby–Bauer test on TCS impregnated PET and PET-β-CD/CTR (LbL) samples against *S. aureus* and *E. coli* with inhibition zone after 24 h of TCS release in PBS at 37 °C. (**B**) Effect of treatment with caffeic acid in solution and loaded in the nPSi-β-CD/CTR microparticles on the ability of HUVECs to form tubular structures in Matrigel. Adapted from [70,73], with permission from Elsevier and MDPI, respectively.

In all reviewed works, the CD/CTR-implant systems showed stronger antibacterial activity than materials without the CD/CTR coating. In the cases in which other biomedical applications were explored, interesting results were also obtained. For example, Guzman–Oyarzo et al. (2022) [73] reported that the controlled release of polyphenols from coated microparticles of nanoporous silicon with β-CD/CTR displayed higher antiangiogenic activity than polyphenols just in solution to treat HUVEC cells. Figure 6B shows the significant reduction in the formation of tubules in the three concentrations when caffeic acid, a polyphenol, was microencapsulated. Authors also reported that coated microparticles presented a more time-controlled antioxidant effect than uncoated samples.

The CD/CTR are biopolymers, which means that they are biodegradable and biocompatible. Regarding biodegradability, a study about it is reported by Vermert et al. (2017) [66]: samples of PLLA coated with HP-β-CD/CTR were immersed in PBS at 37 °C under constant stirring. The virgin PLLA did not reveal any significant weight loss after 180 days, whereas the functionalized PLLA (33%-wt) showed a weight loss of around 30% after 120 days and then stabilization until the end of the experiment. As a consequence, the observed weight loss was therefore attributed to the degradation of CD/CTR polymer coating by hydrolysis in PBS within four months. On the other hand, the biocompatibility of CD/CTR has been studied by using a wide range of cell strains, depending on the application, such as human embryonic lung cells (L132) [9,54], human epithelial embryonic cells [62], human pulmonary microvascular endothelial cells (HPMEC) [56,64], fibroblast cells (NIH3T3) [44], and human umbilical vein endothelial cells (HUVEC) [69,73].

Regarding biological assays using animals, there is a work reported in the literature by Jean-Baptiste et al. (2012) [75]. The authors coated polyester vascular prostheses (PVPs) with HP-β-CD/CTR polymer designed to provide an in situ reservoir for the sustained delivery of antibiotics (rifampin, vancomycin hydrochloride, and ciprofloxacine). Their results showed that coated samples presented excellent biocompatibility, healing, and degradation properties in vitro and in albino Swiss mice (*Mus musculus*) in an animal model. The antimicrobial activity of samples was shown against *S. aureus* and *E. coli.* strains.

It is important to mention that CD/CTR polymers have not only been used as drug-delivery systems, but other interesting applications have also been studied, such as the removal of pollutants in water of heavy metal ions [76,77], dyes [78,79], organic compounds [78–80], and other things. Most recently, CD/CTR has also been utilized for host–guest recognition in sensors of herbicides [81] and antibiotics [82].

5. Pretreatments on the Substrates

As shown in Tables 3–5, different surfaces or substrates have been coated with CD/CTR-based biopolymers to generate controlled drug-release systems. These functionalized surfaces have been used in different applications, such as tissue regeneration [54] and bacterial infections [58], along with medical supplies and surgical materials [60,62], among other things. Here, preparing the surface prior to coating application is essential to determining the properties of the coating, particularly its roughness, adhesion, corrosion resistance and the ability to deliver the therapeutic substances. Then, depending on the substrate to be coated, different surface pretreatments and functionalizations have been carried out in order to achieve a successful coating with the desired properties.

Porous materials are one of the most interesting types of materials for drug-delivery applications. This is due to advanced properties, such as high surface area and high reactivity, among other things. In this sense, several reports have shown porous silicon (PSi) as a promising material for drug delivery. For example, nanoporous and macroporous PSi has been coated with CD/CTR-based coating via in situ polymerization. Herein, the surface has been previously treated by a chemical oxidation step by using H_2O_2 to mechanically stabilize the pore structure [10,67,69,73,83]. Besides, this chemical treatment of PSi, prior to CD/CTR-based coating, is an oxidation process involving different reactions; Si–H bonds can be transformed to Si–OH, Si–O–Si or –Oy-Si–Hx. Thus, the amalgam between the PSi substrates and CD/CTR was generated by hydrogen bonding and the anchoring effect of the porous matrix. Moreover, the CD/CTR coating adhesion on PSi can be enhanced with a chitosan grafting after the PSi chemical oxidation; positive $-NH_3$ of chitosan interacts electrostatically with both negative SiOx groups of the oxidized PSi surface, and negative $-COOH$ of CD/CTR biopolymer [67,69,73].

Other porous materials, such as hydroxyapatite and zeolite, have been functionalized with CD/CTR-based coatings without any substrate pretreatment [34,58]. A similar methodology has been reported for PDVF-based substrates [54,55]. In both cases, hydrogen bonding was the main chemical interaction between substrates and CD/CTR.

In the case of metallic samples, such as CoCr stents and Ti disks, an elaborated pretreatment was necessary to succesfully graft the CD/CTR biopolymer [8,64]. First, samples were mechanically polished, followed by chemical oxidations by using a "piranha solution". Afterward, samples were functionalized with dopamine, which enabled further CD/CTR-based coatings.

On the other side, by use of LbL techniques consisting of alternating physisorption of oppositely charged polyelectrolytes [84], different coatings have been formed on the substrate based on PET textil [9,61,62,70]. Interestingly, raw material activation was necessary for CD-CTR multilayer-based materials on nonwoven PET textile substrates. Such activation ensured the adhesion of the multilayer coating on the textile. This process is called "pad-dry-cure". There are four steps that mainly constitute this process: (i) impregnation of the PET textile into an aqueous solution containing CTR as a crosslinking agent, CD and a catalyst, (ii) roller squeezing, (iii) drying, and (iv) thermofixing (at variable temperature and time) [37]. This process aims at developing an ion exchange textile by forming a coating based on the previously explained polyesterification reaction (Figure 4).

The pad-dry-cure process has also been used for functionalized visceral mesh, and vascular prostheses based on PET substrates [44,56,68], as well as the coating of synthetic thermoplastic polymers such as polypropylene and polyamide, which have been used as artificial abdominal wall implants for the prolonged release of ciprofloxacin and to obtain inguinal meshes with improved antibiotic delivery properties, respectively [57,59]. This methodology has also been used to coat biocompatible synthetic polymeric substrates such as poly-L-lactic acid, which is capable of inducing subclinical inflammation in the host to stimulate collagen formation [66,85].

For the cases of natural textile-based substrates, such as cotton and paper, both direct [60,63] or indirect coating followed by the pad-dry-cure method has been used to form CD-based controlled drug-release systems. In this line, Tabary et al., (2014) proposed the use of a prefunctionalization step based on the oxidation of paper points [65]. The oxidation reaction was done in a nitric acid (HNO_3) and phosphoric acid (H_3PO_4) mixture at room temperature for 12 to 48 h with intermediate stirring with a glass rod. Their results showed that the functionalized oxidized paper point allowed the control of the bioresorption rate of the device, which could be used as a reliable complementary periodontal therapy. In this context, it is important to mention that natural textile-based substrates are mainly composed of cellulose, which implies that the esterification reaction occurs at the -OH functional groups of cellulose (or CDs), resulting in the formation of ester functional groups not present in cellulose. Thus, the detection of these functional groups determines the success of the CD grafting reaction on cellulose-based materials [60].

6. Mechanisms of Release of CD/CTR-Based Biopolymers

In clinical practice, when an implant surgery is performed, systemic treatments with various drugs are used to avoid or reduce possible postoperative complications. The methods consist of preoperative, perioperative, or postoperative administration of antibiotics, antiseptics, or other suitable molecules. Drugs can be administered orally, intravenously, or irrigated at the implantation site [86]. The doses administered and the duration of treatment are intensified in high-risk patients, such as those undergoing reconstructive surgery and/or undergoing radiotherapy treatments [87]. Traditional drug administration treatments, such as the venous or oral route, have poor control over these substances in the blood plasma because the drug concentration level reached is not stable. At the beginning of the administration, the level reaches high values, and then falls rapidly. Consequently, this variation in the concentration of the drug makes traditional treatments ineffective [88]. On the other hand, drugs given systemically can cause unwanted effects. For example, traditionally administered antibiotics may have difficulty penetrating the biofilm of bacteria, so only subinhibitory concentrations are reached at the site of infection, which causes the development of bacterial resistance [89]. Other drugs, such as zafirlukast (ZFL), which is administered orally for capsular contracture in mammary implant surgeries, can produce side effects like potential serious liver poisoning. For this reason, the use of ZFL is still restricted to severe and recurrent contractures [90].

The use of CD/CTR coatings on the implant surface offers a solution to the difficulties involved in the traditional drug-delivery system in surgeries. The release of the drug from the coated implant allows it to achieve a release in situ, that is, in the immediate environment of the implant. Thus, the side effects caused by the drugs can be reduced [59]. Moreover, the controlled delivery system based on CD/CTR coatings allows the drug concentration to be kept as close to the effective level of the treatment, which is below the toxic level and above the minimum of efficacy. In this way, the administration of repeated doses of drugs can be avoided [88].

On the other hand, in the drug-delivery systems based on polymers, the release can be controlled by diffusion, swelling, erosion, and/or external stimulations [91]. To develop and understand the drug-release mechanisms, mathematical models are very useful. In particular, semiempirical mathematical models are easy to use, and the established empirical rules help to explain transport mechanisms. In most cases, drug-diffusional mass transport is the predominant step in the control of drug release, whereas in others, it is present in combination with polymer swelling or polymer erosion [92]. In that sense, the most successfully semiempirical model to explain drug-delivery systems based on CD/CTR biopolymers is the Korsemeyer–Peppas model.

The Korsmeyer–Peppas model is a simple relationship to describe drug release from a polymeric system by using an exponential-type equation. This model analyzes Fickian, and non-Fickian release mechanisms considering the geometric characteristics of the system [93]. It was developed by Korsmeyer et al. (1983) [12], and Ritger and Peppas (1987) [13].

The Korsmeyer–Peppas equation is

$$Q(t)/Q_{\infty} = k_{\mathrm{KP}} t^{n}, \quad (1)$$

where $Q(t)$ is the amount of drug released in a time t and Q_{∞} is the amount of drug released in an infinitely long time; k_{KP} (h^{-n}) is the Korsmeyer–Peppas kinetic constant, which characterizes the drug-matrix system and is also considered the release velocity constant; and n is the exponent that indicates the drug-release mechanism.

The release mechanisms, according to the Korsemeyer–Peppas model, are shown in Table 6. These models can be categorized into five types [93–96]: (1) the quasi-Fickian model indicates that drug diffusion is the predominant phenomenon, but the matrix is partially swollen; (2) the Fickian mechanism (referred to as "case I") means that diffusion is the main present phenomenon; (3) in anomalous transport, the velocity of solvent diffusion and the polymeric relaxation speed possess similar magnitudes; (4) the zero order ("case II") is when the drug is released at a constant rate independent of concentration, and the velocity of solvent diffusion is less than the polymeric relaxation process; (5) in the super case transport, the velocity of solvent diffusion is much higher, causing an acceleration of solvent penetration. This causes tension and breakage of the polymer (erosion).

In this regard, when Korsmeyer–Peppas model was applied to the drug release profiles from porous silicon coated with β-CD/CTR, the calculated mechanism release was quasi-Fickian for ciprofloxacin, prednisolone, florfenicol, and caffeic acid [10,67,69]. However, in the case of pinocembrin, the mechanism release was an anomalous transport due to the strong interaction between this polyphenol and the polymer [69]. Figure 7 shows the polyphenols release profiles, caffeic acid and pinocembrin, from porous silicon coated with β-CD/CTR. On the other hand, results obtained for simvastatin release profile from nanofibers based on HP-β-CD/CTR coating stents suggested that the erosion (super case II transport) was the mechanism release [34].

Although the Korsmeyer–Peppas model is a useful and easy mathematical tool to implement, it may only be used for up to 60% of the released drug, and it has no provisions for an analysis of the remaining 40%. Thus, there is no phenomenological connection with this data [97]. For this reason, it is important to develop mathematical models to adequately study the release kinetics from polymer coatings to liquid media.

Table 6. Release mechanisms for different geometries according to the Korsmeyer–Peppas model.

Release Mechanisms	Geometry	Release Exponent *n*
Quasi-Fickian	Planar (thin films) Cylinders Spheres	$n < 0.5$ $n < 0.45$ $n < 0.43$
Fickian diffusion (case I)	Planar (thin films) Cylinders Spheres	0.5 0.45 0.43
Anomalous transport	Planar (thin films) Cylinders Spheres	$0.5 < n < 1$ $0.45 < n < 1$ $0.43 < n < 1$
Zero order (case II)	Planar (thin films) Cylinders Spheres	1 0.89 0.85
Super case II transport	Planar (thin films) Cylinders Spheres	$n > 1$ $n > 0.89$ $n > 0.85$

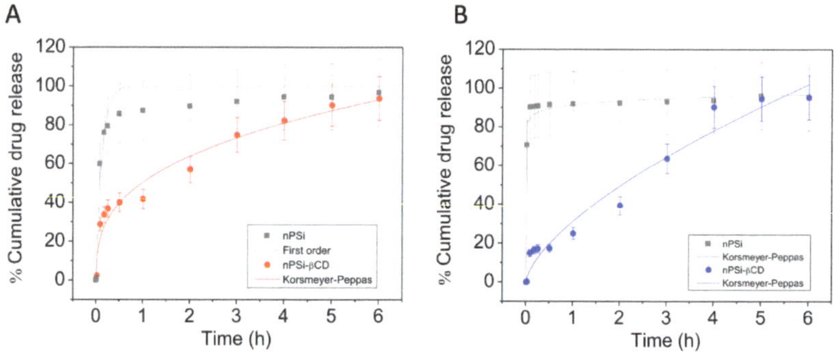

Figure 7. Polyphenols release profiles from porous silicon (control) and porous silicon coated with β-CD/CTR in phosphate-buffered saline (PBS) at 37 °C. (**A**) Caffeic acid, and (**B**) pinocembrin. Adapted from [69], with permission from MDPI.

In that sense, recently, Hernandez–Montelongo et al. coated silicone breast implants with HP-β-CD/CTR loading the rose bengal (RB) dye. This experimental setup was used for developing a mathematical model that covers 100% of the released drug. The proposed model also contemplates a unidirectional recursive diffusion process which follows Fick's second law while considering the convective phenomena from the polymer matrix to the PBS, where the drug is delivered, and the equilibrium of the polymer–liquid drug distribution. Results indicated that diffusion controls the delivery rate; however, as RB concentration increases, the equilibrium plays an increasing role, becoming the controlling mechanism for a longer time [14]. These sophisticated mathematical models also allow for determining the drug-concentration profile in the polymer matrix (Figure 8).

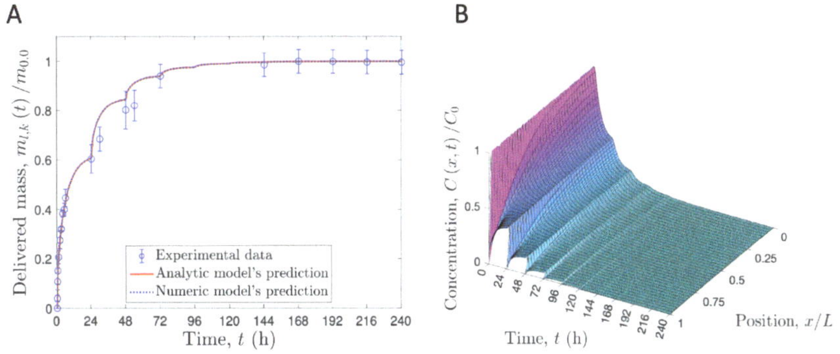

Figure 8. Recursive drug delivery. (**A**) Comparison of the experimental data and prediction for the delivered rose bengal. (**B**) Prediction of the drug concentration profile in the HP-β-CD/CTR matrix. Adapted from [14], with permission from MDPI.

7. Concluding Remarks and Future Perspectives

Postoperative risks of medical implant surgeries, such as bacterial infections, sharp pain, inadequate healing, and other risks, can be reduced by local drug release. In that sense, because CD/CTR are biodegradable, biocompatible, economically feasible, and ecofriendly, they have been successfully used as coatings on implants, and other materials, for drug-delivery applications. The fan of utilized substrates is very wide, which includes plastic implants, porous ceramics and semiconductors, cellulose papers, and metallic devices. Even though the CD/CTR coatings have been obtained in the order of microns on macrostructures, recent works are being focused on the synthesis of nanolayers and the coating of nanomaterials.

Traditionally, the main application of the developed drug-delivery systems, based on CD/CTR biopolymers, was to reduce bacterial infections. Therefore, antibiotics have been the most common drug for loading and releasing in these systems. Current works are centred on alternative molecules like metal ions. As systems evolved, new prominent medical applications were explored, like treatments for restenosis, atherosclerosis, and arterial wall healing. In that sense, the perspective is that more complex biomedical applications are going to be studied. Although the CD/CTR systems are very versatile and can be used as drug delivery for a wide fan of drugs and molecules, it is recommended that one perform experimental tests for loading and releasing new drugs.

On the other hand, diffusion is the principal predominant step in the control of release from drug delivery based on CD/CTR systems; however, other phenomena can be present, such as swelling or erosion. In that sense, the semiempirical model of Korsmeyer–Peppas has been the easiest and most useful mathematical implemented tool for studying the release kinetics of drugs. Nevertheless, this model can only be used to take into account up to 60% of the cumulative drug release. In that sense, to glean deeper insight into the release kinetics, mathematical models for the specific systems are starting to be developed.

In general, this review presented that coatings of CD/CTR biopolymers have been thoroughly proven as excellent drug-delivery systems; consequently, in vivo experiments should be also considered in further studies. In addition, these systems have significant commercial potential to improve the quality of medical implant surgeries.

Author Contributions: Writing original draft preparation, K.E. and J.H.-M.; writing review and editing, K.A.G.-M., R.P. and N.N.; visualization and supervision, M.M.-S. and J.H.-M. All authors have read and agreed to the published version of the manuscript.

Funding: This research was funded by FONDECYT–Chile (Grant Number 11180395), CONICYT PFCHA/DOCTORADO/2017-21172001 (Nelson Naveas) and PFCHA/ DOCTORADO/2015-21151648 (Ruth Pulido), and project PID2020-112770RB-C22, from the Ministerio de Ciencia e Innovacion (Spain).

Institutional Review Board Statement: Not applicable.

Informed Consent Statement: Not applicable.

Data Availability Statement: The data that support the findings of this study are available from the corresponding author upon reasonable request.

Acknowledgments: We recognize PhD programs in "Advanced Materials and Nanotechnologies" from Universidad Autónoma de Madrid (UAM, Spain) and "Ingeniería de Procesos de Minerales" from Universidad de Antofagasta (UA, Chile).

Conflicts of Interest: The authors declare no conflict of interest. The funders had no role in the design of the study, in the collection, analysis, or interpretation of data, in the writing of the manuscript, or in the decision to publish the results.

References

1. Lopes, J.H.; Tabary, N.; Hernandez-Montelongo, J. Editorial: Biomacromolecules Systems Applied to Medical Implants for the Release of Therapeutic Agents. *Front. Bioeng. Biotechnol.* **2022**, *10*, 910203. [CrossRef] [PubMed]
2. Bhatt, S.; Pathak, A.; Grover, P.; Bharadwaj, A.; Bhatia, D.; Tomar, R.; Kaurav, M. Different aspects of polymers—A review article. *Mater. Today Proc.* **2022**, *64*, 1490–1495. [CrossRef]
3. Martel, B.; Weltrowski, M.; Ruffin, D.; Morcellet, M. Polycarboxylic acids as crosslinking agents for grafting cyclodextrins onto cotton and wool fabrics: Study of the process parameters. *J. Appl. Polym. Sci.* **2002**, *83*, 1449–1456. [CrossRef]
4. Narayanan, G.; Shen, J.; Matai, I.; Sachdev, A.; Boy, R.; Tonelli, A.E. Cyclodextrin-based nanostructures. *Prog. Mater. Sci.* **2022**, *124*, 100869. [CrossRef]
5. Iravani, S.; Varma, R.S. Nanosponges for Drug Delivery and Cancer Therapy: Recent Advances. *Nanomaterials* **2022**, *12*, 2440. [CrossRef]
6. Ghorpade, V.S.; Yadav, A.V.; Dias, R.J. Citric acid crosslinked cyclodextrin/hydroxypropylmethylcellulose hydrogel films for hydrophobic drug delivery. *Int. J. Biol. Macromol.* **2016**, *93*, 75–86. [CrossRef]
7. Ghorpade, V.S.; Yadav, A.V.; Dias, R.J. Citric acid crosslinked β-cyclodextrin/carboxymethylcellulose hydrogel films for controlled delivery of poorly soluble drugs. *Carbohydr. Polym.* **2017**, *164*, 339–348. [CrossRef]
8. Pérez-Anes, A.; Gargouri, M.; Laure, W.; Berghe, H.V.D.; Courcot, E.; Sobocinski, J.; Tabary, N.; Chai, F.; Blach, J.F.; Addad, A.; et al. Bioinspired Titanium Drug Eluting Platforms Based on a Poly-β-cyclodextrin–Chitosan Layer-by-Layer Self-Assembly Targeting Infections. *ACS Appl. Mater. Interfaces* **2015**, *7*, 12882–12893. [CrossRef]
9. Junthip, J.; Tabary, N.; Chai, F.; Leclercq, L.; Maton, M.; Cazaux, F.; Neut, C.; Paccou, L.; Guinet, Y.; Staelens, J.N.; et al. Layer-by-layer coating of textile with two oppositely charged cyclodextrin polyelectrolytes for extended drug delivery. *J. Biomed. Mater. Res. Part A* **2016**, *104*, 1408–1424. [CrossRef]
10. Hernandez-Montelongo, J.; Naveas, N.; Degoutin, S.; Tabary, N.; Chai, F.; Spampinato, V.; Ceccone, G.; Rossi, F.; Torres-Costa, V.; Manso-Silvan, M.; et al. Porous silicon-cyclodextrin based polymer composites for drug delivery applications. *Carbohydr. Polym.* **2014**, *110*, 238–252. [CrossRef]
11. Smith, P.A. Carbon Fiber Reinforced Plastics—Properties. *Compr. Compos. Mater.* **2000**, *2*, 107–150. [CrossRef]
12. Korsmeyer, R.W.; Gurny, R.; Doelker, E.; Buri, P.; Peppas, N.A. Mechanisms of solute release from porous hydrophilic polymers. *Int. J. Pharm.* **1983**, *15*, 25–35. [CrossRef]
13. Ritger, P.L.; Peppas, N.A. A simple equation for description of solute release I. Fickian and non-fickian release from non-swellable devices in the form of slabs, spheres, cylinders or discs. *J. Control. Release* **1987**, *5*, 23–36. [CrossRef]
14. Hernandez-Montelongo, R.; Salazar-Araya, J.; Hernandez-Montelongo, J.; Garcia-Sandoval, J.P. Mathematical Modeling of Recursive Drug Delivery with Diffusion, Equilibrium, and Convection Coupling. *Mathematics* **2022**, *10*, 2171. [CrossRef]
15. Bakshi, P.R.; Londhe, V.Y. Widespread applications of host-guest interactive cyclodextrin functionalized polymer nanocomposites: Its meta-analysis and review. *Carbohydr. Polym.* **2020**, *242*, 116430. [CrossRef] [PubMed]
16. Saji, V.S. *Supramolecular Chemistry in Corrosion and Biofouling Protection*; CRC Press: Boca Raton, FL, USA, 2021. [CrossRef]
17. Davis, M.E.; Brewster, M.E. Cyclodextrin-based pharmaceutics: Past, present and future. *Nat. Rev. Drug Discov.* **2004**, *3*, 1023–1035. [CrossRef]
18. Sherje, A.P.; Dravyakar, B.R.; Kadam, D.; Jadhav, M. Cyclodextrin-based nanosponges: A critical review. *Carbohydr. Polym.* **2017**, *173*, 37–49. [CrossRef]
19. Zhang, D.; Lv, P.; Zhou, C.; Zhao, Y.; Liao, X.; Yang, B. Cyclodextrin-based delivery systems for cancer treatment. *Mater. Sci. Eng. C* **2019**, *96*, 872–886. [CrossRef]
20. Ioele, G.; De Luca, M.; Garofalo, A.; Ragno, G. Photosensitive drugs: A review on their photoprotection by liposomes and cyclodextrins. *Drug Deliv.* **2017**, *24*, 33–44. [CrossRef]
21. Saenger, W. Cyclodextrin inclusion compounds in research and industry. *Angew. Chem. Int. Ed. Engl.* **1980**, *19*, 344–362. [CrossRef]
22. Buschmann, H.J.; Denter, U.; Knittel, D.; Schollmeyer, E. The use of cyclodextrins in textile processes—an overview. *J. Text. Inst.* **1998**, *89*, 554–561. [CrossRef]
23. Szente, L.; Fenyvesi, É. Cyclodextrin-enabled polymer composites for packaging. *Molecules* **2018**, *23*, 1556. [CrossRef] [PubMed]

24. Li, Z.; Chen, S.; Gu, Z.; Chen, J.; Wu, J. Alpha-cyclodextrin: Enzymatic production and food applications. *Trends Food Sci. Technol.* **2014**, *35*, 151–160. [CrossRef]
25. Szejtli, J. Introduction and general overview of cyclodextrin chemistry. *Chem. Rev.* **1998**, *98*, 1743–1754. [CrossRef]
26. Tang, W.; Zou, C.; Da, C.; Cao, Y.; Peng, H. A review on the recent development of cyclodextrin-based materials used in oilfield applications. *Carbohydr. Polym.* **2020**, *240*, 116321. [CrossRef]
27. Erdogar, N.; Varan, G.; Varan, C.; Bilensoy, E. Chapter 19—Cyclodextrin-based polymeric nanosystems. In *Drug Targeting and Stimuli Sensitive Drug Delivery Systems*; William Andrew: Norwich, NY, USA, 2018; pp. 715–748. [CrossRef]
28. Parmar, V.; Patel, G.; Abu-Thabit, N.Y. 20—Responsive cyclodextrins as polymeric carriers for drug delivery applications. In *Stimuli Responsive Polymeric Nanocarriers for Drug Delivery Applications, Volume 1*; Woodhead Publishing: Sawston, CA, USA, 2018, pp. 555–580. [CrossRef]
29. Taha, M.; Chai, F.; Blanchemain, N.; Goube, M.; Martel, B.; Hildebrand, H.F. Validating the poly-cyclodextrins based local drug delivery system on plasma-sprayed hydroxyapatite coated orthopedic implant with toluidine blue O. *Mater. Sci. Eng. C* **2013**, *33*, 2639–2647. [CrossRef]
30. Concheiro, A.; Alvarez-Lorenzo, C. Chemically cross-linked and grafted cyclodextrin hydrogels: From nanostructures to drug-eluting medical devices. *Adv. Drug Deliv. Rev.* **2013**, *65*, 1188–1203. [CrossRef]
31. Martel, B.; Ruffin, D.; Weltrowski, M.; Lekchiri, Y.; Morcellet, M. Water-soluble polymers and gels from the polycondensation between cyclodextrins and poly(carboxylic acid)s: A study of the preparation parameters. *J. Appl. Polym. Sci.* **2005**, *97*, 433–442. [CrossRef]
32. García-Fernández, M.J.; Tabary, N.; Martel, B.; Cazaux, F.; Oliva, A.; Taboada, P.; Concheiro, A.; Alvarez-Lorenzo, C. Poly-(cyclo)dextrins as ethoxzolamide carriers in ophthalmic solutions and in contact lenses. *Carbohydr. Polym.* **2013**, *98*, 1343–1352. [CrossRef]
33. Seligra, P.G.; Jaramillo, C.M.; Famá, L.; Goyanes, S. Biodegradable and non-retrogradable eco-films based on starch–glycerol with citric acid as crosslinking agent. *Carbohydr. Polym.* **2016**, *138*, 66–74. [CrossRef]
34. Jahangard, N.; Baghbanian, S.M.; Khaksarmaghami, S. Poly (β-Cyclodextrin-co-citric Acid) Functionalized Natural Nanozeolite: An Eco-Friendly Platform for IB Delivery. *Appl. Sci.* **2022**, *12*, 8241. [CrossRef]
35. Welch, C.M. Tetracarboxylic Acids as Formaldehyde-Free Durable Press Finishing Agents: Part I: Catalyst, Additive, and Durability Studies1. *Text. Res. J.* **1988**, *58*, 480–486. [CrossRef]
36. Yang, C.Q.; Wang, X. Infrared spectroscopy studies of the cyclic anhydride as the intermediate for the ester crosslinking of cotton cellulose by polycarboxylic acids. II. Comparison of different polycarboxylic acids. *J. Polym. Sci. Part A Polym. Chem.* **1996**, *34*, 1573–1580. .:8<1573::AID-POLA22>3.0.CO;2-4. [CrossRef]
37. Martel, B.; Thuaut, P.L.; Bertini, S.; Crini, G.; Bacquet, M.; Torri, G.; Morcellet, M. Grafting of cyclodextrins onto polypropylene nonwoven fabrics for the manufacture of reactive filters. III. Study of the sorption properties. *J. Appl. Polym. Sci.* **2002**, *85*, 1771–1778. [CrossRef]
38. Thi, T.H.H.; Chai, F.; Lepretre, S.; Blanchemain, N.; Martel, B.; Siepmann, F.; Hildebrand, H.F.; Siepmann, J.; Flament, M.P. Bone implants modified with cyclodextrin: Study of drug release in bulk fluid and into agarose gel. *Int. J. Pharm.* **2010**, *400*, 74–85. [CrossRef]
39. Ghoul, Y.E.; Martel, B.; Achari, A.E.; Campagne, C.; Razafimahefa, L.; Vroman, I. Improved dyeability of polypropylene fabrics finished with β-cyclodextrin–citric acid polymer. *Polym. J.* **2010**, *42*, 804–811. [CrossRef]
40. Sharma, Y.C.; Srivastava, V.; Singh, V.K.; Kaul, S.N.; Weng, C.H. Nano-adsorbents for the removal of metallic pollutants from water and wastewater. *Environ. Technol.* **2009**, *30*, 583–609. [CrossRef]
41. Wieszczycka, K.; Staszak, K.; Woźniak-Budych, M.J.; Litowczenko, J.; Maciejewska, B.M.; Jurga, S. Surface functionalization—The way for advanced applications of smart materials. *Coord. Chem. Rev.* **2021**, *436*, 213846. [CrossRef]
42. Thatiparti, T.R.; Shoffstall, A.J.; von Recum, H.A. Cyclodextrin-based device coatings for affinity-based release of antibiotics. *Biomaterials* **2010**, *31*, 2335–2347. [CrossRef]
43. Cyphert, E.L.; Zuckerman, S.T.; Korley, J.N.; von Recum, H.A. Affinity interactions drive post-implantation drug filling, even in the presence of bacterial biofilm. *Acta Biomater.* **2017**, *57*, 95–102. [CrossRef]
44. Vermet, G.; Degoutin, S.; Chai, F.; Maton, M.; Bria, M.; Danel, C.; Hildebrand, H.F.; Blanchemain, N.; Martel, B. Visceral mesh modified with cyclodextrin for the local sustained delivery of ropivacaine. *Int. J. Pharm.* **2014**, *476*, 149–159. [CrossRef] [PubMed]
45. Haley, R.M.; Qian, V.R.; Learn, G.D.; von Recum, H.A. Use of affinity allows anti-inflammatory and anti-microbial dual release that matches suture wound resolution. *J. Biomed. Mater. Res. Part A* **2019**, *107*, 1434–1442. [CrossRef] [PubMed]
46. Chai, F.; Maton, M.; Degoutin, S.; Vermet, G.; Simon, N.; Rousseaux, C.; Martel, B.; Blanchemain, N. In vivo evaluation of post-operative pain reduction on rat model after implantation of intraperitoneal PET meshes functionalised with cyclodextrins and loaded with ropivacaine. *Biomaterials* **2019**, *192*, 260–270. [CrossRef] [PubMed]
47. Romi, R.; Nostro, P.L.; Bocci, E.; Ridi, F.; Baglioni, P. Bioengineering of a Cellulosic Fabric for Insecticide Delivery via Grafted Cyclodextrin. *Biotechnol. Prog.* **2005**, *21*, 1724–1730. [CrossRef] [PubMed]
48. Abdelkader, M.B.; Azizi, N.; Baffoun, A.; Chevalier, Y.; Majdoub, M. Fragrant Microcapsules Based on β-Cyclodextrin for Cosmetotextile Application. *J. Renew. Mater.* **2019**, *7*, 1347–1362. [CrossRef]
49. Wang, Z.; Guo, S.; Zhang, B.; Fang, J.; Zhu, L. Interfacially crosslinked β-cyclodextrin polymer composite porous membranes for fast removal of organic micropollutants from water by flow-through adsorption. *J. Hazard. Mater.* **2020**, *384*, 121187. [CrossRef]

50. Bezerra, F.M.; Lis, M.J.; Firmino, H.B.; da Silva, J.G.; de Cassia Siqueira Curto Valle, R.; Valle, J.A.B.; Scacchetti, F.A.P.; Tessaro, A.L. The Role of β-Cyclodextrin in the Textile Industry—Review. *Molecules* **2020**, *25*, 3624. [CrossRef]
51. Wei, W.; Zhang, X.; Chen, X.; Zhou, M.; Xu, R.; Zhang, X. Smart surface coating of drug nanoparticles with cross-linkable polyethylene glycol for bio-responsive and highly efficient drug delivery. *Nanoscale* **2016**, *8*, 8118–8125. [CrossRef]
52. Shi, Y.; Jiao, H.; Sun, J.; Lu, X.; Yu, S.; Cheng, L.; Wang, Q.; Liu, H.; Biranje, S.; Wang, J.; et al. Functionalization of nanocellulose applied with biological molecules for biomedical application: A review. *Carbohydr. Polym.* **2022**, *285*, 119208. [CrossRef]
53. Sanità, G.; Carrese, B.; Lamberti, A. Nanoparticle Surface Functionalization: How to Improve Biocompatibility and Cellular Internalization. *Front. Mol. Biosci.* **2020**, *7*, 587012. [CrossRef]
54. Boschin, F.; Blanchemain, N.; Bria, M.; Delcourt-Debruyne, E.; Morcellet, M.; Hildebrand, H.; Martel, B. Improved drug delivery properties of PVDF membranes functionalized with β-cyclodextrin—Application to guided tissue regeneration in periodontology. *J. Biomed. Mater. Res. Part A* **2006**, *79A*, 78–85. [CrossRef] [PubMed]
55. Lepretre, S.; Boschin, F.; Tabary, N.; Bria, M.; Martel, B.; Blanchemain, N.; Hildebrand, H.F.; Morcellet, M.; Delcourt-Debruyne, E. Guided tissue regeneration membranes with controlled delivery properties of chlorhexidine by their functionalization with cyclodextrins. *J. Incl. Phenom. Macrocycl. Chem.* **2007**, *57*, 297–302. [CrossRef]
56. Blanchemain, N.; Laurent, T.; Chai, F.; Neut, C.; Haulon, S.; Krump-konvalinkova, V.; Morcellet, M.; Martel, B.; Kirkpatrick, C.J.; Hildebrand, H.F. Polyester vascular prostheses coated with a cyclodextrin polymer and activated with antibiotics: Cytotoxicity and microbiological evaluation. *Acta Biomater.* **2008**, *4*, 1725–1733. [CrossRef] [PubMed]
57. El Ghoul, Y.; Blanchemain, N.; Laurent, T.; Campagne, C.; El Achari, A.; Roudesli, S.; Morcellet, M.; Martel, B.; Hildebrand, H. Chemical, biological and microbiological evaluation of cyclodextrin finished polyamide inguinal meshes. *Acta Biomater.* **2008**, *4*, 1392–1400. [CrossRef]
58. Leprêtre, S.; Chai, F.; Hornez, J.C.; Vermet, G.; Neut, C.; Descamps, M.; Hildebrand, H.F.; Martel, B. Prolonged local antibiotics delivery from hydroxyapatite functionalised with cyclodextrin polymers. *Biomaterials* **2009**, *30*, 6086–6093. [CrossRef]
59. Laurent, T.; Kacem, I.; Blanchemain, N.; Cazaux, F.; Neut, C.; Hildebrand, H.F.; Martel, B. Cyclodextrin and maltodextrin finishing of a polypropylene abdominal wall implant for the prolonged delivery of ciprofloxacin. *Acta Biomater.* **2011**, *7*, 3141–3149. [CrossRef]
60. Cusola, O.; Tabary, N.; Belgacem, M.N.; Bras, J. Cyclodextrin functionalization of several cellulosic substrates for prolonged release of antibacterial agents. *J. Appl. Polym. Sci.* **2013**, *129*, 604–613. [CrossRef]
61. Martin, A.; Tabary, N.; Leclercq, L.; Junthip, J.; Degoutin, S.; Aubert-Viard, F.; Cazaux, F.; Lyskawa, J.; Janus, L.; Bria, M.; et al. Multilayered textile coating based on a β-cyclodextrin polyelectrolyte for the controlled release of drugs. *Carbohydr. Polym.* **2013**, *93*, 718–730. [CrossRef]
62. Martin, A.; Tabary, N.; Chai, F.; Leclercq, L.; Junthip, J.; Aubert-Viard, F.; Neut, C.; Weltrowski, M.; Blanchemain, N.; Martel, B. Build-up of an antimicrobial multilayer coating on a textile support based on a methylene blue–poly(cyclodextrin) complex. *Biomed. Mater.* **2013**, *8*, 065006. [CrossRef]
63. Lavoine, N.; Givord, C.; Tabary, N.; Desloges, I.; Martel, B.; Bras, J. Elaboration of a new antibacterial bio-nano-material for food-packaging by synergistic action of cyclodextrin and microfibrillated cellulose. *Innov. Food Sci. Emerg. Technol.* **2014**, *26*, 330–340. [CrossRef]
64. Sobocinski, J.; Laure, W.; Taha, M.; Courcot, E.; Chai, F.; Simon, N.; Addad, A.; Martel, B.; Haulon, S.; Woisel, P.; et al. Mussel Inspired Coating of a Biocompatible Cyclodextrin Based Polymer onto CoCr Vascular Stents. *ACS Appl. Mater. Interfaces* **2014**, *6*, 3575–3586. [CrossRef] [PubMed]
65. Tabary, N.; Chai, F.; Blanchemain, N.; Neut, C.; Pauchet, L.; Bertini, S.; Delcourt-Debruyne, E.; Hildebrand, H.F.; Martel, B. A chlorhexidine-loaded biodegradable cellulosic device for periodontal pockets treatment. *Acta Biomater.* **2014**, *10*, 318–329. [CrossRef] [PubMed]
66. Vermet, G.; Degoutin, S.; Chai, F.; Maton, M.; Flores, C.; Neut, C.; Danjou, P.E.; Martel, B.; Blanchemain, N. Cyclodextrin modified PLLA parietal reinforcement implant with prolonged antibacterial activity. *Acta Biomater.* **2017**, *53*, 222–232. [CrossRef] [PubMed]
67. Hernández-Montelongo, J.; Oria, L.; Cárdenas, A.B.; Benito, N.; Romero-Sáez, M.; Recio-Sánchez, G. Nanoporous Silicon Composite as Potential System for Sustained Delivery of Florfenicol Drug. *Phys. Status Solidi (b)* **2018**, *255*, 1700626. [CrossRef]
68. Garcia-Fernandez, M.J.; Maton, M.; Benzine, Y.; Tabary, N.; Baptiste, E.J.; Gargouri, M.; Bria, M.; Blanchemain, N.; Karrout, Y. Ciprofloxacin loaded vascular prostheses functionalized with poly-methylbeta- cyclodextrin: The importance of in vitro release conditions. *J. Drug Deliv. Sci. Technol.* **2019**, *53*, 101166. [CrossRef]
69. Guzmán-Oyarzo, D.; Plaza, T.; Recio-Sánchez, G.; Abdalla, D.S.P.; Salazar, L.A.; Hernández-Montelongo, J. Use of nPSi-βCD Composite Microparticles for the Controlled Release of Caffeic Acid and Pinocembrin, Two Main Polyphenolic Compounds Found in a Chilean Propolis. *Pharmaceutics* **2019**, *11*, 289. [CrossRef]
70. Junthip, J.; Tabary, N.; Maton, M.; Ouerghemmi, S.; Staelens, J.N.; Cazaux, F.; Neut, C.; Blanchemain, N.; Martel, B. Release-killing properties of a textile modified by a layer-by-layer coating based on two oppositely charged cyclodextrin polyelectrolytes. *Int. J. Pharm.* **2020**, *587*, 119730. [CrossRef]
71. Kersani, D.; Mougin, J.; Lopez, M.; Degoutin, S.; Tabary, N.; Cazaux, F.; Janus, L.; Maton, M.; Chai, F.; Sobocinski, J.; et al. Stent coating by electrospinning with chitosan/poly-cyclodextrin based nanofibers loaded with simvastatin for restenosis prevention. *Eur. J. Pharm. Biopharm.* **2020**, *150*, 156–167. [CrossRef]

72. Zhang, J.; Qu, L.; Lin, Y.; Guo, Z.; Cai, Z.; Ge, F. The preparation of antibacterial eco-friendly bio-based PTT-based β-cyclodextrin by complexation of copper and zinc ions. *Text. Res. J.* **2021**, *92*, 2800–2807. [CrossRef]
73. Guzmán-Oyarzo, D.; Hernández-Montelongo, J.; Rosas, C.; Leal, P.; Weber, H.; Alvear, M.; Salazar, L.A. Controlled Release of Caffeic Acid and Pinocembrin by Use of nPSi-βCD Composites Improves Their Antiangiogenic Activity. *Pharmaceutics* **2022**, *14*, 484. [CrossRef]
74. Folch-Cano, C.; Yazdani-Pedram, M.; Olea-Azar, C. Inclusion and functionalization of polymers with cyclodextrins: Current applications and future prospects. *Molecules* **2014**, *19*, 14066–14079. [CrossRef] [PubMed]
75. Jean-Baptiste, E.; Blanchemain, N.; Martel, B.; Neut, C.; Hildebrand, H.; Haulon, S. Safety, healing, and efficacy of vascular prostheses coated with hydroxypropyl-β-cyclodextrin polymer: Experimental in vitro and animal studies. *Eur. J. Vasc. Endovasc. Surg.* **2012**, *43*, 188–197. [CrossRef]
76. Li, W.; Liu, H.; Li, L.; Liu, K.; Liu, J.; Tang, T.; Jiang, W. Green synthesis of citric acid-crosslinked β-cyclodextrin for highly efficient removal of uranium (VI) from aqueous solution. *J. Radioanal. Nucl. Chem.* **2019**, *322*, 2033–2042. [CrossRef]
77. Rubin Pedrazzo, A.; Smarra, A.; Caldera, F.; Musso, G.; Dhakar, N.K.; Cecone, C.; Hamedi, A.; Corsi, I.; Trotta, F. Eco-friendly β-cyclodextrin and linecaps polymers for the removal of heavy metals. *Polymers* **2019**, *11*, 1658. [CrossRef] [PubMed]
78. Zhao, D.; Zhao, L.; Zhu, C.S.; Huang, W.Q.; Hu, J.L. Water-insoluble β-cyclodextrin polymer crosslinked by citric acid: Synthesis and adsorption properties toward phenol and methylene blue. *J. Incl. Phenom. Macrocycl. Chem.* **2009**, *63*, 195–201. [CrossRef]
79. Huang, W.; Hu, Y.; Li, Y.; Zhou, Y.; Niu, D.; Lei, Z.; Zhang, Z. Citric acid-crosslinked β-cyclodextrin for simultaneous removal of bisphenol A, methylene blue and copper: The roles of cavity and surface functional groups. *J. Taiwan Inst. Chem. Eng.* **2018**, *82*, 189–197. [CrossRef]
80. Zhou, Y.; Gu, X.; Zhang, R.; Lu, J. Removal of aniline from aqueous solution using pine sawdust modified with citric acid and β-cyclodextrin. *Ind. Eng. Chem. Res.* **2014**, *53*, 887–894. [CrossRef]
81. Tcheumi, H.L.; Tassontio, V.N.; Tonle, I.K.; Ngameni, E. Surface functionalization of smectite-type clay by facile polymerization of β-cyclodextrin using citric acid cross linker: Application as sensing material for the electrochemical determination of paraquat. *Appl. Clay Sci.* **2019**, *173*, 97–106. [CrossRef]
82. Li, L.S.; Zhang, Y.X.; Gong, W.; Li, J. Novel β-cyclodextrin doped carbon dots for host–guest recognition-assisted sensing of isoniazid and cell imaging. *RSC Adv.* **2022**, *12*, 30104–30112. [CrossRef]
83. Naveas, N.; Costa, V.T.; Gallach, D.; Hernandez-Montelongo, J.; Palma, R.J.M.; Garcia-Ruiz, J.P.; Manso-Silvan, M. Chemical stabilization of porous silicon for enhanced biofunctionalization with immunoglobulin. *Sci. Technol. Adv. Mater.* **2012**, *13*. [CrossRef]
84. Richardson, J.J.; Björnmalm, M.; Caruso, F. Technology-driven layer-by-layer assembly of nanofilms. *Science* **2015**, *348*, aaa2491. [CrossRef] [PubMed]
85. Fitzgerald, R.; Bass, L.M.; Goldberg, D.J.; Graivier, M.H.; Lorenc, Z.P. Physiochemical Characteristics of Poly-L-Lactic Acid (PLLA). *Aesthet. Surg. J.* **2018**, *38*, S13–S17. [CrossRef] [PubMed]
86. Jeon, B.S.; Shin, B.H.; Huh, B.K.; Kim, B.H.; Kim, S.N.; Ji, H.B.; Lee, S.H.; Im Kang, S.; Shim, J.H.; Kang, S.M.; et al. Silicone implants capable of the local, controlled delivery of triamcinolone for the prevention of fibrosis with minimized drug side effects. *J. Ind. Eng. Chem.* **2018**, *63*, 168–180. [CrossRef]
87. Barr, S.; Topps, A.; Barnes, N.; Henderson, J.; Hignett, S.; Teasdale, R.; McKenna, A.; Harvey, J.; Kirwan, C.; Collaborative, N.B.S.R. Infection prevention in breast implant surgery—A review of the surgical evidence, guidelines and a checklist. *Eur. J. Surg. Oncol. (EJSO)* **2016**, *42*, 591–603. [CrossRef]
88. Arredondo Peñaranda, A.; Londoño López, M.E. Hydrogels: Potentials Biomaterials for Controlled Drug Delivery. *Rev. Ing. Biomédica* **2009**, *3*, 83–94.
89. Sukhova, I.; Müller, D.; Eisenmann-Klein, M.; Machens, H.G.; Schantz, J.T. Quo vadis? Brustimplantate–aktuelle Entwicklungen und neue Konzepte. *Handchir. Mikrochir. Plast. Chir.* **2012**, *44*, 240–253.
90. Costagliola, M.; Atiyeh, B.S.; Rampillon, F. An innovative procedure for the treatment of primary and recurrent capsular contracture (CC) following breast augmentation. *Aesthetic Surg. J.* **2013**, *33*, 1008–1017. [CrossRef]
91. Wang, N.X.; von Recum, H.A. Affinity-based drug delivery. *Macromol. Biosci.* **2011**, *11*, 321–332. [CrossRef]
92. Siepmann, J.; Siepmann, F. Mathematical modeling of drug delivery. *Int. J. Pharm.* **2008**, *364*, 328–343. [CrossRef]
93. Paarakh, M.P.; Jose, P.A.; Setty, C.; Christoper, G. Release kinetics–concepts and applications. *Int. J. Pharm. Res. Technol.* **2018**, *8*, 12–20.
94. Klech, C.M.; Simonelli, A.P. Examination of the moving boundaries associated with non-fickian water swelling of glassy gelatin beads: Effect of solution pH. *J. Membr. Sci.* **1989**, *43*, 87–101. [CrossRef]
95. Gupta, B.; Chaurasia, U.; Chakraborty, P. Design and development of oral transmucosal film for delivery of salbutamol sulphate. *J. Pharm. Chem. Biol. Sci.* **2014**, *2*, 118–129.
96. Bruschi, M.L. Mathematical models of drug release. In *Strategies to Modify the Drug Release from Pharmaceutical Systems*; Elsevier: Amsterdam, The Netherlands, 2015; pp. 63–86. [CrossRef]
97. Lucht, L.M.; Peppas, N.A. Transport of penetrants in the macromolecular structure of coals. V. Anomalous transport in pretreated coal particles. *J. Appl. Polym. Sci.* **1987**, *33*, 1557–1566. [CrossRef]

pharmaceutics

Article

Application of Box-Behnken Design in the Preparation, Optimization, and In-Vivo Pharmacokinetic Evaluation of Oral Tadalafil-Loaded Niosomal Film

Kawthar K. Abla [1], Amina T. Mneimneh [1], Ahmed N. Allam [2,*] and Mohammed M. Mehanna [3,*]

1 Pharmaceutical Nanotechnology Research Lab, Faculty of Pharmacy, Beirut Arab University, Beirut, Lebanon
2 Department of Pharmaceutics, Faculty of Pharmacy, Alexandria University, Alexandria 21521, Egypt
3 Department of Industrial Pharmacy, Faculty of Pharmacy, Alexandria University, Alexandria 21521, Egypt
* Correspondence: ph.a.allam@gmail.com (A.N.A.); mohamed.mehanna@alexu.edu.eg (M.M.M.); Tel.: +20-1005422491 (A.N.A.); +20-1030651034 (M.M.M.)

Abstract: Benign prostatic hyperplasia (BPH) affects about 90% of men whose ages are over 65. Tadalafil, a selective PDE-5 inhibitor, was approved by FDA for BPH, however, its poor aqueous solubility and bioavailability are considered major drawbacks. This work intended to develop and evaluate oral fast dissolving film containing tadalafil-loaded niosomes for those who cannot receive the oral dosage form. Niosomes were statistically optimized by Box-Behnken experimental design and loaded into a polymeric oral film. Niosomes were assessed for their vesicular size, uniformity, and zeta potential. The thickness, content uniformity, folding endurance, tensile strength, disintegration time, and surface morphology were evaluated for the prepared polymeric film. The optimized niosomes revealed high entrapment efficiency (99.78 ± 2.132%) and the film was smooth with good flexibility and convenient thickness (110 ± 10 μm). A fast release of tadalafil was achieved within 5 min significantly faster than the niosomes-free drug film. The in-vivo bioavailability in rats established that the optimized niosomal film enhanced tadalafil systemic absorption, with higher peak concentration (C_{max} = 0.63 ± 0.03 μg/mL), shorter T_{max} value (0.66-fold), and relative bioavailability of 118.4% compared to the marketed tablet. These results propose that the oral film of tadalafil-loaded niosomes is a suitable therapeutic application that can be passed with ease to geriatric patients who suffer from BPH.

Keywords: Box-Behnken; methylcellulose; niosomes; oral film; tadalafil

Citation: Abla, K.K.; Mneimneh, A.T.; Allam, A.N.; Mehanna, M.M. Application of Box-Behnken Design in the Preparation, Optimization, and In-Vivo Pharmacokinetic Evaluation of Oral Tadalafil-Loaded Niosomal Film. *Pharmaceutics* **2023**, *15*, 173. https://doi.org/10.3390/pharmaceutics15010173

Academic Editor: Ping Hu

Received: 18 November 2022
Revised: 28 December 2022
Accepted: 28 December 2022
Published: 3 January 2023

1. Introduction

Benign prostate hyperplasia (BPH) is one of the most common diseases in aging men and the most common cause of lower urinary tract symptoms (LUTS). Clinically, BPH arises from the tension exerted by the prostate smooth muscle on the prostatic urethra and nearly every man age 65 or older will be affected by it at some point in his life [1]. In addition, many patients do not stand the conventional medications; alpha-blockers and 5-alpha reductase inhibitors, for their adverse effects such as dizziness, postural hypotension, reduced ejaculation, loss of libido, and male infertility [2,3] which creates the need for another molecule. Clinical studies have granted evidence that PDE-5 inhibitors enhance BPH and LUTS symptoms due to the relaxing action of nitric oxide (NO) and the inhibition of prostatic stromal cells proliferation [4,5].

Tadalafil was approved in 2003 by US Food and Drug Administration (FDA) as the first and only PDE5 inhibitor clinically proven to provide sustained efficacy and in 2011, a single 5 mg daily dose was licensed to treat LUTS secondary to BPH with or without erectile dysfunction. Pharmacokinetically, it is known for its long half-life and duration of action (17.5 and 36 h, respectively) in comparison to sildenafil (3.8 and 8 h) and vardenafil (3.9 and 12 h) [6]. Despite the previously mentioned ascendancy, one of the demerits that hinders tadalafil action is its poor bioavailability which was found to be around 35% of the administered dose [7,8]. This is attributed to its low aqueous solubility since it belongs to class II drugs according to the FDA biopharmaceutical classification system [9].

Nanotechnology has emerged as a successful approach to the creation of nanocarriers for distinct diseases [10]. Conventional therapeutics are somehow destined to failure due to problems related to solubility, bioavailability, distribution, or transport through biological membranes. On the other hand, nanocarriers can be designed in a way that leads to manipulative targeting, optimal delivery, and the release of drugs to achieve the desired outcomes [11–13]. Several strategies in the nanotechnology were adopted to enhance tadalafil solubility and dissolution rate [14–18]. Nevertheless, the niosomal approach to enhance tadalafil solubility has not been studied before despite all the merits that characterized this nanoparticulate system.

Niosomes are bi-layered nanocarriers that can be prepared by the addition of non-ionic surfactant to cholesterol in a proper proportion followed by its hydration in aqueous media [19]. Niosomes possess many advantages over other nanocarriers due to their high biocompatibility, biodegradability, high stability, and ease of surface modification. In the bargain is their ability to encapsulate both hydrophilic and hydrophobic drugs in a special geometrical structure thus enhancing the bioavailability of certain agents [20]. It was reported by Aboubaker et al. that glutathione niosomes remarkably improved drug oral bioavailability and hepatic tissue uptake [21].

In any pharmaceutical dosage form, the ultimate goals are to improve patient compliance along with the rapid onset of action, convenient handling, and ease of administration. Oral films have attracted expanding interest in pharmaceutical technology in the last few years due to their supremacies. The use of an orally dissolving, permeable film delivery system can serve as a more efficient route to deliver tadalafil. Oral films are flexible and easy to use, making them a more satisfactory and convenient dosage form when compared to conventional oral dosage forms which advocate patient compliance, specifically for children and elderly patients, or patients with swallowing dysfunction or dysphagia where complete and accurate dosing can be difficult to attain [22,23]. Visser et al. showed that orodispersible films were the most favorite candidates for patients who were nursing home residents [24]. Besides, films can be utilized to overcome bioavailability problems of drugs that are vulnerable to poor aqueous solubility by promoting oromucosal absorption, directly entering the systemic circulation [25].

Moreover, the consolidation of both niosomes and film in one dosage form can provide a lot of merits in enhancing therapeutic outcomes. Allam and Fetih, for example, stated that loading metoprolol tartrate in a niosomal oral film enhanced significantly its bioavailability compared to the marketed tablet dosage form and produced a prolonged effect of the drug with no detected side effects [26]. Herein, combining the features of niosomes with the oral film increases the drug solubility of poorly soluble drugs and creates a formulation with reduced local irritation, uniform dispersion in the targeting site, more reproducible drug absorption, and enhanced bioavailability [27].

In the current piece of work, an attempt has been made to formulate and assess oral film containing tadalafil-loaded niosomes to provide a fast systemic effect by improving tadalafil solubility through a patient-geriatric friendly formulation for those suffering from benign prostatic hyperplasia. Box-Behnken design was purposed to optimize the niosomal formulation. The optimized film containing niosomes was evaluated for its physical and mechanical properties, including surface morphology. Besides, film pharmacokinetics characteristics were appraised in rats against the marketed product.

2. Materials and Methods

Tadalafil ($\geq$98%), polyethylene glycol 400 (PEG 400) (~98%), microcrystalline cellulose EP (Avicel® PH-101), methylcellulose (MC) (~98%), polyethylene-polypropylene glycol (Poloxamer®407), polysorbate 80 (Tween®80), sorbitan monostearate (Span®60), saccharine sodium, and menthol were purchased from Sigma-Aldrich, Steinheim, Switzerland. Fat-free soybean phospholipids with 70% phosphatidylcholine (Lipoid S®75) were kindly gifted from Lipoid AG, Sennweidstrasse, Switzerland. All other reagents and solvents used were of analytical grade.

2.1. Preparation and Statistical Optimization of Tadalafil-Loaded Nanovesicles

2.1.1. Preparation of Tadalafil-Loaded Niosomes

The conventional ether-injection method was applied for the screening of non-ionic surfactants and the preparation of the drug-loaded niosomes as Bendas et al. with modifications [28]. Accurately weighed quantities of three nonionic surfactants (span®60, tween®80, and poloxamer®407) were mixed with lipoid in a 2:1 molar ratio and dissolved in diethyl ether. The resulting solution was injected using a microsyringe at a rate of 1 mL/min into a preheated distilled water which was maintained at 65 °C temperature under stirring until complete solvent removal. The surfactant that produced niosomes with the smallest size, minimal polydispersity index, and optimal zeta potential was selected to be used for niosomes formulation.

The drug-loaded niosomes were prepared by the same procedure where the etheric solution of nonionic surfactant and Lipoid S®75 was mixed with methanol formerly containing the required amount of tadalafil.

2.1.2. Box–Behnken Design (BBD) Experiment

The tadalafil-loaded niosomes were optimized using a Box-Behnken response surface methodology experimental design (Design-Expert® Software Version 11) (3 factors, 3 levels). The independent variables selected were mixing time (X1), non-ionic surfactant to lipid ratio (X2), and the total weight of the preparation components (X3) with their low, medium, and high levels for preparing 15 formulations as given in Table 1. The studied responses were particle size (Y1), polydispersity index (Y2), and zeta potential (Y3). Moreover, 3D response surface graphs were plotted to depict the effects of the predetermined factors on the responses measured.

Table 1. Independent and dependent variables in Box–Behnken design for the optimization of Tadalafil-loaded niosomes.

Independent Variables	**Levels**		
	Low	**Medium**	**High**
X_1 = Mixing time (min)	15	22.5	30
X_2 = Non-ionic surfactant to lipid ratio (w/w)	1:2	1:0.8	2:1
X_3 = Total weight of the preparation (mg)	200	350	500
Transformed values	−1	0	+1
Studied Responses	**Goal**		
Y_1 = Particle size (nm)	Minimize		
Y_2 = Polydispersity index	Minimize		
Y_3 = Zeta potential (mV)	Maximize		

2.1.3. Particle Size, Polydispersity Index, and Zeta Potential

The surface potential, vesicle size, and polydispersity index (PDI) of tadalafil-loaded niosomes were measured at 25 ± 2 °C and 90° scattering angle by Zeta sizer 2000 (Malvern Instruments, England, UK) [15]. The above-mentioned characteristics were measured to aid further in the optimization of the preparation. All measurements were carried out in triplicate, the mean and the standard deviation were computed.

2.1.4. Entrapment Efficiency

Niosomes containing tadalafil were separated from the unloaded free drug by applying Mehanna et al. separation technique [29]. In this indirect method of separation, cooling centrifugation at 15,000 rpm for 60 min at 4 °C was executed (Sigma 3–30KS centrifugation,

Osterode, Germany). The supernatant was separated each time, then combined and assayed spectrophotometrically at 291 nm. The amount of entrapped drugs was attained by deducting the amount of free drugs from the total added drug. The percent of entrapment efficiency (EE %) was then calculated as Equation (1). The results are expressed as the mean of three separate experiments:

$$EE\% = \frac{\text{Total amount of drug} - \text{amount of free drug}}{\text{Total amount of drug}} \times 100 \quad (1)$$

2.2. Preparation and Characterization of Tadalafil-Loaded Noisomal Fast Dissolving Films

2.2.1. Preparation of Tadalafil-Loaded Niosomal Oral Film

Based on literature, methylcellulose (MC) was tested as film-forming material for the preparation of fast dissolving film [26]. Polyethylene glycol 400 was used as a plasticizer, saccharine as a sweetener, and menthol as a flavoring agent. Microcrystalline cellulose MCC (Avicel®) was used as a superdisintegrant owing to its short disintegration time [26]. The solvent casting method was applied for the preparation of the film. Initially, the polymer was dispersed in the casting vehicle (distilled water), followed by the addition of saccharine and menthol. Furthermore, MCC (Avicel®) was levigated with PEG 400 before amalgamation into the polymeric solution. After a volume of tadalafil-loaded niosomes (corresponding to the required dose) was incorporated and mildly mixed with the polymeric solution and the final volume was adjusted to 25 mL with distilled water. Later, the solution was poured on the petri dish (surface area, 19.63 cm^2) and allowed to dry until a constant weight. The patches were cut into 4 cm^2 pieces and stored in a dry place at room temperature to preserve their integrity and elasticity.

2.2.2. Vesicle Size Analysis of the Niosomal Film

Vesicle size of the niosomal film was analyzed after reconstitution. The film was dispersed in deionized water followed by sonication for 10 min. The obtained dispersion was analyzed at 25 ± 2 °C and 90° scattering angle for the determination of average particle size, polydispersity index, and zeta potentials for the reconstituted vesicles using Zeta sizer 2000 (Malvern Instruments, England, UK) [30].

2.2.3. In-Vitro Assessment

The niosomal oral film was characterized for its physical appearance, thickness, weight, and content uniformity. Moreover, surface pH, moisture content, folding endurance, tensile strength, disintegration time, and surface morphology of the prepared polymeric film were evaluated.

The physical appearance was checked via visual inspection of the films. The thickness of the films was measured by a micrometer screw gauge at five different points, followed by calculating their mean value [31].

Weight variation test was performed by determining individual weights of 4 cm^2 pieces from ten randomly selected films using an analytical balance (MC-1 AC210S, Sartorius, Goettingen, Germany) to calculate the average weight and the standard deviation [32].

Content uniformity in the formulated films was computed by dissolving 10 randomly selected in 100 mL phosphate buffer (pH 6.8). The resulting solutions were then filtered, and further dilution was carried out with phosphate buffer to measure their absorbance spectrophotometrically at 291 nm to determine tadalafil content [33].

For determining the surface pH, the niosomal films were allowed to be in contact with distilled water and then measured by a pH digital meter (SED 12,500 V Martini Instruments Co., Ltd., Beijing, China) at room temperature (25 ± 0.2 °C) by bringing the electrode in contact with the film surface and allowing them to equilibrate for about one minute [34].

Percentage moisture content was measured by weighing the films before and after drying them in a hot air oven at 105 ± 5 °C for 2 h to indicate the difference in weight according to the following equation [35]:

$$\% \text{ Moisture content} = \frac{\text{Initial weigh} - \text{final weight}}{\text{initial weight}} \times 100 \quad (2)$$

The mechanical strength was determined through the folding endurance of the prepared films which was computed based on the number of times the film can fold at the same place without breaking [36].

The tensile strength of the prepared oral film was measured using a digital tensile testing machine (Lloyd Instruments Ltd., LR 10K, Bognor Regis, UK). The film was cut into a rectangular shape and the tensile tester was set with a crosshead speed of 35 mm/minute and an initial grip separation of 25 mm. The film was placed vertically between the tensile tester's two clamps which they were pulled apart until the film broke [27]. Tensile strength was calculated as follows [37]:

$$\text{Tensile strength} = \frac{\text{Force at breakge (kg)}}{\text{Area (mm}^2\text{)}} \quad (3)$$

Moreover, the strain (% elongation) was evaluated to detect the stretching and toughness of the prepared polymeric film. The film elongation before breakage is referred to as the strain or percentage elongation which was determined as follows [35]:

$$\% \text{ Elongation} = \frac{\text{Increase in the film length}}{\text{Initial length of film}} \times 100 \quad (4)$$

In-vitro disintegration time was calculated by placing the film into a petri dish containing phosphate buffer (pH 6.8) and swirling it every 10 s. The disintegration time was computed when the film started to disintegrate or break down [26].

Scanning electron microscopy (SEM-JEOL, JSM-840A, Takamatsu, Japan) examined the film surface topography and morphology. The films were mounted on the sample stab using a double-sided adhesive tape and were coated with gold (200A) under reduced pressure for 5 min to enhance the conductivity using an ion sputtering device (JEOL, JFC-1100E, Takamatsu, Japan) [38].

2.2.4. In-Vitro Release Study

The release pattern of tadalafil from the niosomal film was conducted using the beaker method with slight modifications to compare free-drug-containing film [39,40]. A solution of 0.1 N HCl and 2% *w/v* tween®80 (pH 1.2) was used as a dissolution medium as it was previously proved to be a compatible medium for the release of tadalafil [15]. The dissolution medium was placed in a shaking water bath (FALC, WB-MF24, Treviglio, BG, Italy) set at 37 ± 0.5 °C and 100 rpm. Samples were periodically withdrawn at different time intervals and assayed using a UV-visible spectrophotometer (Jasco V-730 spectrophotometer, Heckmondwike, UK) at 291 nm. Samples were replaced with the same volume of fresh dissolution medium to maintain sink condition. The experiment was conducted in triplicates. The amount of drug released at each time interval was calculated, and the cumulative amount of drug released was determined as a function of time to construct the drug release profile graph. The release kinetics of tadalafil-loaded niosomal film was investigated by the curve fitting method to different mathematical models [41].

2.3. *In-Vivo Assessment*

2.3.1. Experimental Animals

Male albino Wistar rats weighed between 130–150 g were used for the in-vivo pharmacokinetic study. Rats were obtained from the animal house of the Faculty of Pharmacy, Beirut Arab University (BAU), Lebanon. Rats were housed in polyacrylic cages under standard animal housing conditions before and during the experiment. The animals had access to water and standard laboratory chow.

Animal handling during the work was carried out following the regulations and guidelines stipulated by the Institutional Animal Care and Use Guidelines (IACUG) at BAU, Lebanon and authenticated by the Ministry of Public Health. All experiments were performed at Beirut Arab University laboratories after obtaining approval from the Investigation Review Board (IRB), number: 2022-0045-P-M-93.

2.3.2. In-Vivo Pharmacokinetic Study

Tadalafil-loaded niosomal oral film and the marketed tablet were evaluated for their pharmacokinetic parameters in male albino Wistar rats. Randomly, the rats were divided into two groups, each of five rats. The first group received the oral film and the second received the marketed tablet. The animals of the first group were pre-anesthetized with ether where a film containing 5 mg of tadalafil was placed in the rat buccal cavity with the help of forceps and a Teflon spatula. The second group received an aqueous oral suspension of the marketed tablet using the gavage technique. Blood samples were withdrawn from the tail vein at predetermined time intervals post-dose. The blood samples were collected in heparinized tubes and subjected to centrifugation (Centurion Scientific, Chichester, UK) at 4500 rpm for 15 min at 4 ± 0.2 °C. The plasma was carefully separated using a micropipette and stored in Eppendorf tubes at −80 ± 5 °C (So-Low, Ultra-Low Freezer, Environmental Equipment, Cincinnati, OH, USA) for further analysis [37].

2.3.3. Extraction of Tadalafil from Plasma

The frozen plasma sample was thawed at room temperature (25 ± 2 °C) for the tadalafil quantification assay. Acetonitrile was added to 100 µL of the thawed plasma sample to precipitate the proteins followed by vortexing the mixture for 5 min. The sample was then centrifuged at 8500 rpm at 4 ± 0.2 °C for 20 min from which 100 µL of the clear supernatant was transferred into a clean vial, filtrated, degassed, and analyzed using reverse-phase high-performance liquid chromatography [42].

2.3.4. HPLC Analysis

Quantitative analysis was carried out using an Agilent technology (Waldbronn, Germany) equipped with C18 column (250 × 4.6 mm I.D), autosampler, pump, and photodiode array detector. An isocratic mobile phase consisting of buffer (potassium dihydrogen orthophosphate) and acetonitrile (1:1 *v/v*) mixture was eluted at a flow rate of 1.2 mL/min at ambient temperature (25 ± 0.5 °C) and the column effluent was detected at 285 nm wavelength with a total run time of 18 min. Tadalafil retention time was found to be 3.18 min. Tadalafil concentration was determined through a calibration curve of plotted peak area versus concentration [43].

2.3.5. Pharmacokinetic Parameters

Tadalafil pharmacokinetics calculations were performed using a non-compartmental approach, applying Kinetica® 4.4.1 SPSS 14 software®. Tadalafil concentration-time curve was used to obtain the tadalafil maximum concentration (C_{max}, µg/mL) and the time of tadalafil maximum concentration (T_{max}, hours). The area under the concentration-time curve from zero to the last analyzed point (AUC_{0-24}, µg.h/mL) was computed using the linear trapezoidal rule and cp/k was added to obtain $AUC_{0-\infty}$, where cp is the last measured concentration and k is the elimination rate constant. $T_{1/2}$ (hour) was determined based on the first order. Fraction (F) of drug absorbed and relative bioavailability were calculated according to the following equations:

$$F = \frac{\text{AUC} * \text{clearance (CL)}}{\text{Amount of drug dose (x)}} \quad (5)$$

$$RB = \frac{AUC\ 0 - t\ (film)}{AUC\ 0 - t\ (reference)} \times 100 \quad (6)$$

2.4. Stability Study

The stability evaluation of the optimized tadalafil-loaded niosomal film was assessed at two distinct storage conditions. Patches of the film were stored in aluminum packages at 25 °C with 50–60% humidity (ordinary conditions) and 40 °C with 75% humidity (accelerated conditions) for twelve weeks, then the content of tadalafil was determined, in addition to other parameters, as weight and thickness [44].

2.5. Statistical Analysis

The obtained results of the two treated groups were expressed as mean ± standard deviation (SD) and compared using a one-way analysis of variance or a two-sided Student's *t*-test for pairwise comparison where results were considered statistically significant if the *p*-value was ≤ 0.05.

3. Results and Discussion

3.1. Box-Behnken Statistical Optimization of Tadalafil-Loaded Niosomal Formulation

Upon applying the ether injection method in the preparation of niosmes, the alteration in temperature between phases governed by the slow injection of the lipid component into the aqueous phase encouraged the swift vaporization of solvent, ensuring spontaneous vesiculation and formation of niosomes [45]. The pre-formulation studies revealed that tween®80 was a suitable non-ionic surfactant as it aided in the production of niosomes with small particle size (147 ± 2.63 nm), PDI (0.331), and ideal zeta potential (−31.3 ± 0.87 mV) compared to poloxamer®407 and span®60 (Table 2). The incorporation of tween® in the lipid bilayers of the vesicles provided control over the shape, size, phase transition temperature, and fluidity of the niosomal vesicle [46]. This result is analogous to Alyami et al. where the particle size of niosomes containing tweens® was smaller than those containing Spans®. The hydrophilic head group of tweens® led to the formation of a thin bilayer and thus a smaller particle size [47].

Table 2. Pre-formulation non-ionic surfactants screening.

Surfactant	Particle Size (nm)	Polydispersity Index	Zeta Potential (mV)
Tween®80	147 ± 2.63	0.331 ± 0.022	−31.3 ± 0.87
Span®60	340 ± 12.06	0.395 ± 0.033	−8.2 ± 0.425
Poloxamer®407	217.1 ± 8.20	0.769 ± 0.088	−39.4 ± 0.624

The results are expressed as ± standard deviation (n = 3).

The present study optimized the preparation of niosomes via ether injection method by applying the Box-Behnken design. Each independent factor was examined at three levels, in addition to their binary interactions and their polynomial effects. The inspected features of the prepared systems were the vesicular size, polydispersity index, and surface charge which are depicted in Table 3. Cubic mathematical models were applied to analyze the relationship between the independent factors and the studied responses (Equations (7)–(9)):

$$Y_1 = +156.55 - 10.935\ A + 29.359\ B + 9.232\ C + 7.390\ AB + 9.925\ AC + 8.463\ BC - 13.476\ A^2 + 55.086\ B^2 + 5.701\ C^2 \quad (7)$$

$$Y_2 = +0.302 - 0.017\ A + 0.203\ B + 0.016\ C + 0.017\ AB + 0.016\ AC - 0.044\ BC - 0.030\ A^2 + 0.178\ B^2 + 0.027\ C^2 \quad (8)$$

$$Y_3 = -29.37 + 0.793\ A - 3.99\ B + 0.343\ C - 0.205\ AB + 0.800\ AC - 0.320\ BC + 1.036\ A^2 - 6.689\ B^2 + 0.741\ C^2 \quad (9)$$

Table 3. Regression analysis for particle size (responses Y_1), polydispersity index (Y_2), zeta potential (Y_3) of tadalafil-loaded niosomes.

Response	Mathematical Model	Adequate Precision	R^2	Adjusted R^2	Predicted R^2	SD	%CV *	*p*-Value **
Y_1	Quadratic	23.772	0.987	0.964	0.796	7.510	4.13	0.0001
Y_2	Quadratic	18.724	0.987	0.965	0.801	0.034	8.69	0.0009
Y_3	Quadratic	19.724	0.988	0.967	0.832	0.865	2.71	0.0001

* Percentage coefficient of variation. ** Significant p-value < 0.05.

As presented in Table 3, the obtained data proposed a quadratic model for the analysis of particle size, PDI, and zeta potential, and the difference between adjusted and predicted R^2 values for the investigated responses was less than 0.2 which indicates a reasonable agreement in the study design. The particle size ranged from 126.80 nm (F14) and 267.70 nm (F6), polydispersity index from 0.224 (F14) and 0.760 (F3) and the zeta potential from −27.80 mV (F14) and −40.00 mV (F3) (Table 4).

Table 4. Box-Behnken design with actual values of the variables *.

Formulation (F)	Mixing Time (min)	Surfactant to Lipid Ratio	Total Weight of the Preparation (mg)	Particle Size (nm)	Polydispersity Index	Zeta Potential (mV)
1	30	1:2	350	145.67 ± 2.34	0.236 ± 0.02	−30.76 ± 3.76
2	22.5	1:0.8	350	153.00 ± 2.78	0.31 ± 0.07	−30.00 ± 7.80
3	22.5	2:1	200	223.10 ± 4.77	**0.760** ± 0.04	**−40.00** ± 8.09
4	22.5	1:0.8	350	157.54 ± 1.26	0.3 ± 1.53	−29.00 ± 3.30
5	15	1:0.8	500	150.90 ± 3.11	0.341 ± 0.06	−28.98 ± 5.81
6	22.5	2:1	500	**267.70** ± 2.29	0.650 ± 0.01	−39.87 ± 7.83
7	22.5	1:2	200	183.90 ± 8.56	0.276 ± 0.05	−31.40 ± 9.52
8	15	1:0.8	200	161.50 ± 6.26	0.288 ± 0.16	−27.98 ± 5.73
9	22.5	1:2	500	194.65 ± 4.76	0.343 ± 1.12	−29.99 ± 7.49
10	15	2:1	350	235.87 ± 7.89	0.660 ± 2.45	−38.87 ± 3.98
11	30	2:1	350	221.76 ± 1.12	0.657 ± 3.12	−37.89 ± 6.17
12	15	1:2	350	189.34 ± 9.32	0.278 ± 0.03	−32.56 ± 8.51
13	22.5	1:0.8	350	159.00 ± 5.21	0.301 ± 3.12	−29.90 ± 8.42
14	30	1:0.8	200	**126.80** ± 2.11	**0.224** ± 0.01	**−27.80** ± 2.91
15	30	1:0.8	500	155.90 ± 4.26	0.341 ± 0.09	−25.60 ± 6.59

* The results are expressed as mean ± standard deviation (n = 3). The bold data represent the upper range and the lower range for each studied parameter.

From the studied independent variables, the total weight of the formulation (X_3) showed minimal correlation and didn't affect the investigated parameters, viz. particle size, PDI, and zeta potential, whether it was at its minimum or maximum the value of the formulation total weight did not possess any effect.

The *p*-values computed in this study were less than 0.05, thus revealing the significant influence of the formulation variables, specifically the time of mixing and surfactant to lipid ratio on the studied responses. The contour plots shown in Figure 1A,B illustrates that upon prolongation of mixing time from 15 to 30 min, both the niosomes particle size and polydispersity index decreased resulting in a more uniform vesicles size distribution. This was parallel to what was reported by Shah et al. where increasing mixing times from 30 to 60 min ensured lower particle sizes and PDI. This comportment may be elucidated by the fact that the short time for mixing is not satisfactory to form complete uniform niosomes [48]. Concerning tween®80 to lipoid® ratio, it was observed that as the non-ionic surfactant increased in the formula composition, the formulation had a larger particle size as in F6, F10, and F11 (Table 4, Figure 1A). The presence of a surfactant with high HLB induces niosomal vesicle size enlargement as the surface free energy reduces upon increasing surfactants hydrophobicity [49]. Howbeit, particle size approached adequate values when an appropriate ratio was optimized (1:0.8) as shown in formulations F5, F14, and F15 with a particle size of 150.90, 126.80, and 155.90 nm, respectively (Table 4).

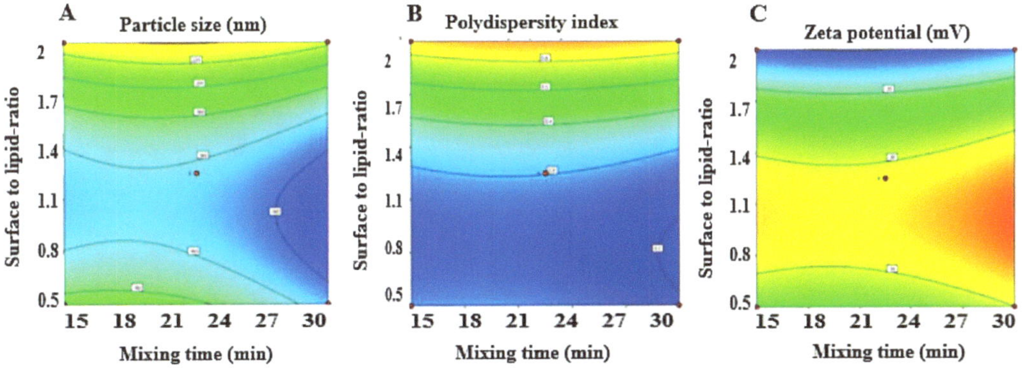

Figure 1. The contour plots of the effect of mixing time (X1) and surfactant to lipid ratio (X2) on particle size (**A**), polydispersity index (**B**), and Zeta potential (**C**) of tadalafil-loaded niosomes. (The red points are the design points).

The zeta potential of the runs ranged between −27.80 mV (F14) and −40.00 mV (F3). These high negatively charged surface particles reflected positively on the stability of the niosomes where the vesicles will tend to repel rather than aggregate. Okore et al. proposed a characteristic line to separate between stable and unstable vesicles, which was roughly taken at either +30 or −30 mV [50]. Sailaja et al. attained kindred outcomes with the preparation of naproxen-loaded niosomes by the ether injection method, where tween®80 was considered the suitable surfactant for such formulation with a zeta potential of −31.9 mV, suggesting its stability [51].

After experimentally executing the different 15 runs, formula (F14) with the smallest particle size (126.80 nm), lowest PDI (0.224), and optimal zeta potential (−27.80 mV) was selected. This formula was obtained with tween®80 to lipoid® molar ratio of 1:0.8, a total weight of 200 mg, and mixed for 30 min. According to the Box Behnken design, the optimal desirable solution for each of the variables and independent factors is illustrated in Figure 2. The data in Table 5 shows a small residual value between the expected and the observed ones for particle size, polydispersity index, and zeta potential. The measured values mirror close concession between the predicted values and the minimal standardized residuals to imply the validity of the developed mathematical model within this design space to interpret the effect of surfactant to lipid ratio, the weight of the formulation, and mixing time on the formulated tadalafil-loaded niosomes.

Table 5. Predicted and observed values of the physicochemical characteristics of the optimized tadalafil-loaded niosomes.

Factor			Optimized Level
X_1 = Mixing time (min)			29.42
X_2 = Surfactant: Lipid (ratio)			0.93
X_3 = Total weight (mg)			243.9
Response	**Expected**	**Observed**	**Residual**
Y_1 = Particle size (nm)	122	126.8	4.8
Y_2 = Polydispersity index	0.178	0.224	0.046
Y_3 = Zeta potential (mV)	−27.68	−27.80	0.12

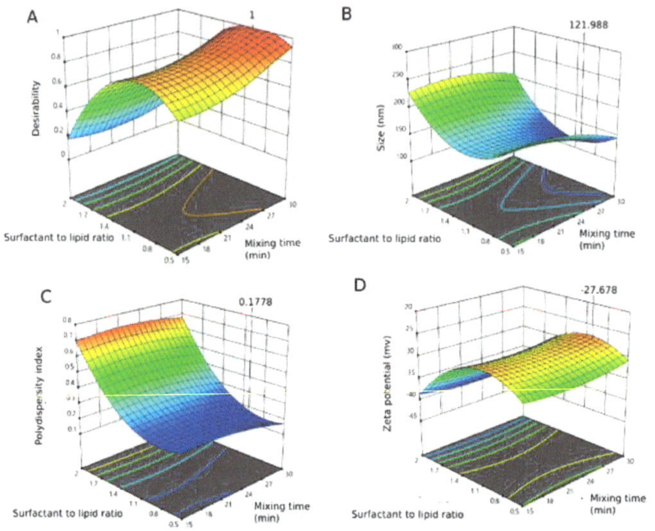

Figure 2. The three-dimensional surface of the desirability function at the factor space (**A**). Individual response is graphed to show the optimum point. Particle size (nm) (**B**), polydispersity index (**C**) and zeta potential (mV) (**D**).

3.2. Entrapment Efficiency

The entrapment efficiency for the optimized prepared niosomal formulation employing the ether injection method was 99.78 ± 2.13%. The high EE of tadalafil in the niosomal preparation indicates the effectiveness of niosomes in solving the poor aqueous solubility of this drug. Similar outcomes were conquered by Sezgin-Bayindir et al. where the EE of candesartan cilexetil-loaded niosomes was high (99.06 ± 1.74%) proving that niosomes can be applied to enhance the aqueous solubility of these drug candidates [52]. The high EE is pretentious by the chain length and size of the hydrophilic head group of the non-ionic surfactant employed. Nonionic surfactants with stearyl (C18) chains display higher entrapment efficiency than those with lauryl (C12) chains. Here the utilization of tween® bearing a long alkyl chain and a large hydrophilic moiety with lipoid® S75 provided this high entrapment efficiency. The relationship between the chain and the entrapment efficiency is controversial, Ruckmani and Sankar showed that tween®80 with a longer saturated alkyl chain than tween®60 and tween®20 exhibited lower entrapment efficiency, which increased from 79.5 ± 0.8% to 82.4 ± 1.4%, and 83.8 ± 1.2% for the latter, respectively, concluding that the lower the HLB value of the surfactant, the lower the entrapment efficiency [46]. However, these results were divergent from those declared by Ahmed et al. which suggested that the lower the HLB of the surfactant, the higher will be the entrapment efficiency [53].

3.3. Vesicle Size Analysis of the Niosomal Film

The average particle size of the reconstituted niosomes was 151 ± 3.09 nm with polydispersity index of 0.341± 0.05, and zeta potential of value 29.9 ± 0.9 mV. The result revealed that there was a non-significant difference in particle size of reconstituted film compared with tadalafil niosomal dispersion ($p > 0.05$). The polydispersity index was narrow indicating a narrow particle size distribution and a good resdispersibility of the film containing tadalafil-loaded niosomes of drug within the nanocarrier in the film [54].

3.4. In-Vitro Assessment of Tadalafil-Loaded Niosomal Oral Film

The formulation should be able to form a film with sufficient elasticity, softness, flexibility, and good physicochemical stability. As a result, these parameters should be evaluated carefully during the development of oral films to assure their effective performance. Studying the quality attributes of a film is a prerequisite that includes assessing properties such as surface morphology, weight, thickness and content variation, surface pH, mechanical strength, moisture content, disintegration time, and in-vitro release [55]. Results of the physical and mechanical properties of tadalafil oral film are presented in Table 6.

Table 6. Physical and mechanical features of tadalafil-loaded niosomal oral film.

Test	Result
Appearance	Transparent and homogenous
Thickness (μm)	110 ± 10 *
Weight variation (mg)	5.74 ± 0.29 **
Content uniformity (*w*/*w*%)	97.82 ± 0.33 **
Surface pH	6.67 ± 0.49 *
Moisture content (%)	3.02 ± 0.60 *
Folding endurance	320 ± 26.47 *
Tensile strength (MPa)	0.079 ± 0.03 *
Elongation (%)	6.66 ± 0.12 *
Disintegration time (seconds)	30.27 ± 5.06 *

The results are expressed as mean ± standard deviation (* n = 3 and ** n = 10).

According to the visual inspection and morphological features, the prepared tadalafil-loaded niosomal film was elegant, transparent, flexible, homogenous, and smooth which indicates the good dispersion of the niosomes within the film and the viability of the preparation method [56].

The film thickness should be evaluated since it is related directly to the quantity of the drug within the film. A suitable thickness is also crucial for the comfortable application of the oral film. The optimal thickness should be between 50 and 1000 μm to be suitable for oral administration [57]. As tadalafil film thickness was around 110 ± 10 μm, it would be convenient for oral use. These results are in agreement with previously reported data on film thickness, which was around 160 μm [58].

Similarly, determining the weight variation of the film is necessary to ensure the consistency of the film preparation, repeatability of the technique, as well as drug uniformity [59]. The average weight of the films was around 5.74 mg with a small standard deviation value (±0.29 mg) signifying the chance for non-uniformity in tadalafil content which was also confirmed by the content uniformity testing.

Content uniformity is performed to determine drug content in the individual oral patch and to check the reproducibility of the technique. Tadalafil content was almost the same among the prepared films ~97.82%. This result was coherent with another study in which the film contained metoclopramide and methylcellulose as a polymer and displayed content uniformity of around 95% [60]. These values are accepted according to USP27 which specifies that the content should be between 85% and 115% with less than 6% standard deviation [61].

A film that has inappropriate pH either toward basic or acidic medium may induce damage to the mucosal layer lining the oral cavity leading to patient discomfort. The mean value of surface pH of tadalafil film was 6.67 ± 0.49, with a non-significant difference ($p > 0.005$), which is within the range of the oral cavity pH (6.4–6.8), thus the film is less likely to be irritant to the oral mucosal membrane [62].

The moisture content affects the friability, brittleness, and stability of oral films. Many factors are responsible for increasing the film moisture level as the solvent system, the drug hygroscopicity, the excipients in the formula, and the manufacturing techniques. The moisture content of the prepared tadalafil-loaded niosmal film was 3.02 ± 0.60% which is considered within the acceptable range (<5%) [63]. This result was analogous to the Linku and Sijimol investigation where the moisture content of the prepared polymeric film varied between 1.1% and 3.84% [64].

Folding endurance is carried out to estimate the mechanical properties of the film. In another word, it is performed to detect the flexibility of the film to ensure it can be administrated without breakage. The film has a great mechanical strength when it requires more than 300 time folding to break and develop visible cracks [65]. The folding endurance of tadalafil film was about 320, indicating good flexibility which is indirectly related to the appropriate concentration and dispersion of the methylcellulose within the fabricated formula.

An ideal oral film should display an adequately high tensile strength to be able to withstand normal handling. Despite this, a very high rigid film is not desired, because it could retard the drug release from the polymer matrix. The prepared niosomal oral film had an average tensile strength of 0.79 ± 0.03 MPa which is in line with the previously prepared polymeric film which has a tensile strength value of 0.78 ± 0.05 MPa [66]. The percentage elongation of the prepared film was 6.66 ± 0.12% which is considered ideal for the polymeric film. These data suggested that polyethylene glycol 400, which was used as a plasticizer, was able to reduce the glass transition temperature of methylcellulose and promoted its plasticity and flexibility. This temperature is one of the most vital properties that determine chain mobility of polymer in which the polymer transforms from hard, glassy material to soft, rubbery material with accepted tensile strength and percentage elongation [67].

The disintegration time is the time needed by the film to disperse or disintegrate when it comes in contact with the saliva. The film thickness and weight affect greatly the physical properties of the film. In general, the disintegration time ranges from 5 to 30 s to allow faster drug release and fast oromucosal absorption [61]. The disintegration time of the prepared film was 30.31 ± 3.64 s, which is considered rapid and acceptable compared with niosomal films prepared by Allam and Fetih, where they showed disintegration times ranging from 38 to 180 s [26].

The surface morphology of the formulated film was examined using SEM to clarify its feature. As illustrated in Figure 3, the film showed a continuous, smooth, and homogenous surface. Besides, niosomes vesicles can be visualized in the niosomal film with spherical and smooth surface without any aggregation and the nanometric size range signifying successful incorporation of the selected niosomes within the optimized film. A similar result was observed in Arafa et al. study where SEM images of the prepared propolis-based oral film showed spherical niosomes and smooth features of the film [68].

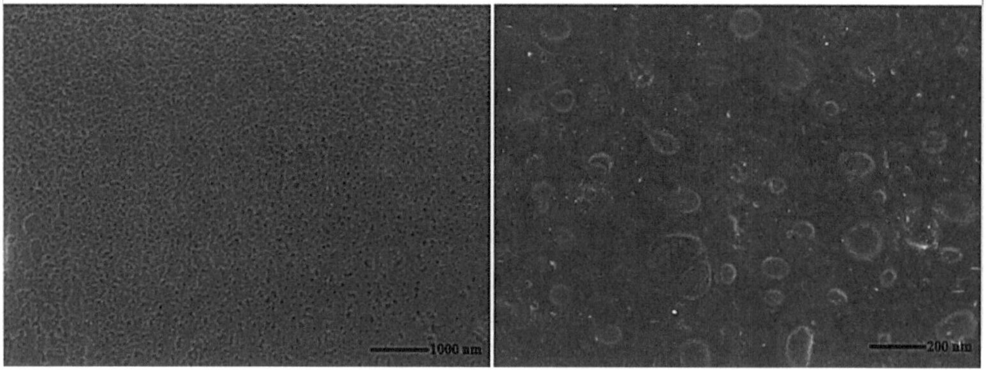

Figure 3. Scanning electron microscope images of oral tadalafil niosomal film.

3.5. In-Vitro Release of Tadalafil from the Optimized Niosomal Film

The percentage of tadalafil released from the formulated niosomal film in comparison with its release from the film without niosomes is illustrated in Figure 4. The drug in the niosomal film demonstrated a fast release within 5 min (22.65 ± 1.432%), significantly greater than that from the film alone (7.72 ± 6.782%, $p < 0.05$). Comparable verdicts were reported by Khan et al. where a burst release of ceftriaxone and rifampicin from all the niosomal formulations was detected at the beginning of the dissolution testing compared with drugs alone [69].

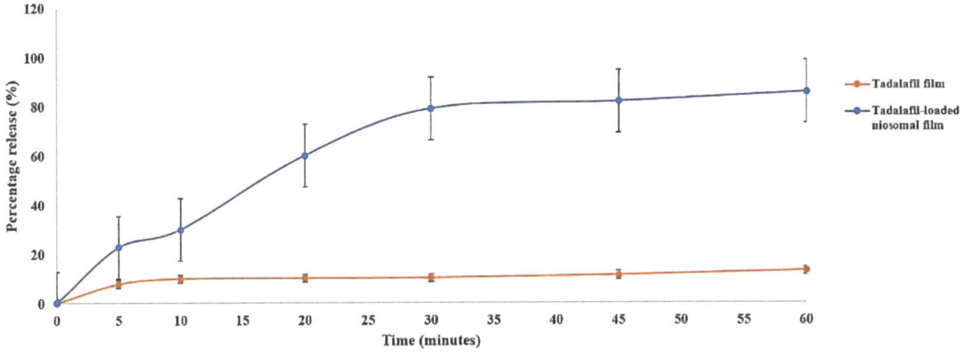

Figure 4. In-vitro percentage release (%) of tadalafil from the niosomal film in comparison with its release from the marketed tablet as function of time (minutes).

In the present study, the release of tadalafil in both formulations increased with the progress of the study. After 30 min the niosomal film provided 78.95 ± 1.117% release of tadalafil, whereas it reached only 10.21 ± 6.012% from the film ($p < 0.05$). The water solubility of MC utilized created porosity in the film, allowing the surrounding solvent to penetrate the film, thus accelerating its dissolving, similar results to what was attained by Auda et al. [51]. Additionally, employing microcrystalline cellulose (Avicel®) added faster disintegration of the formulation and hence rapid initial release. These data were in agreement with those of Serrano et al. as the disintegration time was enhanced when higher amounts of Avicel® were employed [70].

The pattern of release continued in a controlled manner; the tadalafil percentage release was 81.94 ± 0.234% at 45 min and reached 85.76 ± 3.123% at the end of the one-hour study. As for the release from the film without niosomes, it was significantly less with 11.30 ± 2.765 and 13.04 ± 3.665% at 45 and 60 min, respectively ($p < 0.05$). The controlled release template was achieved by the incorporation of the drug into the niosomal structures. Niosomes delay the release of the encapsulated drugs due to the presence of lipids in their composition. The existence of lipids decreases the niosomes membrane fluidity by lessening the leakage and permeability of the drugs [71]. Similar data was endorsed by Shailaja and Shreya, as a formulation containing tween 80 showed an optimal release profile of naproxen from the niosomes with 88.9 ± 0.71% after 12 h [51].

In this study, the oral niosomal film provided a dual release pattern characterized by a fast-dissolving profile at the beginning of the experiment yielded by the film components and a controlled one for the remaining time assured by niosomes.

To investigate the release kinetics of tadalafil from the niosomal film, different mathematical release models were adapted, namely, Higuchi, Hixson-Crowell, Korsmeyer-Peppas, first-order, and zero-order models. From the outcomes, it was noticed that tadalafil release from the niosomal film fitted into the Korsmeyer-Peppas model displaying a linear relationship ($R^2 = 0.9986$). The release exponent 'n' corresponding to the mechanism of drug release was 0.472, indicating that it falls within the range of Fickian diffusion [72]. These inputs were coherent with those of Sadeghi et al. where the release of lysozymes from the niosomes followed the Korsmeyer-Peppas model and n was 0.33, thus quasi-Fickian diffusion determined the drug release mechanism [73]. In this study niosomes as a nanocarrier are considered as s drug reservoir since it was able to control the release of tadalafil governed by the small size of the formulation and lipophilicity of lecithin employed that retarded the release.

3.6. *In-Vivo Pharmacokinetic Assessment*

The plasma concentration versus time curves and pharmacokinetic parameters of tadalafil after a single dose administration (oral film and the marketed tablet) are illustrated in Figure 5 and Table 7. Animals who received tadalafil film orally displayed a plasma level-time profile characterized by significantly higher peak concentration (C_{max}) with a larger area under the curves ($AUC_{0–24}$ and $AUC_{0–\infty}$) compared with those that received the marketed tablets ($p \leq 0.05$). Additionally, at studied time points, the mean tadalafil plasma concentrations were higher in rats treated with the investigated formula than in those treated with the marketed tablet. Moreover, tadalafil-loaded niosomal film exhibited a significantly shorter T_{max} value (0.66 fold) compared to the marketed tablet ($p < 0.05$). The relative bioavailability of the formulation upon comparison with the marketed tablet was 118.4%, indicating that the oral film improved tadalafil bioavailability.

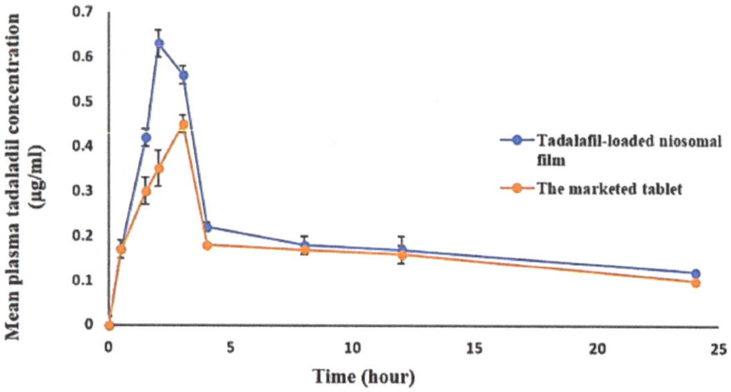

Figure 5. Mean tadalafil plasma concentration versus time after single dose administration of the optimized niosomal oral film and the marketed tablet in two groups of rats.

Table 7. Tadalafil pharmacokinetics parameters after niosomal oral film and marketed tablet administration.

Pharmacokinetic Parameters *	Oral Niosomal Film	Marketed Tablet	p-Value
C_{max} (µg/mL)	0.63 ± 0.03	0.45 ± 0.04	0.001
$AUC_{0–24}$ (µg.h/mL)	4.82 ± 0.51	4.07 ± 0.26	0.01
$AUC_{0–\infty}$ (µg.h/mL)	8.90 ± 1.54	7.02 ± 0.83	0.009
K elimination (h^{-1})	0.029 ± 0.001	0.034 ± 0.001	0.05
F	0.71	0.63	0.05
T_{max} (h)	2 ± 0.5	3 ± 0.5	0.0001
$t_{1/2}$ (h)	23.87 ± 4.1	20.05 ± 3.2	0.0003
Relative bioavailability (%)	118.4		

* Data are the mean value ± standard deviation (n = 4).

These findings can be credited to many reasons, first, the presence of tadalafil within the niosomes as a nanocarrier enhanced its solubility as well as its dissolution rate compared to the marketed product [35]. Furtherly, the rapid disintegration of the niosomal oral film in the saliva caused faster tadalafil absorption via the buccal mucosa, therefore reaching higher plasma concentrations more rapidly than that in the control group through pre-gastric absorption. Furtherly, it is worth mentioning that oral mucosa is highly vascularized, which helps in rapidly achieving tadalafil therapeutic serum concentration [37]. Thereby, the route of administration is the key factor for ameliorating drug bioavailability. In support of this statement, Wong et al. showed that despite griseofulvin being encapsulated within fast-dissolving microparticles, the formulation failed to enhance the drug bioavailability when it was administrated orally through oral gavage technique [74]. The nanosized drug particles adhesiveness feature could also prolong the residence time of the drug on the mucosal surfaces along with the gastrointestinal tract, providing more time for drug absorption and reducing erratic and variable absorption [42]. The nanosized nanocrystalline cellulose-based orally-dispersible film was also responsible for the rapid release, absorption, and enhanced donepezil bioavailability in other literature [75]. Furthermore, the incorporation of tween®80 in the oral film formulation might increase tadalafil permeability, owing to its ability to emulsify dispersion and to interact with the mucosal surface to form mixed surfactant-membrane micelles, thereby boosting the drug absorption fraction [76].

3.7. Stability

The optimized tadalafil-loaded niosomal film was stable when stored under ordinary and accelerated conditions, where a non-significant alteration in thickness and weight of the film was observed (Table 8). The content of tadalafil was fairly stable ranging from 97.82 ± 0.33% at the beginning to 95.45 ± 2.13% and 94.89 ± 2.34% at the end of the experiment for ordinary and accelerated conditions, respectively (Figure 6). Similar outcomes were observed by Nishimura et al. were the content of prochlorperazine in the oral disintegrating film containing microcrystalline cellulose, polyethlene glycol, and hydroxypropylmethyl cellulose as the polymeric materials was almost constant regardless of storage conditions [77].

Table 8. Assessment of stability parameters; thickness and weight of tadalafil-loaded oral niosomal film.

	Thickness (μm) *				Weight (mg) *			
Conditions	**Zero Week**	**4 Weeks**	**8 Weeks**	**12 Weeks**	**Zero Week**	**4 Weeks**	**8 Weeks**	**12 Weeks**
Ordinary	110 ± 10	106.45 ± 11.32	105.89 ± 3.43	104.44 ± 2.01	5.74 ± 0.29	5.7 ± 1.98	5.66 ± 1.02	5.59 ± 1.89
Accelerated	110 ± 10	105.65 ± 08.35	104.78 ± 7.67	104.18 ± 1.95	5.74 ± 0.29	5.64 ± 3.99	5.34 ± 4.98	5.31 ± 2.94

* Each value was assessed as mean ± SD (n = 3).

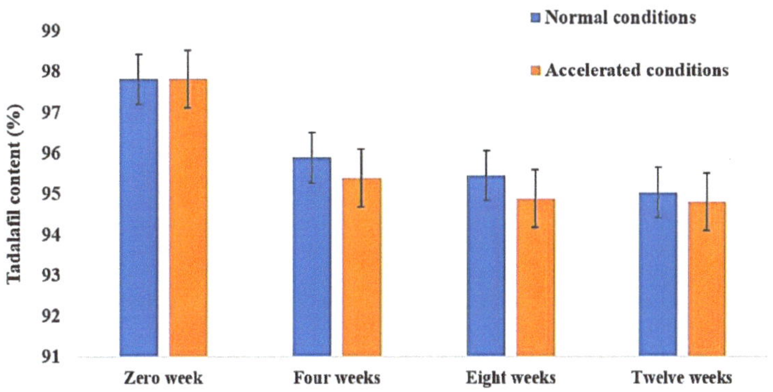

Figure 6. Tadalafil content in the oral niosomal film after storage under different conditions. Each value represents mean ± SD (n = 3).

4. Conclusions

A new generation of tadalafil-loaded surfactant-based vesicle was prepared by ether injection method, optimized using the Box–Behnken Design, and showed unique characteristics such as small vesicular size, unimodal size distribution, and efficient zeta potential. The prepared niosomal dispersions were then successfully loaded into oral polymeric film composed of methylcellulose. The optimized film showed acceptable mechanico-physical characteristics including neutral pH, low moisture content, uniform drug distribution, rapid disintegration, and accepted tensile strength. The film showed a smooth and homogenous surface structure signifying the successful incorporation of the selected niosomal formulation into the polymeric film. Niosomal film displayed also a rapid release of tadalafil within 5 min, which was statistically higher than that of the marketed tablet. Moreover, the in-vivo bioavailability evaluations in rats clarified that the optimized niosomal oral film augmented tadalafil systemic absorption and increased its maximum concentration significantly in comparison to the market tablet. Therefore, polymeric oral film loaded with niosomal tadalafil formulation can be a convenient and economical approach to boost tadalafil absorption and represents a palatable and stable dosage method that can be easily administrated by geriatric patients who suffer from benign prostatic hyperplasia.

Author Contributions: Conceptualization, writing—review, editing, project administration and supervision, M.M.M.; methodology, software, investigation, and writing—original draft preparation, K.K.A. and A.T.M.; validation, formal analysis, resources, data curation and visualization, A.N.A. All authors have read and agreed to the published version of the manuscript.

Funding: This research received no external funding.

Institutional Review Board Statement: The animal study protocol was approved by the Institutional Review Board of Beirut Arab University (number: 2022-0045-P-M-93/2022).

Informed Consent Statement: Not applicable.

Data Availability Statement: The data presented in this study are available upon request from the corresponding author.

Conflicts of Interest: The authors declare no conflict of interest.

References

1. Chapple, C.R.; Roehrborn, C.G.; McVary, K.; Ilo, D.; Henneges, C.; Viktrup, L. Effect of Tadalafil on Male Lower Urinary Tract Symptoms: An Integrated Analysis of Storage and Voiding International Prostate Symptom Subscores from Four Randomised Controlled Trials. *Eur. Urol.* **2015**, *67*, 114–122. [CrossRef] [PubMed]
2. Yu, Z.-J.; Yan, H.-L.; Xu, F.-H.; Chao, H.-C.; Deng, L.-H.; Xu, X.-D.; Huang, J.-B.; Zeng, T. Efficacy and Side Effects of Drugs Commonly Used for the Treatment of Lower Urinary Tract Symptoms Associated with Enign Prostatic Hyperplasia. *Front. Pharmacol.* **2020**, *11*, 658. [CrossRef] [PubMed]
3. Ventura, S.; Oliver, V.L.; White, C.W.; Xie, J.H.; Haynes, J.M.; Exintaris, B. Novel Drug Targets for the Pharmacotherapy of Benign Prostatic Hyperplasia (BPH). *Br. J. Pharmacol.* **2011**, *163*, 891–907. [CrossRef]
4. Tan, Y.K.; Pearle, M.S.; Cadeddu, J.A. Rendering Stone Fragments Paramagnetic with Iron-Oxide Microparticles to Improve the Efficiency of Endoscopic Stone Fragment Retrieval. *Curr. Opin. Urol.* **2012**, *22*, 144–147. [CrossRef] [PubMed]
5. Tinel, H.; Stelte-Ludwig, B.; Hütter, J.; Sandner, P. Pre-Clinical Evidence for the Use of Phosphodiesterase-5 Inhibitors for Treating Benign Prostatic Hyperplasia and Lower Urinary Tract Symptoms. *BJU Int.* **2006**, *98*, 1259–1263. [CrossRef] [PubMed]
6. Porst, H. IC351 (Tadalafil, Cialis): Update on Clinical Experience. *Int. J. Impot. Res.* **2002**, *14*, S57–S64. [CrossRef]
7. Toque, H.A.; Priviero, F.B.M.; Teixeira, C.E.; Claudino, M.A.; Baracat, J.S.; Fregonesi, A.; De Nucci, G.; Antunes, E. Comparative Relaxing Effects of Sildenafil, Vardenafil, and Tadalafil in Human Corpus Cavernosum: Contribution of Endogenous Nitric Oxide Release. *Urology* **2009**, *74*, 216–221. [CrossRef]
8. Bruzziches, R.; Francomano, D.; Gareri, P.; Lenzi, A.; Aversa, A. An Update on Pharmacological Treatment of Erectile Dysfunction with Phosphodiesterase Type 5 Inhibitors. *Expert Opin. Pharmacother.* **2013**, *14*, 1333–1344. [CrossRef]
9. Su, M.; Xia, Y.; Shen, Y.; Heng, W.; Wei, Y.; Zhang, L.; Gao, Y.; Zhang, J.; Qian, S. A Novel Drug-Drug Coamorphous System without Molecular Interactions: Improve the Physicochemical Properties of Tadalafil and Repaglinide. *RSC Adv.* **2019**, *10*, 565–583. [CrossRef]
10. Mehanna, M.M.; Abla, K.K.; Domiati, S.; Elmaradny, H. Superiority of Microemulsion-Based Hydrogel for Non-Steroidal Anti-Inflammatory Drug Transdermal Delivery: A Comparative Safety and Anti-Nociceptive Efficacy Study. *Int. J. Pharm.* **2022**, *622*, 121830. [CrossRef]
11. Mehanna, M.M.; Abla, K.K.; Elmaradny, H.A. Tailored Limonene-Based Nanosized Microemulsion: Formulation, Physicochemical Characterization and in-Vivo Skin Irritation Assessment. *Adv. Pharm. Bull.* **2020**, *11*, 274–285. [CrossRef]
12. Mehanna, M.M.; Abla, K.K. SiRNA Nanohybrid Systems: False Hope or Feasible Answer in Cancer Management. *Ther. Deliv.* **2022**, *13*, 109–133. [CrossRef] [PubMed]
13. Alwattar, J.K.; Mneimneh, A.T.; Abla, K.K.; Mehanna, M.M.; Allam, A.N. Smart Stimuli-Responsive Liposomal Nanohybrid Systems: A Critical Review of Theranostic Behavior in Cancer. *Pharmaceutics* **2021**, *13*, 355. [CrossRef]
14. Vinesh, V.; Sevukarajan, M.; Rajalakshmi, R.; Thulasi Chowdary, G. Enhancement of Solubility of Tadalafil by Cocrystal Approach. *Int. Res. J. Pharm.* **2013**, *4*, 218–223. [CrossRef]
15. Mehanna, M.M.; Mneimneh, A.T.; Domiati, S.; Allam, A.N. Tadalafil-Loaded Limonene-Based Orodispersible Tablets: Formulation, in Vitro Characterization and in Vivo Appraisal of Gastroprotective Activity. *Int. J. Nanomed.* **2020**, *15*, 10099–10112. [CrossRef]
16. Mehanna, M.M.; Alwattar, J.K.; Habchi, R. Electrohydrodynamic Atomization, a Promising Avenue for Fast-Dissolving Drug Delivery System: Lessons from Tadalafil-Loaded Composite Nanofibers. *J. Appl. Pharm. Sci.* **2020**, *10*, 33–45. [CrossRef]
17. Badr-Eldin, S.M.; Elkheshen, S.A.; Ghorab, M.M. Inclusion Complexes of Tadalafil with Natural and Chemically Modified β-Cyclodextrins. I: Preparation and in-Vitro Evaluation. *Eur. J. Pharm. Biopharm.* **2008**, *70*, 819–827. [CrossRef]

18. Mehanna, M.M.; Motawaa, A.M.; Samaha, M.W. Tadalafil Inclusion in Microporous Silica as Effective Dissolution Enhancer: Optimization of Loading Procedure and Molecular State Characterization. *J. Pharm. Sci.* **2012**, *101*, 2271–2280. [CrossRef] [PubMed]
19. Mehanna, M.M.; Mneimneh, A.T. Formulation and Applications of Lipid-Based Nanovehicles: Spotlight on Self-Emulsifying Systems. *Adv. Pharm. Bull.* **2021**, *11*, 56–67. [CrossRef] [PubMed]
20. Bhardwaj, P.; Tripathi, P.; Gupta, R.; Pandey, S. Niosomes: A Review on Niosomal Research in the Last Decade. *J. Drug Deliv. Sci. Technol.* **2020**, *56*, 101581. [CrossRef]
21. Aboubakr, E.M.; Mohammed, H.A.; Hassan, A.S.; Mohamed, H.B.; El Dosoky, M.I.; Ahmad, A.M. Glutathione-Loaded Non-Ionic Surfactant Niosomes: A New Approach to Improve Oral Bioavailability and Hepatoprotective Efficacy of Glutathione. *Nanotechnol. Rev.* **2021**, *11*, 117–137. [CrossRef]
22. Slavkova, M.; Breitkreutz, J. Orodispersible Drug Formulations for Children and Elderly. *Eur. J. Pharm. Sci.* **2015**, *75*, 2–9. [CrossRef]
23. Hoffmann, E.M.; Breitenbach, A.; Breitkreutz, J. Advances in Orodispersible Films for Drug Delivery. *Expert Opin. Drug Deliv.* **2011**, *8*, 299–316. [CrossRef]
24. Visser, J.C.; Wibier, L.; Mekhaeil, M.; Woerdenbag, H.J.; Taxis, K. Orodispersible Films as a Personalized Dosage Form for Nursing Home Residents, an Exploratory Study. *Int. J. Clin. Pharm.* **2020**, *42*, 436–444. [CrossRef]
25. Jadhav, Y.G.; Galgatte, U.C.; Chaudhari, P.D. Overcoming Poor Solubility of Dimenhydrinate: Development, Optimization and Evaluation of Fast Dissolving Oral Film. *Adv. Pharm. Bull.* **2018**, *8*, 721–725. [CrossRef]
26. Allam, A.; Fetih, G. Sublingual Fast Dissolving Niosomal Films for Enhanced Bioavailability and Prolonged Effect of Metoprolol Tartrate. *Drug Des. Dev. Ther.* **2016**, *10*, 2421–2433. [CrossRef]
27. Abd El Azim, H.; Nafee, N.; Ramadan, A.; Khalafallah, N. Liposomal Buccal Mucoadhesive Film for Improved Delivery and Permeation of Water-Soluble Vitamins. *Int. J. Pharm.* **2015**, *488*, 78–85. [CrossRef]
28. Bendas, E.R.; Abdullah, H.; El-Komy, M.H.M.; Kassem, M.A.A. Hydroxychloroquine Niosomes: A New Trend in Topical Management of Oral Lichen Planus. *Int. J. Pharm.* **2013**, *458*, 287–295. [CrossRef]
29. Mehanna, M.M.; Motawaa, A.M.; Samaha, M.W. Nanovesicular Carrier-Mediated Transdermal Delivery of Tadalafil: I- Formulation and Physicsochemical Characterization. *Drug Dev. Ind. Pharm.* **2015**, *41*, 714–721. [CrossRef]
30. Liu, C.; Chang, D.; Zhang, X.; Sui, H.; Kong, Y.; Zhu, R.; Wang, W. Oral Fast-Dissolving Films Containing Lutein Nanocrystals for Improved Bioavailability: Formulation Development, in Vitro and in Vivo Evaluation. *AAPS PharmSciTech* **2017**, *18*, 2957–2964. [CrossRef]
31. Bala, R.; Khanna, S.; Pawar, P.; Arora, S. Orally Dissolving Strips: A New Approach to Oral Drug Delivery System. *Int. J. Pharm. Investig.* **2013**, *3*, 67. [CrossRef]
32. Panraksa, P.; Jantrawut, P.; Tipduangta, P.; Jantanasakulwong, K. Formulation of Orally Disintegrating Films as an Amorphous Solid Solution of a Poorly Water-Soluble Drug. *Membranes* **2020**, *10*, 376. [CrossRef]
33. El-Feky, Y.A.; Mostafa, D.A.; Al-Sawahli, M.M.; El-Telbany, R.F.A.; Zakaria, S.; Fayez, A.M.; Ahmed, K.A.; Alolayan, E.M.; El-Telbany, D.F.A. Reduction of Intraocular Pressure Using Timolol Orally Dissolving Strips in the Treatment of Induced Primary Open-Angle Glaucoma in Rabbits. *J. Pharm. Pharmacol.* **2020**, *72*, 682–698. [CrossRef]
34. Auda, S.H.; El-Badry, M.; Ibrahim, M.A. Design, Formulation and Characterization of Fast Dissolving Films Containing Dextromethorphan. *Dig. J. Nanomater. Biostruct.* **2014**, *9*, 133–141.
35. Londhe, V.; Shirsat, R. Formulation and Characterization of Fast-Dissolving Sublingual Film of Iloperidone Using Box-Behnken Design for Enhancement of Oral Bioavailability. *AAPS PharmSciTech* **2018**, *19*, 1392–1400. [CrossRef]
36. Kathpalia, H.; Patil, A. Formulation and Evaluation of Orally Disintegrating Films of Levocetirizine Dihydrochloride. *Indian J. Pharm. Sci.* **2017**, *79*, 204–211. [CrossRef]
37. Elshafeey, A.H.; El-Dahmy, R.M. Formulation and Development of Oral Fast-Dissolving Films Loaded with Nanosuspension to Augment Paroxetine Bioavailability: In Vitro Characterization, Ex Vivo Permeation, and Pharmacokinetic Evaluation in Healthy Human Volunteers. *Pharmaceutics* **2021**, *13*, 1869. [CrossRef]
38. Maheswari, K.M.; Devineni, P.K.; Deekonda, S.; Shaik, S.; Uppala, N.P.; Nalluri, B.N. Development and Evaluation of Mouth Dissolving Films of Amlodipine Besylate for Enhanced Therapeutic Efficacy. *J. Pharm.* **2014**, *2014*, 520949. [CrossRef]
39. Kulkarni, P.; Rawtani, D. Application of Box-Behnken Design in the Preparation, Optimization, and in Vitro Evaluation of Self-Assembly–Based Tamoxifen- and Doxorubicin-Loaded and Dual Drug–Loaded Niosomes for Combinatorial Breast Cancer Treatment. *J. Pharm. Sci.* **2019**, *108*, 2643–2653. [CrossRef]
40. Shilakari Asthana, G.; Sharma, P.K.; Asthana, A. In Vitro and In Vivo Evaluation of Niosomal Formulation for Controlled Delivery of Clarithromycin. *Scientifica* **2016**, *2016*, 6492953. [CrossRef]
41. Allam, A.N.; Naggar, V.F.; El Gamal, S.S. Preparation, Formulation and physicochemical characterization of chitosan/acyclovir co-crystals. *Pharm. Dev. Technol.* **2013**, *18*, 856–865. [CrossRef] [PubMed]
42. Alsofany, J.M.; Hamza, M.Y.; Abdelbary, A.A. Fabrication of Nanosuspension Directly Loaded Fast-Dissolving Films for Enhanced Oral Bioavailability of Olmesartan Medoxomil: In Vitro Characterization and Pharmacokinetic Evaluation in Healthy Human Volunteers. *AAPS PharmSciTech* **2018**, *19*, 2118–2132. [CrossRef]
43. Bojanapu, A.; Subramaniam, A.T.; Munusamy, J.; Dhanapal, K.; Chennakesavalu, J.; Sellappan, M.; Jayaprakash, V. Validation and Method Development of Tadalafil in Bulk and Tablet Dosage Form by RP-HPLC. *Drug Res.* **2014**, *65*, 82–85. [CrossRef]

44. Moin, A.; Gangadharappa, H.W.; Adnan, M.; Rizvi, S.M.; Ashraf, S.A.; Patel, M.; Abu Lila, A.S.; Allam, A.N. Modulation of drug release from natural polymer matrices by response surface methodology: In vitro and in vivo evaluation. *Drug. Design Dev. Ther.* **2020**, *14*, 5325–5336. [CrossRef]
45. Ravalika, V.; Sailaja, A.K. Formulation and Evaluation of Etoricoxib Niosomes by Thin Film Hydration Technique and Ether Injection Method. *Nano Biomed. Eng.* **2017**, *9*, 242–248. [CrossRef]
46. Ruckmani, K.; Sankar, V. Formulation and Optimization of Zidovudine Niosomes. *AAPS PharmSciTech* **2010**, *11*, 1119–1127. [CrossRef]
47. Alyami, H.; Abdelaziz, K.; Dahmash, E.Z.; Iyire, A. Nonionic Surfactant Vesicles (Niosomes) for Ocular Drug Delivery: Development, Evaluation and Toxicological Profiling. *J. Drug Deliv. Sci. Technol.* **2020**, *60*, 102069. [CrossRef]
48. Shah, P.; Goodyear, B.; Haq, A.; Puri, V.; Michniak-Kohn, B. Evaluations of Quality by Design (QbD) Elements Impact for Developing Niosomes as a Promising Topical Drug Delivery Platform. *Pharmaceutics* **2020**, *12*, 246. [CrossRef]
49. Ruckmani, K.; Jayakar, B.; Ghosal, S.K. Nonionic Surfactant Vesicles (Niosomes) of Cytarabine Hydrochloride for Effective Treatment of Leukemias: Encapsulation, Storage, and in Vitro Release. *Drug Dev. Ind. Pharm.* **2000**, *26*, 217–222. [CrossRef]
50. Okore, V.C.; Attama, A.A.; Ofokansi, K.C.; Esimone, C.O.; Onuigbo, E.B. Formulation and Evaluation of Niosomes. *Indian J. Pharm. Sci.* **2011**, *73*, 323–328. [CrossRef]
51. Sailaja, A.K.; Shreya, M. Preparation and Characterization of Naproxen Loaded Niosomes by Ether Injection Method. *Nano Biomed. Eng.* **2018**, *10*, 174–180. [CrossRef]
52. Sezgin-Bayindir, Z.; Antep, M.N.; Yuksel, N. Development and Characterization of Mixed Niosomes for Oral Delivery Using Candesartan Cilexetil as a Model Poorly Water-Soluble Drug. *AAPS PharmSciTech* **2014**, *16*, 108–117. [CrossRef] [PubMed]
53. Guinedi, A.S.; Mortada, N.D.; Mansour, S.; Hathout, R.M. Preparation and Evaluation of Reverse-Phase Evaporation and Multilamellar Niosomes as Ophthalmic Carriers of Acetazolamide. *Int. J. Pharm.* **2005**, *306*, 71–82. [CrossRef] [PubMed]
54. Shen, B.D.; Shen, C.Y.; Yuan, X.D.; Bai, J.X.; Lv, Q.Y.; Xu, H.; Dai, L.; Yu, C.; Han, J.; Yuan, H.L. Development and Characterization of an Orodispersible Film Containing Drug Nanoparticles. *Eur. J. Pharm. Biopharm.* **2013**, *85*, 1348–1356. [CrossRef] [PubMed]
55. Shanmugam, S. Oral Films: A Look Back. *Clin. Pharmacol. Biopharm.* **2016**, *5*, 1–3. [CrossRef]
56. Wadetwar, R.N.; Ali, F.; Kanojiya, P. Formulation and Evaluation of Fast Dissolving Sublingual Film of Paroxetine Hydrochloride for Treatment of Depression. *Asian J. Pharm. Clin. Res.* **2019**, *12*, 126–132. [CrossRef]
57. Sevinç Özakar, R.; Özakar, E. Current Overview of Oral Thin Films. *Turk. J. Pharm. Sci.* **2021**, *18*, 111–121. [CrossRef]
58. Vijaykumar, G.; Koyyada, K.; Rao, K.R.S.S. Design, Evaluation and Comparitive Studies of Oral Thin Films of Alendronate. *Int. J. Pharm. Anal. Res.* **2016**, *5*, 95–107.
59. Karki, S.; Kim, H.; Na, S.-J.; Shin, D.; Jo, K.; Lee, J. Thin Films as an Emerging Platform for Drug Delivery. *Asian J. Pharm. Sci.* **2016**, *11*, 559–574. [CrossRef]
60. Auda, S.H.; Mahrous, G.M.; El-Badry, M.; Fathalla, D. Development, Preparation and Evaluation of Oral Dissolving Films Containing Metoclopramide. *Lat. Am. J. Pharm.* **2014**, *33*, 1027–1033.
61. Irfan, M.; Rabel, S.; Bukhtar, Q.; Qadir, M.I.; Jabeen, F.; Khan, A. Orally Disintegrating Films: A Modern Expansion in Drug Delivery System. *Saudi Pharm. J.* **2016**, *24*, 537–546. [CrossRef]
62. Singh, H.; Kaur, M.; Verma, H. Optimization and Evaluation of Desloratadine Oral Strip: An Innovation in Paediatric Medication. *Sci. World J.* **2013**, *2013*, 395681. [CrossRef] [PubMed]
63. Nair, A.B.; Kumria, R.; Harsha, S.; Attimarad, M.; Al-Dhubiab, B.E.; Alhaider, I.A. In Vitro Techniques to Evaluate Buccal Films. *J. Control. Release* **2013**, *166*, 10–21. [CrossRef] [PubMed]
64. Linku, A.; Sijimol, J. Formulation and Evaluation of Fast Dissolving Oral Film of Anti-Allergic Drug. *Asian J. Pharm. Res. Dev.* **2018**, *6*, 5–16. [CrossRef]
65. Mukherjee, D.; Bharath, S. Design and Characterization of Double Layered Mucoadhesive System Containing Bisphosphonate Derivative. *ISRN Pharm.* **2013**, *2013*, 1–10. [CrossRef] [PubMed]
66. Talekar, S.D.; Haware, R.V.; Dave, R.H. Evaluation of Self-Nanoemulsifying Drug Delivery Systems Using Multivariate Methods to Optimize Permeability of Captopril Oral Films. *Eur. J. Pharm. Sci.* **2019**, *130*, 215–224. [CrossRef] [PubMed]
67. Foroughi-Dahr, M.; Mostoufi, N.; Sotudeh-Gharebagh, R.; Chaouki, J. Particle Coating in Fluidized Beds. In *Reference Module in Chemistry, Molecular Sciences and Chemical Engineering*; Elsevier: Amsterdam, The Netherlands, 2017; pp. 1–89. ISBN 978-0-12-409547-2.
68. Arafa, M.G.; Ghalwash, D.; El-Kersh, D.M.; Elmazar, M.M. Propolis-Based Niosomes as Oromuco-Adhesive Films: A Randomized Clinical Trial of a Therapeutic Drug Delivery Platform for the Treatment of Oral Recurrent Aphthous Ulcers. *Sci. Rep.* **2018**, *8*, 2459. [CrossRef] [PubMed]
69. Khan, D.H.; Bashir, S.; Khan, M.I.; Figueiredo, P.; Santos, H.A.; Peltonen, L. Formulation Optimization and in Vitro Characterization of Rifampicin and Ceftriaxone Dual Drug Loaded Niosomes with High Energy Probe Sonication Technique. *J. Drug Deliv. Sci. Technol.* **2020**, *58*, 101763. [CrossRef]
70. Serrano, D.R.; Fernandez-Garcia, R.; Mele, M.; Healy, A.M.; Lalatsa, A. Designing Fast-Dissolving Orodispersible Films of Amphotericin b for Oropharyngeal Candidiasis. *Pharmaceutics* **2019**, *11*, 369. [CrossRef]
71. Rasul, A.; Khan, M.I.; Rehman, M.U.; Abbas, G.; Aslam, N.; Ahmad, S.; Abbas, K.; Shah, P.A.; Iqbal, M.; Al Subari, A.M.A.; et al. In Vitro Characterization and Release Studies of Combined Nonionic Surfactant-Based Vesicles for the Prolonged Delivery of an Immunosuppressant Model Drug. *Int. J. Nanomed.* **2020**, *15*, 7937–7949. [CrossRef]

72. Danyuo, Y.; Ani, C.J.; Salifu, A.A.; Obayemi, J.D.; Dozie-Nwachukwu, S.; Obanawu, V.O.; Akpan, U.M.; Odusanya, O.S.; Abade-Abugre, M.; McBagonluri, F.; et al. Anomalous Release Kinetics of Prodigiosin from Poly-N-Isopropyl-Acrylamid Based Hydrogels for the Treatment of Triple Negative Breast Cancer. *Sci. Rep.* **2019**, *9*, 3862. [CrossRef] [PubMed]
73. Allam, A.N.; Mehanna, M.M. Formulation, physicochemical characterization and in-vivo evaluation of ion-sensitive metformin loaded-biopolymeric beads. *Drug. Dev. Ind. Pharm.* **2016**, *42*, 497–505. [CrossRef] [PubMed]
74. Wong, S.M.; Kellaway, I.W.; Murdan, S. Fast-Dissolving Microparticles Fail to Show Improved Oral Bioavailability. *J. Pharm. Pharmacol.* **2010**, *58*, 1319–1326. [CrossRef]
75. Anjireddy, K.; Karpagam, S. Micro and Nanocrystalline Cellulose Based Oral Dispersible Film; Preparation and Evaluation of in Vitro/in Vivo Rapid Release Studies for Donepezil. *Braz. J. Pharm. Sci.* **2020**, *56*, 1–17. [CrossRef]
76. Bharti, K.; Mittal, P.; Mishra, B. Formulation and Characterization of Fast Dissolving Oral Films Containing Buspirone Hydrochloride Nanoparticles Using Design of Experiment. *J. Drug Deliv. Sci. Technol.* **2019**, *49*, 420–432. [CrossRef]
77. Nishimura, M.; Matsuura, K.; Tsukioka, T.; Yamashita, H.; Inagaki, N.; Sugiyama, T.; Itoh, Y. In Vitro and in Vivo Characteristics of Prochlorperazine Oral Disintegrating Film. *Int. J. Pharm.* **2009**, *368*, 98–102. [CrossRef]

MDPI AG
Grosspeteranlage 5
4052 Basel
Switzerland
Tel.: +41 61 683 77 34

Pharmaceutics Editorial Office
E-mail: pharmaceutics@mdpi.com
www.mdpi.com/journal/pharmaceutics